FOUNDATIONS OF PROFESSIONAL NURSING

Katherine Renpenning, MScN, a graduate of the University of Saskatchewan–Saskatoon and the University of British Columbia–Vancouver, is a nursing consultant whose career has focused primarily on the utility of self-care deficit nursing theory in improving nursing practice and nursing education. Her client base has included governments, professional nursing associations, schools of nursing, acute and long-term care, and community health agencies in Canada, the United States, and worldwide.

Susan Gebhardt Taylor, PhD, MSN, FAAN, is a graduate of Alverno College, Milwaukee, Wisconsin, and Catholic University of America, Washington, DC. She is professor emeritus, Sinclair School of Nursing, University of Missouri–Columbia. She is the recipient of the Alumna of the Year award from Alverno College, the Missouri Tribute to Nurses—Nurse Educator Award, Kemper Fellowship for Teaching Excellence, and the University of Missouri Alumni Association Faculty award.

Judith M. Pickens, PhD, RN, is a graduate of Marymount College, Salina, Kansas, and has done graduate work at the University of Missouri–Columbia and Arizona State University, Tempe, Arizona. She has been an assistant professor/clinical associate professor in psychiatric-mental health (P-MH), teaching clinical and theory courses at the undergraduate and post-master's level. She has extensive clinical expertise and has served as a clinical care coordinator and director of nurses in the behavioral health field.

FOUNDATIONS OF PROFESSIONAL NURSING
CARE OF SELF AND OTHERS

Katherine Renpenning, MScN

Susan Gebhardt Taylor, PhD, MSN, FAAN

Judith M. Pickens, PhD, RN

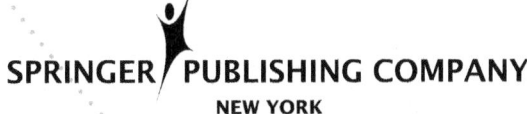

SPRINGER PUBLISHING COMPANY
NEW YORK

Springer Publishing Company, LLC
11 West 42nd Street
New York, NY 10036
www.springerpub.com

Acquisitions Editor: Elizabeth Nieginski
Senior Production Editor: Kris Parrish
Composition: Westchester Publishing Services

ISBN: 978-0-8261-3364-9
e-book ISBN: 978-0-8261-3365-6
Instructor's Manual ISBN: 978-0-8261-3369-4
Instructor's PowerPoints ISBN: 978-0-8261-3368-7

Instructor's Materials are available to qualified adopters by contacting textbook@springerpub.com

16 17 18 19 20 / 5 4 3 2 1

The author and the publisher of this Work have made every effort to use sources believed to be reliable to provide information that is accurate and compatible with the standards generally accepted at the time of publication. Because medical science is continually advancing, our knowledge base continues to expand. Therefore, as new information becomes available, changes in procedures become necessary. We recommend that the reader always consult current research and specific institutional policies before performing any clinical procedure. The author and publisher shall not be liable for any special, consequential, or exemplary damages resulting, in whole or in part, from the readers' use of, or reliance on, the information contained in this book. The publisher has no responsibility for the persistence or accuracy of URLs for external or third-party Internet websites referred to in this publication and does not guarantee that any content on such websites is, or will remain, accurate or appropriate.

Library of Congress Cataloging-in-Publication Data

Names: Renpenning, Katherine McLaughlin, author. | Taylor, Susan G., author. | Pickens, Judith M., author.
Title: Foundations of professional nursing : care of self and others / Katherine Renpenning, Susan Gebhardt Taylor, Judith M. Pickens.
Description: New York, NY : Springer Publishing Company, LLC, [2016] | Includes bibliographical references and index.
Identifiers: LCCN 2016000737| ISBN 9780826133649 (hardcopy : alk. paper) | ISBN 9780826133656 (ebook)
Subjects: | MESH: Nursing Process | Health Behavior | Patient Education as Topic | Nursing
Classification: LCC RT51 | NLM WY 100.1 | DDC 610.73—dc23 LC record available at https://lccn.loc.gov/2016000737

Special discounts on bulk quantities of our books are available to corporations, professional associations, pharmaceutical companies, health care organizations, and other qualifying groups. If you are interested in a custom book, including chapters from more than one of our titles, we can provide that service as well.

For details, please contact:
Special Sales Department, Springer Publishing Company, LLC
11 West 42nd Street, 15th Floor, New York, NY 10036-8002
Phone: 877-687-7476 or 212-431-4370; Fax: 212-941-7842
E-mail: sales@springerpub.com

Printed in the United States of America by McNaughton & Gunn.

CONTENTS

FOREWORD

Self-care describes in a practical, person-centered way what we should all be doing to maintain our health, wellness, and well-being. Through self-care, people can remain healthy into their seventh, eighth, and ninth decades. They can better manage their minor ailments and delay or even prevent chronic "lifestyle" diseases, such as heart attack, stroke, diabetes, and cancers. In addition to these individual, personal benefits, self-care can relieve the pressure on health care systems and contribute substantially to their sustainability.

It is important to note that self-care does not mean no care, nor does it imply that individuals are simply left to look after themselves. Rather, an overarching aim of self-care is to move away from overdependence on overburdened health care systems and toward empowering people—with the appropriate tools, support, and knowledge—to take better care of themselves.

Within today's health care systems, nurses have a particular role to play as respected professionals, and they are valued for their personal approach, friendliness, skill, efficiency, and accessibility. They are seen as easier to interact with than doctors—as attentive, caring, and closer to patients. Nurses are believed to have an important role in providing patients with supplementary information and reassurance, thereby softening the medical setting. Patients need support with self-management of established medical conditions, and nurses can play an increased role in this direction.

However, self-care exists substantially beyond the scope of health care systems—at home and in communities, well before the health care system itself is called upon. To achieve sustainable health (and health care) systems for the future, societies must reshape demand for health services, reducing the disease burden by helping people stay healthy and empowering them to manage their health within the home and community environments. Cultural norms, urban planning, the environment, choices in food and drink, the manner in which children are parented and educated, personal development throughout our lives, and many other factors must evolve in mutually supportive ways to create a new age of healthy behaviors. All this will lead to new opportunities and new roles for nurses in the community setting.

With much at stake and many changes underway or needed, the International Self-Care Foundation (ISF) is delighted to welcome this new book, *Foundations of Professional Nursing: Care of Self and Others*. We commend the authors for the breadth and scope of their work. The exploration of the place of nursing in self-care needs to be made a priority. Self-care needs to be a part of people's lives, integrated into families, communities, organizations, and society. As we move toward this goal, nurses can play a pivotal role.

David E. Webber, PhD
President, ISF
London, England

FOREWORD

The science of self-care, which is the major premise of this important new book, is one of the multiple ways of explicitly *thinking nursing*. Some would argue—and I tend to agree—that the science of self-care is embedded in all other ways of thinking nursing. The most widely known ways of thinking nursing include the conceptual models and derived middle-range theories developed by Dorothy Johnson, Imogene King, Myra Levine, Betty Neuman, Dorothea Orem, Martha Rogers, Callista Roy, and their colleagues. Thus, this book will be useful to all nurses—both practicing nurses and nurse researchers.

An important aspect of the science of self-care is that the individual person—the patient as self-care agent or nurse as his or her own self-care agent—is not alone in managing health, from experiences of high-level wellness to dying. Similarly, families and communities are not alone in managing health at the level of the family system or the community system. Nurses, along with the individual's family members and friends, the nuclear family's extended members and friends, and the community's external partners in health, are crucial members of a health care team that removes barriers to and facilitates the individual's continuing therapeutic self-care. Clearly, self-care is a collaborative enterprise. Furthermore, no one is alone in providing care to dependent others.

Nurses have always excelled in providing direct care for others in need and in providing access to care by other members of health care teams. *In an ideal world, every individual would have his or her own nurse as the point of entry into the health care system, as would every family and every community.* The science of self-care is *the* paradigm that provides the conceptual, theoretical, and empirical rationale for that position.

Perhaps the most important contribution of this book is that *thinking nursing* must come before *doing nursing*. For too long in the history of the profession and discipline of *nursology* (a recently revived term from the 1970s), nurses have been taught how to do nursing without an explicit framework for thinking nursing. The science of self-care provides an innovative, timely, and highly useful framework for thinking nursing. In this book, Katherine Renpenning, Susan Gebhardt Taylor, and Judith Pickens have translated that rather abstract framework into a practical one, with formats for all phases of the nursing process.

It is my honor to have been invited to write a foreword for this book, conceived and written by Renpenning and Taylor, with contributions by Pickens. Renpenning and Taylor are major scholars who have taken up Dorothea Orem's pioneering endeavors in articulating the science of self-care. They, along with Judith Pickens, have produced an eminently readable book that is both a tribute to Orem and a creative and practical extension of her work. Anyone who reads this book will have no doubt about the meaning of *thinking nursing*.

Jacqueline Fawcett, PhD, RN, ScD (hon), FAAN
Professor, Department of Nursing
University of Massachusetts–Boston

PREFACE

Occurring within health care worldwide, and with the burgeoning volume of and ease of access to information and instruction about how to do things, there are likewise evolving requirements for nursing knowledge and skill. In addition to technical competence, contemporary nursing practice requires a framework for decision making that integrates the science of self-care, nursing sciences, and knowledge developed in other disciplines to answer nursing questions. The focus of this book is on providing such a framework and illustrating its usefulness in multiple situations of nursing practice.

The Robert Wood Johnson Foundation (RWJF) is challenging society to participate in building a "Culture of Health" (2014 President's Message), empowering people to live healthier lives. The building of this culture consists of two parts. The first is community action that is aimed at social determinants of health and public education about a healthy lifestyle and prevention of illness. Second, and equally important, is a workforce of health care providers who are knowledgeable about helping people acquire knowledge, make appropriate decisions, and acquire the capabilities to engage in self-care. In another related initiative, on September 14, 2015, the American Academy of Nursing (AAN) recommended in a policy brief that designers of electronic health records (EHRs) and others associated with production and distribution move to include social and behavioral determinants of health in those EHRs. The essence of these two initiatives has long been the goal of the nursing profession, and specific strategies related to this goal are addressed in this text.

Nursing, in many ways, is caught in the groundswell of change that is affecting the whole health care industry. The profession has experienced adaptive, transformative, and evolutionary change, bringing us to where we are today. It has long been recognized that nurses play a valued role in society. At the same time, nurses continue to struggle with *who they are* as a profession and with *how they describe, define,* and *clarify* the primary contributions that they make in an interprofessional environment. It is true that health care professionals, including nurses, often have little or no awareness of the paradigm or paradigms that guide what they do, and often continue to practice primarily from within the medical model. This is evident when looking at many of the items that are used to represent outcomes of nursing practice. It has been found that when nurses have a clear understanding of the unique role of nursing within the interdisciplinary health care system and are able to explain it to others, patient care improves and burnout and work-related stress can be reduced.

Self-care and other similar concepts, such as self-management of chronic illness and symptom management, are the frequent focus of current health care literature. These concepts are broad and understood differently depending on the disciplinary lens being used. Many disciplines have contributed to the knowledge and science of self-care, including, but not limited to, psychology, medicine, social work, anthropology, and nursing. This not only enriches the knowledge base but also may contribute to multiple ways of viewing and understanding this concept that is central to health care. This work will specifically focus on how nurses can understand and use the science of self-care to guide professional nursing practice.

We draw heavily on the work of early nursing theorists, viewing these theories as complementary rather than competitive, and also draw on the theoretical work that has occurred within other disciplines. In presenting the science of self-care, the work done by Dorothea Orem and colleagues is foundational, as Orem was the first nurse scientist to develop theoretical formulations that provided a direction for explicating the components of self-care and linking self-care and nursing. The work provided by Orem scholars is a well-developed, comprehensive theory of nursing practice, the tenets of which are central to this book and to contemporary nursing practice.

The chapters in Part I provide some historical background, helping us understand where we came from and how we got to where we are. Only by knowing the past can we understand the present. Through an analysis of nursing cases, developments in the science of self-care, nursing sciences, and related disciplines, nursing scholars identified the elements of concern in nursing practice and a framework illustrating the relationships among those elements. Systems thinking is discussed as the basis for analyzing the complex interrelationships among these elements associated with nursing practice.

Part II is concerned with exploration of the meaning of these elements for accomplishing self-care, and with the role of nursing in facilitating action when working with individuals. A structure and process for collecting and analyzing data about the relationships among conditioning factors—such as health state, social determinants of health, family system factors, and actions required to promote health, well-being, and development—is introduced. This is followed by the introduction of a structure to assess the self-care capabilities required by dependent people. A comparison of what is required and the capability to act is the basis for prescribing nursing action—helping patients acquire capabilities to accomplish self-care and/or dependent care or acting on their behalf. Construction of the collaborative patient–nursing action system is followed by a discussion about production and control operations that are associated with effective implementation of this action system and evidence-based practice. This includes discussion of the nurse as both a caregiver and a manager. The organizational responsibilities associated with the practice of nursing include a discussion about the framework for practice, the recording system, and the impact that the recording system can have on determining nursing-sensitive outcomes, developing standards of practice, and using employment review standards.

In Part III, the use of the conceptual framework is extended to the consideration of nursing and the family and nursing and the community. A discussion of the family as a system is followed by an examination of the family as a conditioning factor. The family unit as the focus of concern is also explored. The community as a system is introduced, and levels of systems- and community-based nursing are explored in relation to data collection and analysis. Models for population health programs are introduced, including the integration of nursing within these models. Chapters 13 and 14 address legal and ethical concerns along with self-care issues for the practitioner.

Appendices are included, which illustrate use of the framework and articulation of the science of self-care and nursing in a variety of clinical situations. ***Qualified instructors may obtain access to ancillary materials, such as an Instructor's Manual and PowerPoints, by contacting textbook@springerpub.com.***

Katherine Renpenning
Susan Gebhardt Taylor
Judith M. Pickens

ABOUT THIS BOOK

You are reading this book, or taking this course, because you are interested in professional nursing. Begin by exploring your personal concepts and ideas about nursing and how you came to think that way. Take time to reflect on and discuss the questions presented here:

- Being a nurse, how do you describe nursing?
- Where did you get your images of nursing from: books, television, family members, or personal experiences?
- What motivated you to become a nurse?
- What is health? What is well-being? What does it mean to be sick?
- What is self-care? Examine your daily practices. Evaluate their effectiveness. What knowledge did you use to decide what to do and to evaluate the outcomes?
- What does this tell you about nursing? How do you see yourself in the future? Do you think of nursing as work, a calling, knowledge, or something else?

Thinking about nursing and how nurses came to be independent practitioners is essential for understanding the importance of the profession of nursing to health care, as well as providing the basis for forming an image and appreciation of self as nurse. The nurse's world is not often like that described in novels and seen in films and on television. It is not a world of glamour. No longer does the nurse carry a lamp, as Florence Nightingale did during the Crimean War—a depiction that has long served as the symbol of a trained nurse. Nightingale, however, does stand as a prototype for the modern nurse and nurse scientist. Nurses no longer wear starched white uniforms and caps that they were designated to wear when they went to school. Many of the old trappings that identified the person as a nurse are gone; they are replaced with only an identification badge and a professional demeanor. The modern nurse is highly respected, trusted, and caring. Professional nurses are well educated, critical thinkers and leaders.

An increasing number of men and more mature, nontraditional students are entering the nursing workforce from a variety of educational and experiential backgrounds, bringing diversity of thought and varied ways of interaction to the profession. The number of specialties within nursing and types of roles for nurses is ever increasing. Nurses are professionally licensed and have an independent, legally defined scope of practice; that is, nurses are legally responsible for their own actions when acting as nurses.

The focus of nursing has traditionally been on caring for and taking care of people in sickness and in health; in the hospital, home, and community. The locus of care is shifting from the acute care setting to community-based and home settings. Nursing roles are changing to include case management, care transition/coordination, community liaison, transplant coordination, health care advocacy, health education, tele-nursing, and so forth. As these many changes occur, it is imperative that one develop a conceptual model, because in order to *do* nursing, one must first learn to *think* nursing.

Since you became a nurse—even if it was only a few months ago—the world has changed. The environment within which you are living and working is changing. And you have decided to change. Change theory and concepts have meaning both personally and professionally. Knowing different change modalities will give you ways to develop appropriate strategies to meet contemporary challenges. Being an agent of change is an essential characteristic of the professional nurse. The nurse is to be involved at all levels of practice, from changing the way he or she approaches and cares for an individual patient to changing at the unit and institutional levels. Through professional nursing organizations, the nurse can be involved at even broader levels.

Throughout this text, we will use the term *patient* to refer to the recipient of nursing. This is the term used by the American Nurses Association (ANA) in the revised Code of Ethics. They use the term *patient*, which according to them refers to "client or consumers of health care as well as to individuals or groups" (American Nurses Association, 2015, p. xi).

MEET MRS. SMITH

As you move forward on your journey to enhance your clinical skills and gain advanced education, Mrs. Smith will be with you, giving you ways to think about the new concepts and helping you look freshly at familiar ones.

Mrs. Smith is a 65-year-old divorced woman with one son, 30 years old and unmarried, who lives in the same city and has a supportive relationship with his mother. She is physically described as being tall, lean, and having a sallow skin tone and dark hair. She recently retired from working as an administrative assistant in a small company. While working there, she became computer proficient. She has her own computer and Wi-Fi at her home. She lives and functions independently in the family home where she has lived for 35 years. She makes her own decisions about finances and other personal matters and has been doing so since her divorce 20 years ago. She participates in several group activities, such as playing bridge with friends. She describes herself as spiritual but not religious. She speaks English and can read and write, though an idiopathic tremor makes writing difficult for her. She is confident that she will be able to manage any changes in her system of living as she ages. She has not had regular check-ups by a practitioner since she was insured through her employer. She is a U.S. citizen and on her 65th birthday registered for Medicare. She has a supplemental insurance plan with AARP.

While working in her house one day, she fell and fractured the head of the right femur. She was able to call first responders and was transported to the hospital where surgery would be performed. X-rays revealed that in addition to a hip fracture, Mrs. Smith had osteoporosis. This probably was a problem contributing to her current health situation.

As you progress through the book, you will come to know Mrs. Smith as a person and as a member of a family and a community. You will think about the complex system that is Mrs. Smith and develop a more refined nursing lens to look at the evolving profession of nursing and health care.

References

American Nurses Association. (2015). *Code of ethics with interpretive statements*. Silver Spring, MD: Author.

PART I

THE WORLD OF THE NURSE

Recognizing that there is an increased emphasis on self-care in the health services industry, how does nursing fit into this? Much of the nursing research related to self-care addresses what people should do and what health care providers should teach. Other nurse scholars have looked at motivation, decision making, and similar isolated variables in relation to self-care and the meaning they have to nursing practices. We view nursing as a complex system of action that incorporates patient variables, nurse variables, and the action and interactions among those variables. This view has led to moving beyond a needs-based approach toward specifying the self-care actions that are required not only to meet basic human needs but also to achieve the goals of health, well-being, and promotion of development. Looking backward at our history helps us understand our present and be able to contemplate our future. Nursing has evolved from care given by good-meaning people to a profession with a science base. Knowledge of where the profession of nursing began and how it has evolved and changed throughout the ages provides the basis for understanding the goals and processes of the profession. It also provides the nurse with an appreciation and valuing of what nursing is, what nurses do, how nurses think, and their place in society.

CHAPTER 1

NURSING

Profession and Discipline

Nursing is both a profession and a discipline. The *profession* encompasses the responsibilities, standards of action, and the structure of the work of nurses. It defines the place of nursing within the social and political milieu. The *discipline* refers to the body of knowledge that informs nursing actions and relationships. Together, the practice of nursing is formed and informed.

The landscape of health care and nursing is changing dramatically and at an increasingly rapid pace, which is often referred to as an *evolution of convergence* (de Chardin, 1959) or an *accelerating evolution* (Rogers, 1986). One needs to look backward at our history to understand our present and to be able to contemplate our future. Many disciplines use theories of evolution to explain not only how we (the universe, organisms, civilization, people) got to where we are but also to where we may be going. This movement has not been easy. There are issues that endure to this day. With this background, the professional nurse is able to participate more fully in giving impetus to the future development of health care for the health and well-being of the individual as well as for social groups and communities. Globalization is changing the face of health care and how we interact both within our own social groups and between groups.

OBJECTIVES

After reading this chapter, the learner will be able to:

1. Describe the characteristics of a profession
2. Differentiate between the profession of nursing and the discipline of nursing
3. Explain how four major types of change have influenced development of the nursing profession

4. Evaluate the role of care and caring in the nursing profession today
5. Demonstrate understanding of how general systems theory has been applied in various nursing theories
6. Discuss complexity theory and how it relates to nursing
7. Describe the process of the development of nursing knowledge
8. Differentiate between explicit and tacit knowledge
9. Analyze the relative value of different ways and patterns of knowing within the discipline of nursing

KEY CONCEPTS   profession • discipline • types of change • care/caring • General Systems Theory • complexity • explicit knowledge • tacit knowledge • patterns of knowing • structure of the discipline of nursing

PROFESSION

The professions are an example of the establishment of structured relationships with allocation of tasks. A profession arises when any trade or occupation transforms itself through "the development of formal qualifications based upon education, apprenticeship, and examinations, the emergence of regulatory bodies with powers to admit and discipline members, and some degree of monopoly rights" (Bullock & Trombley, 1999, p. 689).

A profession requires specialized education, knowledge, training, and ethics. Although professionals make their living in what they do, this paid work is often more than just a job alone. Whatever the profession, those who are in it are expected to meet and maintain common standards. In nursing, these standards are established by the professional organizations and legislative bodies. Professions are, ideally, made up of people with high ethical standards and who have special knowledge and skills. Nurses who practice nursing with a healthy sense of professionalism are aware of the relationship between what they know and what they do. The professional nurse has a language through which to communicate facts, ideas, and questions about nursing. The professional nurse understands both the practical and the scientific aspects of nursing. He or she will take actions, such as continuing education, formal education, or participation in discussion groups, that are needed to pursue a career in nursing. A *career* is an individual's journey through learning, work, and other aspects of life and is considered a person's life's work. It usually requires special learning that includes individualized components that develop abilities beyond those of which training is capable. A career may not mean stability of work, as it encourages one to take risks. The risks are often internal and therefore planned, such as returning to school. Getting your BSN is a step in the journey, a step up the career ladder.

The organization of health care is a topic of great discussion at this time. The role and scope of nursing within systems of health care are undergoing critical examination. This organization occurs within a particular political system based only partly on the person's need for assistance. How the profession of nursing will evolve is undetermined. Given the rapidity of change and evolution, it is impossible to predict what the nursing profession will look like in the future. With the aim of nurses probably having some control or influence over the direction of change, knowledge of the evolution through the centuries can lead to an understanding of the fundamental principles and values that guided and still guide nurses. These become the foundation for nursing in the future. How did we get to this—to becoming a profession?

Change

There are four types of change that are important to health care and nursing: evolution, adaptation, transformation, and globalization. These types of change are considered in relationship to the development of nursing. See Box 1.1 for a brief description of each of these types of change.

EVOLUTION

The entire universe is constantly evolving. Advances in technology have made it possible for us to understand what this changing universe looks like and how it is affecting the human condition. Nursing is concerned with human people. But people do not exist and live separate from the environment. There is constant, and perhaps simultaneous, interaction between the person and the environment that is a part of the process of evolution. A number of nursing scholars base their work on the ideas of interaction and adaptation. Roy (2009) views nursing as an adaptive

---

BOX 1.1   Description of Types of Change

Evolution

- A dynamic, unfolding, and irreversible process of change with increasing complexity involving all aspects of life

Adaptation

- The process by which an organism or a social institution becomes better suited to its environment, accomplished by change in the organism and/or the environment; the change may be temporary or may become evolutionary over time

Transformation

- A deliberate rather than an evolutionary process of changing something or someone completely for the better

Globalization

- Sometimes viewed as an evolutionary development, characterized by growing connectivity between people and nations, and the emergence of global institutions

system. Rogers (1970, 1992) and Parse (1987, 1992) focus on the simultaneity of interaction between the person and the environment. We humans tend to believe that we are in control of our world, if not the universe. Technology and the increased knowledge that comes with it are showing us that we do, in fact, have some—albeit at this time limited—ability to influence the direction of the change. Some of this may be temporary change but others have the potential to be evolutionary. In a work of fiction, Brown (2013) portrays the effects of the changing world on population growth, describes the consequences of overpopulation on health and social structures, and presents options for changing the outcomes for society, including genetic modifications that will either halt or greatly slow down this overpopulation. The recognition and resolution (or nonresolution) of such dilemmas will face society and challenge our views of person and caring in both the near and extended future. The more we understand the processes of evolution, the better we will be able to respond.

Evolution is simply the way biological, chemical, and physical processes proceed, while science is concerned with mechanisms of action and interaction of events at the physical level. Evolution is basically a learning process, that is, "a trial-and-error process that produces a progressive accumulation of knowledge" (Heylighen, 2007, p. 1).

This implies a specific evolutionary dynamic with a nonarbitrary directional process—that is, what has evolved cannot be un-evolved. A broader meaning of evolution includes dynamic change in all aspects of living. Evolution is a dynamic, unfolding process of increasing complexity. The organisms we see around us have their present characteristics because of their evolution in past circumstances. The idea that human beings have an evolved nature as well as a cultural nature is now being studied by anthropologists and others. They propose that the answer to the question regarding human behavior—is it nature or nurture?—will be shown to be both with an identifiable interconnection between them, with human behavior explained as a product of both culture and evolution (Barna, 2013).

The contemporary view of the world is that of a dynamic, open-ended system in which some events are, in principle, unpredictable. The universe seems to be inherently relational (Barbour, 1997). "Complex dynamic systems, whether physical, chemical, biological, social or personal, are … driven from … [states of] equilibrium" to a point/time when they bifurcate with the possibility of self-organization or they "leap abruptly into new states of increasing order and complexity" (Delio, 2008, p. 18). The process of evolution has a pattern of "crisis and renewal" (p. 19). This relates to the cosmos, the biosphere, and sociocultural revolutions in human history, each of which gives rise to "new, more organized and more inclusive forms of life" (p. 19). Knowledge of the processes of evolution and its path and extent is growing exponentially. What is happening has been described as accelerating evolution; that is, there is more change occurring at a more rapid pace now than in the past and changes will occur with even greater rapidity as we go into the future. Not only understanding what went on in the past but also attempting to influence the path to the future are increasing, with mixed results. Evolution can best be represented as a monotonous (always increasing, one directional) function, although the speed of the corresponding advance is variable, with ups and downs that may give an impression of periodicity, but—most importantly—a strong tendency toward acceleration.

The evolution of care/caring

"Evolution"

Now the times change, the ancient lore gives way
Or meets the keen, relentless test of science.
As blacksmith grew to engineer, and barber became surgeon,
The kindly neighbor now is nurse: and studied skill
Adds to the art of friendly ministration.

—Anonymous (1930, p. 455)

The profession of nursing as we experience it today evolved from minimally organized caring in prehistoric times through centuries where there were levels of greater organization and specialization of caring. Persons begin life dependent on their mothers and the mothers' social group. Within these groups, the pattern of care varied by historic time and by culture.

In early Neolithic Vietnam, a young man survived from early adolescence into adulthood while being completely paralyzed from the waist down and with very limited use of his upper body. Dependent on others for meeting his most basic needs, his survival was only possible because of the high-quality, dedicated, and time-consuming care he received (Tilley, 2012). Looking after those who are unable to look after themselves is a behavior that defines what it is to be human. Furthermore, "without a sense of caring, there can be no sense of community" (D'Angelo, n.d.).

Anthropologist Margaret Mead was once asked what she considered the earliest evidence of civilization. She answered that it was a human thigh bone with a healed fracture that had been excavated from a 15,000-year-old site. For an early human being to have survived a broken femur, living through the months that were required for the bone to heal, the person had to have been cared for—sheltered, protected, and brought food and drink. "While other animals care for their young and injured, no other species is able [or chooses to] to devote as much time and energy to caring for the most frail, ill, and dying of its members" (Byock, 2012).

Evidence suggests that health-related care has been practiced within the human family at least for the past 100,000 years, and some biologists even claim that caregiving was essential to human evolution. Certainly, our response to the health needs of others embodies a wealth of information about ourselves and our community, reflecting cultural norms and values; collective knowledge, skills, and experience; socioeconomic organization; and access to the resources that allow the support of someone experiencing disability.

Care is operationally defined by archeologists as the provision of assistance to an individual experiencing pathology who would otherwise have been unlikely to survive to the age he or she did. Archeologists infer health-related care provision from physical evidence that an individual survived with, or recovered from, a disease or injury that was likely to have resulted in serious disability. What health care comprised depended on the nature of the disability, the context in which it occurred, and care recipient characteristics. Tilley (2012) viewed care as either *direct support* (e.g., providing resources, nursing, and physical therapy) or *accommodation of difference* (e.g., strategies that enable a level of participation in social and/or economic activity). Care may begin as support and be changed to accommodation as an individual recovers (but is left with some disability)—or vice versa. Historical care can only be inferred with reference to what is known about the contemporary social, cultural, economic, and physical environments. What constitutes health, disease, and disability is understood very differently in diverse cultures and at various points in time. In relation to understanding caregiving from the historical aspect, questions might consider what options were likely available for caring, which appear to have been adopted, and why; a comparison of the potential costs and benefits of choices available and those selected; what the ability to provide care suggests about group organization, practice, and history; and what the decision to give care, as well as the type and extent of care given, suggests about general norms and values of the group (Tilley, 2012). Questions of interest about the recipient of care begin with knowing the normal role of the person within the sociocultural context. What was the likely impact of disability on the care recipient's ability to fulfil this role? What alternative roles were available? What sort of personality characteristics might have been needed to manage pathology-imposed limitations? What sort of personality might have inspired others to support or accommodate this particular individual's needs, possibly in difficult circumstances? Throughout history, as knowledge regarding people, disease, effects of environment on health, germ theory, and other events changed, our concepts of care and caring also changed.

There are many representations of care. Care is considered the basis of all the helping professions, of which nursing is one. Some nursing scholars consider caring to be the essence of nursing, the central focus of the profession. There are a number of dimensions related to care that are of importance to nurses: care, caring about, caring for, and taking care of. Although they are all aspects or elements of nursing, they are not exclusive to nursing and manifest themselves in different ways.

> *Too often we underestimate the power of a touch, a smile, a kind word, a listening ear, an honest compliment, or the smallest act of caring, all of which have the potential to turn a life around.*
>
> —Buscaglia (n.d.)

Although each case of care is unique, there is a fundamental principle to be observed in all cases of health-related care: recognition that care is the product of agency. Human agency is the power or capacity of a person to act. Caregiving is an intentional, goal-directed response to a perceived health crisis, and it often consists of complex, interrelated, continuously refined, and negotiated behaviors carried out over time. The decisions reached in relation to giving and receiving care hold the key to interpretation of the event and focus on which of the likely choices made contributed to achieving the care outcomes.

Care is intrinsically emotive and value laden. Care and caring are the subjects of study by nurse scientists; they are also used by educated practitioners of nursing. Their work is important in understanding the dimensions of care. Recent studies make the dimensions of care and caring more explicit. Our understanding of care and caring has evolved from understanding human feelings of affection and connection to recognition of the difference between and complementarity of caring for and caring about. The work done by nurse scientists and philosophers has further made these dimensions known, as well as identified actions of the nurses that manifest and enable care (Finfgeld-Connett, 2008).

EVOLUTION AND CHANGE IN NURSING AND HEALTH CARE

As described earlier, evolution is change over time that becomes permanent. Adaptation is reversible change, like the chameleon changes color as it enters a different environment. Much of what has occurred in nursing relative to change is adaptation. Over time, some adaptive changes may become evolutionary. However, many changes in roles and scope of practice could be either undone or enhanced with legislation. As the evolution of care/caring was happening, so also was the evolution of the actions and knowledge base of the caregivers or healers. The practice and knowledge guiding it were not and are not separate one from the other. Knowledge must guide practice, and practice must contribute to the development of knowledge. Over the history of health care and nursing, this knowledge development led to the development of nursing as a unique area of practice with an identifiable body of knowledge.

The assignment of functions related to caring and healing were culturally based. With the passing of time, these functions were separated and in many cultures they became associated with gender-specific roles. A gendered division of labor describes a set of institutionalized arrangements in which certain forms of work are allocated to women and others are allocated to men. Most late 20th-century anthropologists believed that all societies practiced some form of gendered division of labor, although the content of the work assigned to men and women varied widely from group to group and from place to place. Even as gendered divisions of labor drew women and men into intimate, independent patterns of engagement, the activities generally assigned to women and men were not equally valued. This is true of nursing and medicine. There has been significant change in the gender specificity of caring/healing work in recent decades. The value of division of labor has been skewed to the healing functions as opposed to the caring functions. As science comes to know more about the interrelatedness of caring and healing, the roles and functions of practitioners change. Development of caring components remained experiential for centuries and lagged behind the development of the healing sciences. The development of nursing was closely associated with religious groups and responsibilities. The evolution of the profession of nursing is associated with these culturally, socially, and religiously assigned roles and functions. Included in the evolution of the profession is the development and emergence of a unique body of knowledge, which is an essential characteristic of a profession.

Change is both a process and a product, that is, it is a process of becoming different or making something or somebody different; however, the product of change is an altered way of thinking or a shift from one state, stage, or phase to another, something different. Change is generally considered reversible and can be done purposefully by manipulating aspects of open dynamic systems. Theories of open, dynamic systems are given consideration in many of the sciences that are foundational to nursing. The concept of complex dynamic systems is of major importance in nursing. When nursing scholars were formalizing conceptual models, systems theory was a common element in all their works. Peplau (1991) looked at nursing from the perspective of interpersonal systems. King's (1981) Theory of Goal Attainment comprised personal, interpersonal, and social systems. Neuman (1980) took a broader view of systems and placed nursing within that perspective. Roy (2009) identified a person as an adaptive system. Orem (2001) worked from the perspective of action systems. Common to all was the understanding of and use of principles of and elements from General Systems Theory. A contemporary view of the nursing process is now expanded to contain recognition of the complexities and unpredictability of outcomes hoped/planned for.

The basic analytical tool is still that of systems theory enhanced with the greater recognition of the people, interactions, and processes shown in Figure 1.1. The theory was proposed by von Bertalanffy (1968).

A related model is a model of communication and control (Weiner, 1948) or cybernetics. It explains the system process of information exchange between two elements of a system. An example of its use in nursing is seen in King's work (1981).

Adaptation and *transformation,* two terms that are associated with change, describe the outcome of change. Adaptation is the process where an organism or a social institution becomes better suited to its habitat. This change can be either temporary or evolutionary, and it may be accomplished by a change in the organism or a change in the environment or habitat. There are many instances where nurses assist people in adapting to something, such as changing health conditions, or in adjusting to different situations, conditions, or to a new environment. Adaptation is the focus of Roy's theory. From this perspective, adaptation, the positive response to or coping with environmental changes, is the goal of nursing and it results in the outcome of health (Roy, 2009).

The adaptation of organisms tracks changes in the environment, but there will generally be a slight lag between the two. A feature will be adaptive now so long as the present environment is relevantly similar to the ancestral environment. What organisms have become is a result of adapting to things that happened in the past. The organisms we see around us have their present characteristics because of their evolution in past circumstances. For example, resistant strains of bacteria became

FIGURE 1.1　General Systems Theory Basic Model

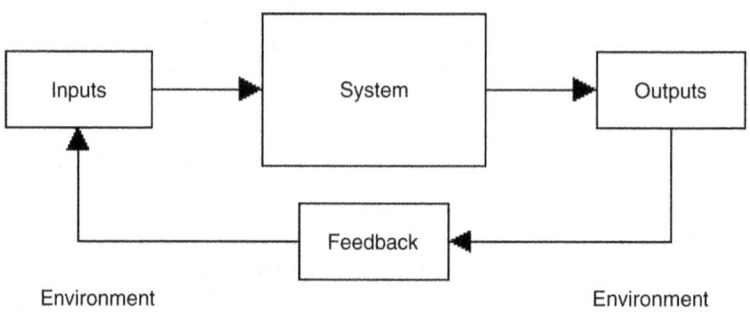

Adapted from von Bertalanffy (1968).

resistant because of the changes to their environment in the past. When new anti-bacterial drugs are introduced, the changes in the bacteria will no longer be adaptive and they will begin to change and evolve as their environment changes. The overuse of antibiotics in people and animals, often for conditions for which the drugs are either ineffective or not needed, is seen as a driving force in the development of resistant bacteria that are often referred to as *super bugs*. The evolutionary cycle for bacteria is comparatively short, leading to a major health care crisis with significant personal, ethical, and societal dimensions. Genetics acts in combination with an organism's environment and experiences to influence development and behavior. Genes may be activated or inactivated, as determined by a cell's or organism's intra- or extracellular environment. For example, genes play a role in determining human height, whereas an individual's nutrition and health during childhood also have a large effect.

Manipulation of any part of the system will produce changes in the other parts. Although some of these changes may be planned and intended, there is always the possibility of unintended consequences. Since all the conditions and aspects of the system are seldom known, the change in one condition may have an outcome that could not be predicted with the available information. For example, drug manufacturers rigorously test their product to create a therapeutic physiological or biochemical change within the person; however, adverse reactions or the absence of a response in the patient are known to occur. Change is a constant in our world; in fact, in the entire universe. The person who initiates or activates the change through action is referred to as a *change agent*. Nurses are often urged to be change agents for individuals, organizations, and broader systems. The purpose of nursing is to create or assist in change related to health and self-care.

Transform means to change somebody or something completely, especially to improve that person's or thing's appearance or usefulness for the better. Transformation is the result of a deliberate rather than evolutionary process. Activities within the health care arena are specifically designed to transform the system.

GLOBALIZATION

Globalization is sometimes viewed as an evolutionary process, which is one of the outcomes of contemporary change (Modelski, 2007). Globalization is characterized by two complementary processes, both of which take place at the planetary (not universal) scale: (a) growing connectivity between people and nations; and (b) the emergence of global institutions. Connections form within social groups when members of the group contribute to meeting the needs of the group and have their own needs met partly by others in the group. It is this basic connection at the heart of human societies that is changing and beginning to be radically reformed (Gore, 2013, p. 60). Globalization of health care is occurring and will only be more a factor in the near future. What is driving this globalization? Several trends of importance are:

- The emerging of a "deeply interconnected global economy" (p. 7)
- A planetwide electronic communication and transportation grid
- Connecting people to rapidly expanding volumes of data

- Increasingly intelligent devices
- Radically different "balance of political, economic and military power" (p. 7)
- Rapid unsustainable growth in populations
- Revolutionary new sets of science technologies, for instance, genetic engineering (Gore, 2013)

The world in which we live and act is changing. Some of this change is evolutionary, and some is more transient. To some extent, we humans can influence both evolution and adaptation or transformative changes. Our ability to do so is accelerating at a rapid pace.

COMPLEXITY

One aspect of our world shaping what we do and how we do it is that of complexity. Scientists and philosophers believe that all things are connected. There are many ways to look at these connections. String theory, the theory of everything, chaos theory, and relationship theories are a few. The one theory commonly used in health care to describe what is happening and how it is organized is systems theory. The complex health care environment presents formidable challenges, as transformations in care processes are designed and implemented.

Complexity involves movement in nonlinear and interactive modalities with unpredicted outcomes that are often realized. Organizations are described as "ever-changing collections of individuals, systems and processes that are dynamic in their interactions" (Hast, DiGioia, Anthony, Thompson, & Wolf, 2013, p. 44) or collections of individuals interacting with their environment in ways that are interconnected and unpredictable. Health care organizations are complex adaptive systems where there is constant molding, adapting to the environment, and emerging into new levels of practice as expertise and local experience allow. Interactions are difficult to predict and control and are robust, unique, and innovative. Rich communication networks exist both among and between complex adaptive systems. Interactions are dependent on the scope of individuals involved in an organization and result in tremendous variability in outcomes. Change occurs as individuals, conditions in the organization, patterns of interaction among individuals, and connections are made through networks of individual agents. Concepts that are relevant to complexity include self-organization; emergence; system characteristics, including information flow; and sense making. As an individual makes changes, new patterns emerge (self-organization and emergence) and characteristics of the system begin to change. The people use their knowledge and imagination to derive new meaning from the perceived patterns. This sense making becomes the basis for considering change, reframing the situation, or generating research questions (Geary & Schumacher, 2012).

Much of what is viewed within the nursing and organization literature regarding complexity is speculative. Metaphors form the basis for much of this. It is not science until it is verified, that is, quantifiable. There is much good learning that comes from ways of knowing, in addition to science (Phelan, 2001). A refined view of nursing through an integrated theoretical perspective enhances the individual's ability to do sense making.

What does knowledge of complexity have to do with nursing? First, it leads nurses to value themselves as complex individuals with a need for self-reflection and understanding. It may help in avoiding an expectation of simple solutions to complex questions. But more importantly, it gives direction to understanding the care needs of individuals within the contexts of self, family, community, and environment. Finding patterns and assigning meaning is/should be a deliberate process. Frequent experiences with similar phenomena may lead to habitual behavior, which may be efficient in practice but may limit the nurse's ability to personalize care and participate in organizational change. The nurse desiring to be a change agent must learn about complex adaptive systems and develop skill in identifying system characteristics.

DISCIPLINE

Disciplinary knowledge is the basis for the profession. The evolution of the profession of nursing is associated with culturally and socially assigned roles and functions. The evolution of the profession includes the development and emergence of a unique body of knowledge, which is an essential characteristic of a profession. Discipline refers to the structured body of knowledge that is unique to nursing and informs its profession and practice.

The development of the knowledge base began experientially; that is, the caregiver/healer tried something that seemed reasonable to him or her. That could be something that someone else had tried with success or something congruent with religious belief. If the action affected the situation positively, it would be repeated in future similar situations. If the result was undesirable, something else might be tried or the situation might be viewed as not amenable to intervention. Many of the decisions were formed within a particular situation. One's view of human beings is crucial to one's approach to health care.

Interaction with other groups, such as nomadic tribes, enhanced the sharing and aggregation of knowledge, a beginning of what we now see as the beginning of the globalization of health care. Methods of communication began to rely less on the oral tradition and more on forms of written communication. The sharing of experiential knowledge was cross-cultural. As the domestication of pack animals and the development of shipping technology increased the capacity for prehistoric people to carry heavier loads over greater distances, cultural exchanges and trade developed rapidly. Soon after the Roman conquest of Egypt in 30 BCE, regular communications and trade between China, Southeast Asia, India, the Middle East, Africa, and Europe blossomed on an unprecedented scale. The eastern trade routes from the earlier Hellenistic powers and the Arabs that were a part of the Silk Road were inherited by the Roman Empire. "Some studies indicate that the Black Death, which devastated Europe in the late 1340s, may have reached Europe from Central Asia (or China) along the trade routes of the Mongol Empire" (Hays, 2005). The flow of culture and goods continues to this day. Western medical practices have a significant influence on Eastern cultures' delivery of care, predominantly through the development of science and technology. In recent decades, Eastern traditions have been driving a renewed interest in alternative medicine or caring practices; for example, meditation and acupuncture (Hansen, 2012; Kuzmina & Mair, 2008).

The Discipline of Nursing Is Developing Through Research and Science

Humans have an unrelenting desire to know. As knowledge accumulated over time, thinkers in many social groups were developing ways to verify knowledge or establish truth. Over time, common agreement on methods of knowing emerged. The methods of science provided verifiable information. No one person can be credited as the inventor of the scientific method. Rather than being invented, it was recognized and developed as the natural method of obtaining reliable knowledge. Many authors trace the beginning of the scientific method and experimenting back to ancient artisans, Greeks, Arabs, Spaniards, and others (Scientific Method History, n.d.).

Aristotle (384–322 BCE), one of history's noted original thinkers, was the first to devise methods for trying to arrive at reliable knowledge based on observation. Roger Bacon (1214–1294), drawing on the writings of Muslim scientists, described a repeating cycle of observation, hypothesis, experimentation, and verification. Current methods of science and the development of knowledge merge elements of philosophical thinking and methods of science.

Knowing connotes that one has a solid base on which to structure an action or way of being. That base is knowledge, but in order to gain knowledge one has to employ a process known as learning. Throughout your journey into professional nursing, you will build a knowledge base and master technologies that enable you to both think and do nursing. The use of conceptual maps and an understanding of the value or meaning of tacit knowledge as well as explicit knowledge will be important as you move forward from being a novice or a beginner to being a competent nurse and, eventually, an expert. A cognitive map (also known as a *mental map* or *mental model*) is a type of mental representation that serves an individual to acquire, code, store, recall, and decode information about the relative locations and attributes of phenomena in their everyday or metaphorical spatial environment. The development of your own cognitive map is a function of both explicit knowledge/learning and tacit knowing/learning.

Explicit knowledge is both formal and systematic. It can be easily communicated and shared. Typically, it has been documented, expressed, and recorded as words, numbers, codes, mathematical and scientific formulae, and musical notations. Explicit knowledge is easy to communicate, store, and distribute and it is the knowledge found in books, on the web, and through other visual and oral means. You gain explicit knowledge through formal learning and self-education.

Tacit knowledge, on the other hand, is not so easily expressed. It is highly personal, hard to formalize, and difficult to communicate to others. It may also be impossible to capture. The challenge is to identify which elements of tacit knowledge can be captured and made explicit—while accepting that some tacit knowledge just cannot be captured. For tacit knowledge that cannot be captured, the goal is to connect the possessors of tacit knowledge with the seekers of that knowledge. Tacit knowledge consists of beliefs, ideals, values, schemata, and mental models that are deeply ingrained in us and that we often take for granted. Although difficult to articulate, this cognitive dimension of tacit knowledge shapes the way we perceive the world. It involves learning and skill but not in a way that can be written down. On this account, knowledge, or embodied knowledge, is characteristic of the expert, who acts, makes judgments, and so forth, without discernibly reflecting on the principles or rules involved. The expert works without having a theory of his or her work; he or she just performs skillfully without deliberation or focused attention. The transfer of tacit knowledge requires close interaction and the buildup of shared understanding and trust among experts and knowledge-seekers. This is one of the reasons for nursing students to have clinical experiences with seasoned nurses.

There is much tacit knowledge used in nursing. It is acquired through practice and interacting with expert nurses. For such knowledge to have meaning, it is interpreted within a well-defined theoretical structure of nursing. Much of what is viewed or thought of as tacit knowledge can, in fact, be communicated and become explicit knowledge through sharing in interviews, conducting research, writing case studies, and so on. Do not be satisfied when someone tells you, "We've always done it this way." Ask for explanations: Ask "why." With tacit knowledge, people are often unaware of the knowledge they possess or how it can be valuable to others. Effective transfer of tacit knowledge generally requires extensive personal contact, regular interaction, and trust. This kind of knowledge can only be revealed through practice in a particular context and transmitted through social networks. To some extent, it is "captured" when the knowledge holder joins a network or a community of practice (Smith, 2003).

CONTEMPORARY WAYS OF KNOWING IN NURSING

Gathering information in a methodical way is an early stage of the scientific method. Evidence refers to what is known about the phenomenon of concern, gathered through a thorough review and synthesis of the literature and incorporating what is known experientially. Evidence is (or should be) based in experimental research to the extent possible. This evidence can be the basis for evaluating a clinical practice or problem. This method has limitations for knowing in nursing practice. Hence, other ways of knowing and methods of knowledge development beyond those of experiential and experimental knowledge are being used in the development of nursing knowledge today.

Although much emphasis is placed on the development and use of scientific knowledge, humans come to know in other ways. "In preparation for the future, both nurses and nursing students must understand how to learn rather than how to hoard knowledge, how to critique rather than how to accept, how to expand rather than how to contract" (Silva, Sorrell, & Sorrell, 1995).

An early formulation of how nurses know, extending beyond the scientific, was Carper's (1978) fundamental patterns of knowing in nursing: empirics, esthetic, personal knowing, and ethics. Though presented as discrete categories, they are now viewed as integrated and interrelated ways of knowing, encompassing both the science and the art of nursing. *Empirics* refers to scientific and factual knowledge and *esthetics* refers to the art of nursing and creative knowledge, whereas *ethics* deals with the moral component of nursing. Personal knowing is the relational component and therapeutic engagement with the patient; knowledge develops from reflection (McGovern, Lapum, Clune, & Martin, 2013).

KNOWLEDGE DEVELOPMENT THROUGH CASE STUDIES

The use of cases to develop knowledge is well known. In the field of ethics, this is known as *casuistry*. Casuistry is reasoning that is used to resolve moral problems by extracting or extending theoretical rules from particular instances and applying these rules to new instances. In nursing and medicine, case studies are used in the clinical setting for knowledge and synthesis. New ideas often emerge when the science behind the case is reviewed. The identification of patterns or aberrations in collected case studies can lead to questions for research.

In nursing, case studies are used to teach clinical decision making and critical thinking skills. An example of a collection of cases for use in nursing is *Winningham's Critical Thinking Cases in Nursing: Medical–Surgical, Pediatric, Maternity, and Psychiatric* (Harding, Snyder, & Preusser, 2013). The scholarly tradition of using comparative cases to generate new knowledge is not yet established in nursing. This may be due, in part, to the fact that nursing cases have traditionally been categorized according to the medical paradigm (e.g., medical, surgical, etc.). They have also been categorized by location of service—community, acute care, home care—and occasionally by population—adult, child, family. To be useful in generating new knowledge, the analysis of nursing cases should reflect the structure of the discipline of nursing, examining nursing-sensitive variables. Nursing-sensitive indicators refer to things that respond to nursing interventions. They may be aspects of patient care that are directly related to the quality and quantity of nursing care. Some indicators identified in the literature include "hospital rates of decubitus ulcer, failure to rescue, infections due to medical care, acute myocardial infarction (AMI) mortality, congestive heart failure mortality, and pneumonia mortality" (Furukawa, Raghu, & Shao, 2010). As you proceed through this text and your curriculum, you will be introduced to other ways of identifying nurse-sensitive outcomes and their measurement.

The Structure of the Discipline

NURSING'S METAPARADIGM

Acknowledging that nursing has a particular body of knowledge, how would we describe or circumscribe that knowledge? Fawcett (1984) formalized what has come to be known as nursing's metaparadigm concepts, namely person, health, environment, and nursing. These concepts have been generally accepted within the discipline. The literature is replete with analysis, descriptions, and commentaries about these. The one that needs the most definition is the concept of nursing. In the next few chapters, we explore a structure or theory that includes and expands on the concept of nursing that is congruent with and complementary to the evolving views of health, well-being, and self-care.

To begin, the structure of the discipline (Figure 1.2) lays out the relationship of areas of knowledge that inform nursing science and the field of nursing itself.

Relevant non-nursing sciences indicate the bodies of knowledge that help us understand the science of nursing. The categories identified in the diagram are neither exclusive nor inclusive. Many categories of basic knowledge could be used. As science progresses, new designations are being introduced that have relevance

FIGURE 1.2   The Structure of the Discipline

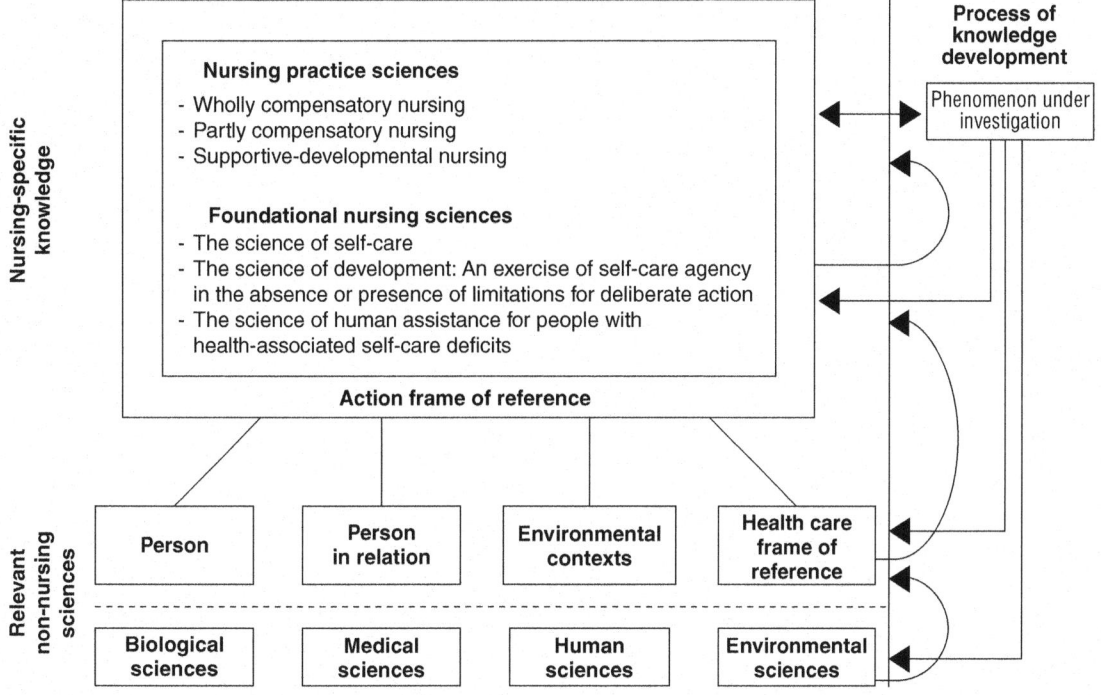

Source: Renpenning, Taylor, Bekel, and Denyes (2004).

for nursing science and practice. These provide us with knowledge that is needed to understand and work with people, people in relation, environmental contexts, and the health care frame of reference. This structure is built on the premise that all knowledge is ultimately related; though each discipline has a particular focus, knowledge has meaning across boundaries (Taylor & Renpenning, 2011, p. 20). Nursing-specific knowledge is within an action frame of reference. The significance of this and descriptions of the identified categories are developed in future chapters. Clearly, to be interdisciplinary requires that the person have clear understanding of the focus and processes of the discipline they represent.

LEARNING ACTIVITIES

1. Diagram a system indicating and labeling elements, boundaries, and relationships. Show how a change in one element would lead to change in another.
2. Explain the significance of distinguishing between profession and discipline.
3. Formulate in your own words a brief paragraph that reflects your understanding of the structure of the discipline of nursing as represented in Figure 1.2.

References

Anonymous. (1930). Evolution. *The American Journal of Nursing, 30*(4). Retrieved from http://www.jstor.org.proxy.mul.missouri.edu/stable/3411166

Barbour, I. (1997). *Issues in science and religion.* London, UK: SCM Press.

Barna, M. (2013). Anthropology faculty explore links between evolution and human behavior. *Mizzou Weekly, 35*(4).

Brown, D. (2013). *Inferno.* New York, NY: Doubleday.

Bullock, A., & Trombley, S. (1999). *The new Fontana dictionary of modern thought.* London, UK: HarperCollins.

Buscaglia, L. (n.d.). Retrieved from www.goodreads.com/quotes/tag/caring

Byock, I. (2012). *The best care possible: A physician's quest to transform care through the end of life.* New York, NY: Avery/Penguin Group.

Carper, B. (1978). Fundamental patterns of knowing in nursing. *Advances in Nursing Science, 1*(1), 13–23.

D'angelo, A. (n.d.). Retrieved from www.brainyquote.com/quotes/authors/a/anthony_j_dangelo.html

de Chardin, P. T. (1959). *The phenomenon of man* (B. Wall, Trans.). New York, NY: Harper. (Original work published 1955).

Delio, I. (2008). *Christ in evolution.* Maryknoll, NY: Orbis Books.

Fawcett, J. (1984). The metaparadigm of nursing: Present status and future refinements. *Journal of Nursing Scholarship, 16*(3), 77–87. doi:10.1111/j.1547-5069.1984.tb01393.x

Finfgeld-Connett, D. (2008). Meta-synthesis of caring in nursing. *Journal of Clinical Nursing, 17,* 196–204.

Furukawa, M. F., Raghu, T. S., & Shao, B. B. M. (2010). Electronic medical records, nurse staffing, and nurse-sensitive patient outcomes: Evidence from California hospitals, 1998–2007. *Health Services Research, 45*(4), 941–962. doi:10.1111/j.1475-6773.2010.01110.x

Geary, C. R., & Schumacher, K. L. (2012). Care transitions: Integrating transition theory and complexity science concepts. *Advances in Nursing Science, 35*(3), 236–248. doi:10.1097/ANS.0b013e31826260a5

Gore, A. (2013). *The future: Six drivers of global change.* New York, NY: Random House.

Hansen, V. (2012). *The silk road: A new history.* New York, NY: Oxford University Press.

Harding, M. M., Snyder, J. S., & Preusser, B. A. (2013). *Winningham's critical thinking cases in nursing: Medical-surgical, pediatric, maternity, and psychiatric* (5th ed.). St. Louis, MO: Mosby.

Hast, A. S., DiGioia, I., Anthony, M., Thompson, D., & Wolf, G. (2013). Utilizing complexity science to drive practice change through patient- and family-centered care. *Journal of Nursing Administration, 43*(1), 44–49. doi:10.1097/NNA.0b013e31827860db

Hays, J. N. (2005). *Epidemics and pandemics: Their impacts on human history.*

Heylighen, F. (2007). Accelerating socio-technological evolution: From ephemeralization and stigmergy to the global brain. In G. Modelski, T. Devezas, & W. Thompson (Eds.). *Globalization as an evolutionary process: Modeling global change.* London, UK: Routledge.

King, I. M. (1981). *A theory for nursing: Symptoms, concepts, process.* New York, NY: John Wiley & Sons.

Kuzmina, E. E., & Mair, V. H. (2008). *The prehistory of the Silk Road.* Philadelphia, PA: University of Pennsylvania Press.

McGovern, B., Lapum, J., Clune, L., & Martin, L. S. (2013). Theoretical framing of high-fidelity simulation with Carper's fundamental patterns of knowing in nursing. *Journal of Nursing Education, 52*(1), 46–49. doi:10.3928/01484834-20121217-02

Modelski, G. (2007). Globalization as an evolutionary process. In G. Modelski, T. Devezas, & W. Thompson (Eds.), *Globalization as an evolutionary process: Modeling global change* (pp. 11–29). London, UK: Routledge.

Neuman, B. (1980). The Betty Neuman health-care systems model: A total person approach to patient problems. In J. P. Riehl & C. Roy (Eds.), *Conceptual models for nursing practice* (2nd ed., pp. 119–134). New York, NY: Appleton-Century-Crofts.

Orem, D. E. (2001). *Nursing: Concepts of practice*. St. Louis, MO: Mosby.

Parse, R. (1987). *Nursing science: Major paradigms, theories and critiques*. Philadelphia, PA: W. B. Saunders.

Parse, R. R. (1992). Human becoming: Parse's theory of nursing. *Nursing Science Quarterly, 5*, 35–42.

Peplau, H. E. (1991). *Interpersonal relations in nursing: A conceptual frame of reference for psychodynamic nursing*. New York, NY: Springer Publishing Company.

Phelan, S. E. (2001). What is complexity science, really? *Emergence: Complexity and organization, 3*(1), 120–136. doi:10.1207/S15327000EM031_08 Retrieved from https://faculty.unlv.edu/phelan/Phelan_What%20is%20complexity%20science.pdf

Renpenning, K., Taylor, S., Bekel, G., & Denyes, J. (2004). Structure of the discipline of nursing within foundational and nursing specific knowledge. Paper presented at the 8th World Congress Self-Care Deficit Nursing Theory. September 29–October 3, 2004. Ulm, Germany.

Rogers, M. E. (1970). *An introduction to the theoretical basis of nursing*. Philadelphia, PA: F. A. Davis.

Rogers, M. E. (1986). Science of unitary beings. In V. M. Malinski (Ed.), *Explorations on Martha Rogers' science of unitary human-beings* (pp. 3–8). Norwalk, CT: Appleton-Century-Crofts.

Rogers, M. E. (1992). Nursing science and the space age. *Nursing Science Quarterly, 5*, 27–33.

Roy, C. (2009). *The Roy adaptation model* (3rd ed.). Upper Saddle River, NJ: Prentice Hall Health.

Scientific Method History. (n.d.). Retrieved from www.scientificmethod.com/sm5_smhistory.html

Silva, M. C., Sorrell, J. M., & Sorrell, C. D. (1995). From Carper's patterns of knowing to ways of being: An ontological philosophical shift in nursing. *Advances in Nursing Science, 18*(1), 1–13.

Smith, M. K. (2003). Michael Polanyi and tacit knowledge. *The Encyclopedia of Informal Education*. Retrieved from http://infed.org/mobi/michael-polanyi-and-tacit-knowledge

Taylor, S. G., & Renpenning, K. (2011). *Self-care science, nursing theory, and evidence-based practice*. New York, NY: Springer Publishing Company.

Tilley, L. (2012). The bioarchaeology of care. *The SAA Archaeological Record, 12*(3). Retrieved from http://onlinedigeditions.com/display_article.php?id=1078681

von Bertalanffy, L. (1968). *General system theory: Foundations, development, applications* (rev. ed., 1976). New York, NY: George Braziller.

Weiner, N. (1948). *Cybernetics, or control and communication in the animal and the machine*. Cambridge, MA: MIT Press.

CHAPTER 2

HEALTH, WELL-BEING, AND SELF-CARE

The evolution of health care is shifting from a major focus on cure to an ever-expanding emphasis on health promotion and disease prevention, self-care, symptom management, and self-management of chronic illness. Topol (2012, 2015), a renowned cardiologist and professor of genomics, suggested in a March 2013 televised interview that it will be the patient who will drive the greatest changes in health care in the near/foreseeable future. Although there will be increased reliance on technologies for the diagnosis and monitoring of patients' medical status, there also will be a greater need for individual involvement and responsibility in personal care and decision making, that is, in self-care.

The terms *self-care, symptom management*, and *self-management* of chronic illness are often used interchangeably. Depending on the context, the reference may be to the person taking primary responsibility for health in an effort to reduce health care costs, encouraging the person to take increased responsibility for living a healthier life, or helping the person to learn management strategies related to chronic illness. The philosophical foundations and cultural understanding and expression of these terms vary. In this chapter, these variations are explored as we begin the discussion of the meaning of self-care in relation to nursing practice and the development of nursing science. Concepts of health and well-being are explored as a frame for understanding self-care in general and the place of the nurse and nursing knowledge within these broader fields.

OBJECTIVES

After reading this chapter, the learner will be able to:

1. Describe the evolution of the meaning of the concept of health
2. Distinguish between health and well-being

21

3. Examine the role of social determinants of health in the health and well-being of individuals, families, and social groups
4. Define health promotion and discuss related theories
5. Define primary, secondary, and tertiary prevention and provide examples of each
6. Differentiate among self-care, symptom self-management, and self-management of chronic illness
7. Analyze factors associated with a growing focus on self-care in today's health care environment
8. Describe initiatives that are underway worldwide to promote self-care
9. Identify models that address chronic illness and discuss the significance of these models
10. Discuss the importance of cultural variations in the understanding and expression of self-care

KEY CONCEPTS health • well-being • self-care • social determinants of health • health promotion • levels of prevention • symptom self-management • self-management of chronic illness

EVOLUTION OF THE CONCEPT OF HEALTH

The ancient Greeks viewed health holistically, encompassing the overall effects of environmental factors in combination with habits of living such as exercise, food, and other lifestyle routines. Medical science developed slowly with an increasing focus in the Western world on physical health. This changing emphasis during the 1700s and 1800s led to increased reliance on medical treatments with decreased importance placed on the individual's contribution to health through self-care (Saylor, 2004; Stanhope & Lancaster, 2012). During the early to mid-1900s, the medical model continued to evolve and to dominate, with the absence of physical and/or mental disease becoming the conventional definition of health. In the late 1900s and early 2000s, the importance of self-care again reemerged in the overall context of "political activism" (Stanhope & Lancaster, 2012, p. 378) and in the emerging understanding of a "positive idea of health" (p. 378). For some, this has meant emphasis on lay initiatives to enhance self-care and symptom management, whereas for others it has signified helping people and their health care providers develop collaborative working relationships.

Nursing's Understanding of Health

Florence Nightingale, from the preface of *Notes on Nursing, What It Is and What It Is Not*, stated that "Every day sanitary knowledge, or the knowledge of nursing, or in other words, of how to put the constitution in such a state as that it will have no disease, or that it can recover from disease … is recognized as the knowledge which everyone ought to have …" (Nightingale, 1859). This perspective represented an understanding of health as primarily the absence of and recovery from disease, although Nightingale also recognized environmental factors that influenced the disease or health state. These environmental factors included ventilation and warming, "health" of houses, noise, proper food, bed and bedding, light, and cleanliness. This was one of the first representations of an environmental theory of health.

From a very early time, nurses have understood health from a holistic, integrated perspective, and they have recognized that health and illness are closely related. Early nursing theorists described individuals as unitary systems that function as a whole, with mind and body dimensions, including biological, psychological, social, and spiritual (Saylor, 2004). Orem (1971) described these dimensions as inseparable and continually interacting with one another. The American Holistic Nurses' Association and other nursing theorists continue to advance understanding of the interconnection of these dimensions.

CONTEMPORARY VIEWS OF HEALTH AND WELL-BEING

Health

The understanding of what it means to "be healthy" has evolved over the years. The original 1948 World Health Organization (WHO) definition of *health* was "a state of complete physical, mental and social well-being and not merely the absence of disease or infirmity" (WHO, 1946). Although this definition has been criticized for being unrealistic, since no one can achieve complete well-being, it signified a major shift from a disease perspective to a more holistic view. The meaning of health has further developed to embody the impact that social determinants have on health; that is, how conditions such as circumstances of birth, income, social status, education, age, gender, and other such factors influence health. Social determinants of health also include wider systems such as social norms, policies, and political systems (WHO, 2016).

The movement toward broadening the understanding of health has taken place over the past several decades. It was spearheaded by the Alma Ata declaration, which was the outcome of a conference sponsored by the WHO and the United Nation Children's Fund (UNICEF; 1978). The declaration was the first document of its kind to have so many countries recognize the link between social and economic development and health, and to emphasize the importance of social, educational, and financial involvement in achieving health-related goals. The conference established the goal of "health for all" to be achieved by the year 2000.

After the Alma Ata conference, the first international conference on health promotion was held in Ottawa, Canada, and the Ottawa Charter for Health Promotion was drafted (WHO, 1986). This charter identified health as a resource that enabled people to achieve a state of physical, mental, and social well-being. In addition to meeting needs and achieving aspirations as components of health, it recognized the requirement to change or to cope with the environment. In addition, it identified eight conditions and resources that are essential to health: peace, shelter, education, food, income, a stable ecosystem, sustainable resources, and social justice and equity. Health and social professionals were charged with advocating to society

---

BOX 2.1 Millennium Development Goals

- Eradicate extreme poverty and hunger
- Achieve universal primary education
- Promote gender equality and empower women
- Reduce child mortality
- Improve maternal health
- Combat HIV/AIDS, malaria, and other diseases
- Ensure environmental sustainability
- Develop a global partnership for development

Source: Millennium Development Goals (2000). Reprinted with the permission of the United Nations.

---

at large the importance of economic and political issues in overall health and well-being.

The goals of Alma Ata and the principles of the Ottawa Charter are still relevant and actively provide direction for both health promotion and development of related government policies. In 2000, 191 member nations of the United Nations (UN) signed a document titled "Millennium Development Goals" (2000), which included eight goals to be achieved by the year 2015. A summary of progress toward these goals is reported in the Millennium Development Goals Report (2015), and areas that continue to present major concern are identified. See Box 2.1 for these goals, which are ongoing.

These goals do not only apply to developing nations. They also have importance in developed nations, as the impact of social determinants of health are experienced in these countries as well, along with little or no evidence of action taken by governments and societies to address these concerns.

An indication of the need for similar goals in developed countries is the health initiative that was launched in 2010 by the U.S. Department of Health and Human Services, Healthy People 2020. These goals follow and build upon the earlier initiative, Healthy People 2010. See Box 2.2 for the major goals that were identified in Healthy People 2020.

When seeking to accomplish any or all of these goals, it is important to consider cultural variations in perspectives on health. All cultures have beliefs about health that guide actions that people in the culture are willing to take or will do to promote health. For example, most Western societies such as the United States view disease as caused by microorganisms in the natural world. People in other societies may view disease as a result of supernatural forces. The approach to treatment in these diverse cultures will be very different. Therefore, strategies that are designed to achieve broad health goals will also need to vary among cultures. It is also important to remember that many, if not most, societies today, especially in the West, are multicultural, so it is essential not to assume, but rather to assess, cultural values and beliefs regarding health.

BOX 2.2   Goals of U.S. Healthy People 2020

- Attain high-quality, longer lives free of preventable disease, disability, injury, and premature death;

- Achieve health equity, eliminate disparities, and improve the health of all groups;

- Create social and physical environments that promote good health for all; and

- Promote quality of life, healthy development, and healthy behaviors across all life stages.

Source: Centers for Disease Control and Prevention (2011).

One measurement of health that has been explored extensively concerns the relationship between income and active life expectancy. Several studies explored active life expectancy interpreted as meaning states of health, for example, with and without functional limitations. *Healthy* was considered as being able to conduct usual physical movements without help, and complete tasks necessary for ordinary independent living. Examples of data included measurements of eating, dressing, bathing, walking a certain distance, and being able to go up and down stairs. Health professionals often include these items when exploring health issues with patients. Active life expectancy appears to favor urban over rural life. The reason for this was suggested to be better access to health services and higher socioeconomic status (SES). When active life expectancy rather than simply longevity is measured, there is no gender difference. Women may live longer but the length of active life expectancy is not statistically different for women as compared to men (Papavlassopulos & Keppler, 2011).

The idea of health promotion is emerging as an important approach in health care, and it will become even more important in the future. *Health promotion* has been defined as "the process of enabling people to increase control over, and to improve, their health. It moves beyond a focus on individual behavior toward a wide range of social and environmental interventions" (WHO, n.d.). A variety of theoretical models have been proposed to guide health promotion interventions. These theoretical models for health promotion are presented in Table 2.1.

This table is not meant to be exhaustive, but rather is a representative sample of theories that can be used, singularly or in combination, for the purpose of health promotion. The majority of these theories are summarized in Raingruber (2014).

Salutogenic Theory is identified in Table 2.1 as an ecological model of health promotion. This theoretical framework proposes that health promotion be studied not from the perspective of pathogenesis, risk factors, and disease prevention, but from the perspective of salutogenesis, that is, from the perspective of the origins of health (Antonovsky, 1996). Within this framework, generalized resistance resources help a person cope with and manage life, with the outcome of a strong sense of coherence. The sense of coherence develops over time as people are exposed to a

TABLE 2.1 Examples of Theoretical Models to Guide Health Promotion		
Behavioral Change Theories	**Ecological Theories and Models**	**Nursing Models and Theories**
• Health Belief Model (Rosenstock, Strecher, & Becker, 1988) • Social Cognitive (or Learning) Theory (Bandura, 1989) • Self-Determination Theory (Deci & Ryan, 1991) • Transtheoretical Model/ Stages of Change (Prochaska & DiClemente, 1982)	• Social Ecological Models (Bronfenbrenner, 1979; derived from Systems Theory) • Salutogenic Theory (Antonovsky, 1996) • Life Course Health Development Model (Halfon & Hochstein, 2002)	• Environmental Theory (Nightingale, 1859) • Transcultural Theory of Care (Leininger, 1976) • Self-Care Deficit Nursing Theory (Orem, 1971, 2001) • Goal Attainment Theory (King, 1981) • Health Promotion Model (Pender, 1982) • Model of Self-Care for Health Promotion in Aging (Leenerts, Teel, & Pendleton, 2002)

Adapted from Raingruber (2014).

variety of experiences, both stressful and nonstressful. A person with a strong sense of coherence would:

> —wish to, be motivated to, cope (meaningfulness)
> —believe that the challenge is understood (comprehensibility)
> —believe that resources to cope are available (manageability).
> (Antonovsky, 1996, p. 15)

Antonovsky's hypothesis is that a strong sense of coherence facilitates a movement toward health. And if so, it provides a powerful theoretical guide for both research and action related to health promotion. This theoretical approach is an alternative to one originating in disease. It may also be helpful to a further understanding of the construct of well-being.

Well-Being

Well-being and health are often spoken of and studied together. However, they should also be considered separately, as health has a different theoretical base than well-being. Health can be considered the "*state* of a person that is characterized by soundness or wholeness of developed human structures and of bodily and mental functioning" (Orem, 2001, p. 186). Conditions related to health can be measured objectively, although there may be discrepancies between these objective measures and a person's perception of being healthy.

Well-being, on the other hand, is purely subjective. It is used in the sense of a person's "perceived condition of existence. . . . a state characterized by experiences of contentment, pleasure, and kinds of happiness; by spiritual experiences; by movement toward fulfillment of one's self-ideal; and by continuing personalization" (Orem, 2001, p. 186).

One way in which well-being has been studied is through what has been called *preference theory* and *happiness research;* that is, exploring choices people make in reference to well-being and in relation to what people say makes them happy. For example, Papavlassopulos and Keppler (2011) studied what they called "subjective well-being" to incorporate both of these theoretical perspectives into their research. They found that experiencing subjective well-being included being able to maximize the time of positive experience, and minimizing the time that negative feelings were experienced. They also found that people who were better educated were better decision makers and had more choices available to them in relation to pursuing feelings of well-being. These findings have implications for economic policy, suggesting that it should focus on enrichment of quality of life, not merely on productivity. This, in turn, suggests that the economic value of one person cannot have more influence in the formulation of public policy than that of another. However, as with all allocation of funding and government policies, there are competing interests as demonstrated in the lack of progress worldwide relative to "achieving health for all."

As nurses, we must ask ourselves the following questions: What are the implications of these goals and conceptions of health and well-being for nursing practice? What knowledge and skills do nurses require to play a part in achieving these goals? How can we best help people cope with these issues in daily living? How are individual health-related self-care systems affected by the issues involved?

Self-Care

The idea and practice of self-care is as old as humanity. Historically, self-care was the primary paradigm of health care for individuals, families, and communities. People assumed responsibility for their own and others' care, because they had either few or no other options. With the advent of medical and technological approaches, self-care took a secondary role and people often became passive recipients of care. The health care system became increasingly paternalistic, with physicians as the experts taking the primary role, which was to cure illness, rather than to prevent disease or promote health. In many ways, although self-care is the historical foundation of health care, it has generally not been included in the formal system (International Self-Care Foundation [ISF], n.d.). And yet, in the real world, self-care remains the underpinning of a person's overall health and well-being. See Figure 2.1 for a depiction of the place of self-care in a person's overall health care system. The figure shows a pyramid with self-care as the foundation. The three commonly understood levels of prevention used in this figure to create the pyramid include primary (disease prevention), secondary (early detection and treatment of disease to reduce impact), and tertiary (management of chronic disease and rehabilitation) levels.

The limited acknowledgement of self-care in the health care systems of the 19th through the mid-20th centuries, especially in Western civilized countries, is rapidly and dramatically changing. For one thing, paternalistic models of care are expensive. See Figure 2.2 for cost relative to the basic practices that people use in their daily lives compared with the cost of formal health care.

People worldwide are becoming better educated, have extensive access to health information through the Internet and other resources, and typically want more choice and control in most areas of their life, including health care. A vast

FIGURE 2.1   Place of Self-Care in a Person's Overall
Health Care System

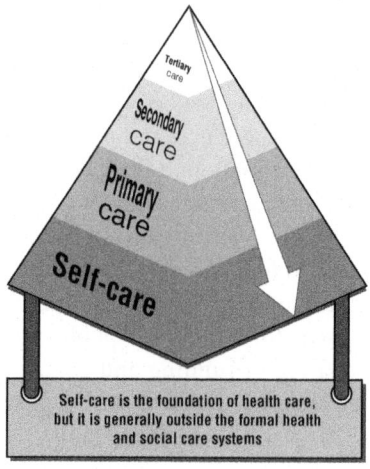

Adapted from ISF (n.d.).

FIGURE 2.2   The Inverse Cost of Health Care

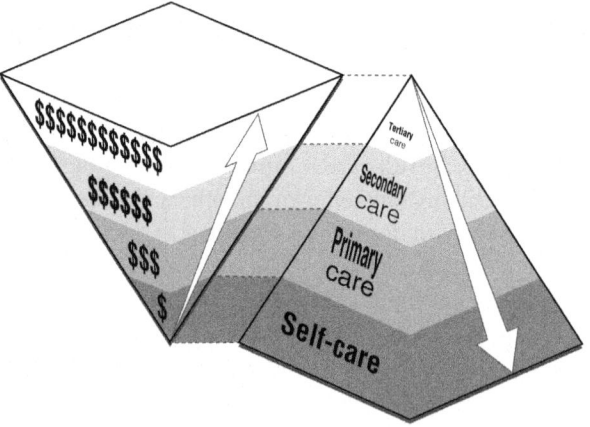

Adapted from ISF (n.d.).

amount of self-help literature is available. As a result, people are becoming active participants in addressing their health care concerns as opposed to being more passive recipients.

Some authors have cited the increasing prevalence and/or awareness of chronic illness worldwide as a significant factor affecting the growing emphasis on self-care (Richard & Shea, 2011; Wilkinson & Whitehead, 2009). The economic burden of chronic illness is exorbitant. In the United States, it is projected that the cumulative loss attributed to cardiovascular disease, chronic respiratory disease, cancer, diabetes, and mental illness will approximate $4.7 trillion over the next two decades. This amount represents 75% of global gross domestic product (GDP) in 2010 (Bloom et al., 2011). In a comparable trend, approximately 70% to 80% of health care costs in Europe are spent on care of chronic conditions. As a result, it has been suggested that the long-term sustainability of the European health care system will depend on shifting focus from illness care to health promotion, in addition to improved management of chronic illness (Economist Intelligence Unit, 2012). Some of these chronic conditions, such as cardiovascular disease, chronic respiratory disease, and diabetes, are considered, to some extent, lifestyle conditions that are at least somewhat preventable through better self-care, for example, taking steps to address smoking and obesity (ISF, n.d.). At least partially as a result of these factors, there is increasing focus on patient-centered or person-focused care, with growing understanding of the critical role that self-care plays in the overall management of health and well-being throughout the life cycle.

Important initiatives to promote incorporation of self-care into formal health care systems are underway. In the United Kingdom, self-care was emphasized in the National Health Services (NHS) Plan as one of the major components of a patient-centered health system (Department of Health, 2005). In addition, the ISF (n.d.) is a registered UK Charity that was founded specifically to advocate for issues related to self-care worldwide. Included in this initiative are efforts to develop evidence-based concepts and practices related to self-care, and to help advance the role of self-care in overall health care policy. A related but independent organization, ISF Hong Kong, was established in 2013 with its focus on Greater China. Thailand, with a higher-than-average regional prevalence of noncommunicable diseases and HIV/AIDS, along with an aging population (Deerochanawong & Ferrario, 2013), continues to take a leadership role in self-care. The second International Conference on Prevention and Management of Chronic Conditions was held concurrently with the 11th World Congress of Self-Care Deficit Nursing Theory in Bangkok in 2011, and many research and health initiatives are in progress.

Other related activities in the United Kingdom include the Social Dimensions of Health Institute in Scotland, which supports a comprehensive conceptualization of health that includes well-being, social participation, and societal inclusion. The Alliance for Self-Care Research (n.d.) is a consortium associated with the Institute that fosters research and further development of self-care knowledge and science.

Self-care is evolving as a key concept in the development of Canadian health policy (McCormack, 2003). As early as 1974, the Lalonde Report was published, suggesting that medical services were not the most important factors in determining a person's health. Four other influential factors were identified: lifestyle, environment, human biology, and health care organizations. These factors were believed to be interdependently responsible for the health of individuals (Hancock, 1986). The Lalonde Report is considered a rudimentary precursor to the Alma Ata declaration previously discussed. Self-care has continued to play a central role in the development of Canadian health policy, and a health care delivery system based on self-care has been recommended (McCormack, 2003).

No formal governmental or national strategy in the United States is directed toward self-care. From a philosophical perspective, a self-care focus can be discerned in initiatives toward prevention and self-management of illness. The primary U.S. goal is to improve population health through individual practitioner- and community-based programs such as those that increase immunizations, stop smoking, and decrease obesity rates. The strategies identified do not specifically include self-care (Soto, 2013). In the Medicare program in the United States, part B covers diabetes outpatient self-management training to teach a person how to cope with and manage diabetes. It includes tips for eating healthy, being active, monitoring blood sugar, taking medication, and reducing risks. Medicare may cover up to 10 hours of initial diabetes self-management training (DMST; Medicare.gov, n.d.)

An important development in the United States in the late 1990s was the creation and advancement of the Chronic Care Model (Bodenheimer, Wagner, & Grumbach, 2002; Wagner, 1998). Developers of this model acknowledge that a significant amount of care for chronic conditions takes place outside of the formal health care system. The focus of the model is on connecting active, well-informed patients who have chronic conditions with proactive health care teams. Elements identified as essential for any initiative that is designed to address chronic care include, among others, community resources, the health care system, and patient self-management (Singh & Ham, 2006). A derivative of the Chronic Care Model is the health care pyramid developed by Kaiser Permanente, a not-for-profit integrated health plan. This pyramid has health promotion and population-wide prevention as the foundation, with the subsequent levels of supported self-care, disease management, and case management. Approximately 80% of people with a chronic medical condition fall into the category of individuals who can learn, with the right support, to actively participate in their own care and management of their medical condition, thus preventing complications and slowing worsening of the condition (Economist Intelligence Unit, 2012; Singh & Ham, 2006). These and other chronic care models provide potential guidance for health care in the United States and worldwide.

Thus far, we have talked about self-care without actually defining what it means. There are multiple definitions with a variety of emphases to be found in the literature. Providing a very broad context, the WHO has defined *self-care* in health as referring to "the activities individuals, families and communities undertake with the intention of enhancing health, preventing disease, limiting illness, and restoring health. These activities are derived from knowledge and skills from the pool of both professional and lay experience. They are undertaken by lay people on their own behalf, either separately or in participative collaboration with professionals" (WHO, 1983).

It is noted that this and many definitions of self-care focus mainly on primary and secondary health promotion, as well as disease prevention. A definition provided by the UK Department of Health expands this definition to include not only maintaining good physical and mental health, and meeting social and psychological needs, but also caring for "minor ailments and long-term conditions; and maintain(ing) health and wellbeing after acute illness or discharge from hospital" (Department of Health, 2005).

According to the WHO and U.S. Centers for Disease Control and Prevention (CDC; cited in Schulman-Green et al., 2012), chronic illnesses such as cardiovascular disease, cancer, and diabetes are among the most widespread and most expensive of all worldwide health problems, are the main reason that adults seek health care, and are the foremost cause of death and disability in the United States. At least in part as a result of fiscal concerns related to the economic burden of chronic illness, governmental health policies, in general, have encouraged greater involvement of people with chronic illness in self-management of their disease process, with a focus on self-care. Another factor affecting the current emphasis on self-care, as alluded to earlier, may be a changing perception of health care providers as the experts who provide care to one of active participation on the part of both providers and recipients of care. The role of health care providers in this emerging health care environment is to "support and empower patients" as they take greater responsibility in managing their own health (Richard & Shea, 2011, p. 255).

A wealth of articles in recent literature, the vast majority of them by nurses, address symptom self-management across all spectrums of disease processes. Some examples of these approaches include exploration of strategies that people may use to manage symptoms of non-metastatic prostate cancer (Hsiao, Moore, Insel, & Merkle, 2014), schizophrenia (Kennedy, Schepp, & O'Connor, 2000), and che-motherapy-induced peripheral neuropathy in breast cancer (Speck et al., 2012). Other articles address an evaluation of interventions that are designed to increase symptom self-management capabilities, for example, of auditory hallucinations (Buccheri, Trygstad, Buffum, Lyttle, & Dowling, 2010), diabetes (Garcia, Brown, Horner, Zuniga, & Arheart, 2015), and multiple sclerosis (Plow, Bethoux, McDaniel, McGlynn, & Marcus, 2014).

A similar approach to symptom self-management is that of self-management of chronic illness, which has resulted in development of important models, includ-ing the Chronic Disease Self-Management Program (CDSMP) at Stanford Univer-sity in the United States (Lorig, Sobel, Ritter, Hobbs, & Laurent, 2001). Symptom management has been addressed primarily within the nursing literature, whereas self-management of chronic illness resides within the broader interprofessional perspective. A metasynthesis of literature related to self-management from the viewpoints of people living with a chronic illness resulted in three processes, one of which is activating resources (Schulman-Green et al., 2012). The idea of acti-vating resources suggests an interdisciplinary focus, which includes coordination of family members, friends, health care providers, and community resources and services from a social service perspective. Potential community resources include medical, psychosocial, spiritual, and financial components. Tasks and skills related to engaging with these resources include communicating with all types of health care providers, coordinating services, identifying and accessing psychological re-sources, participating in a spiritual community, finding social support, and manag-ing social and/or environmental challenges (p. 141). Nurses and physicians should be involved in supporting not only self-management of chronic illness but also social workers, psychologists, psychiatrists, chaplains, nutritionists, naturopaths, physical therapists, and other health care professionals. Involving all of these mul-tidisciplinary aspects will facilitate holistic care of the individual patient (p. 142). Positive outcomes have been reported as a result of self-care/self-management programs (Ory et al., 2013).

Similar programs have been developed across cultures and across disease states, for example, Illness Management and Recovery (IMR) implemented in Denmark for people with severe mental illness (Dalum et al., 2011), the Health and Recovery Peer Program (HARP) (Druss et al., 2010), and the Wellness Recovery Action Plan (WRAP) commonly used with people with serious mental illness in the United States (Copeland, 1997). Although these initiatives primarily involve lay people, the principles and practices of the recovery movement and associated concepts of self-management and self-care have been embraced by mental health clinicians and researchers (Lucock et al., 2011; Seed & Torkelson, 2012; Williams & Tufford, 2012).

In discussing the multiple definitions and meanings of self-care, it is important to consider cultural variations. For example, a study of 248 Hispanic men and women with diabetes and with low SES reported that, compared with men, women were less likely to receive support, encountered more barriers, had less self-efficacy, and were less adherent to diabetic protocols (Mansyur, Rustveld, Nash, & Jibaja-Weiss, 2015). The authors concluded that lack of support was a major barrier for Hispanic women with diabetes. From a cultural perspective, Hispanic women may put their families before themselves, believing that it would be selfish to buy food to support a diabetic diet since others in the family may not like it, and financial resources may be limited. Findings from this study suggest that Hispanic men with diabetes may be more likely than women to receive support in pursuing healthy lifestyles and managing their diabetes. The family is also important in Chinese culture. Caring for the sick is viewed as a moral obligation in the tradition of Confucius. Thus, self-care may be valued so that care can be provided to other family members. Also, accepting care from others is to allow them to fulfill their moral obligation of providing care (Tao, Songwathana, Isaramalai, & Wang, 2014).

A few studies have found that self-care is generally poor among some ethnic minorities as compared with Caucasians (e.g., Dickson, McCarthy, Howe, Schipper, & Katz, 2013; Suarez, 1992). However, it is important to consider how self-care is measured in these studies. For example, African American women with AIDS who also had children who were HIV positive would have scored poorly on traditional measures of self-care such as healthy eating, sleep, exercise, and reducing stress. These women actually redefined self-care, to be compatible with their complex lives, as spiritual/religious practices, accessing support from extended family, especially other women, and the actual act of mothering, which gave them a sense of meaning and hope for the future (Shambley-Ebron & Boyle, 2006). The core values of spirituality/religion, support of extended family, and use of nonmedical healing methods (e.g., "kitchen medicine") were also identified in another study (Becker, Gates, & Newsom, 2004, p. 2070).

Further indications of cultural differences are diet and lifestyle. For example, a low sodium diet may be difficult to follow, especially in some ethnic groups, for people with a medical diagnosis of heart failure. One participant in the study by Dickson et al. (2013) stated, "In my culture, women do the cooking . . . I have a daughter . . . she prepares the meals for me and I eat what she prepares" (p. 115). In a study by Jang, Toth, and Yoo (2012), Korean Americans were believed to be adherent to a low sodium diet, because they responded positively to a study item stating, "I watch that I do not eat canned soups or TV dinners" (p. 251). The authors noted that, although the participants reported that they do not eat canned soups or TV dinners, they may not understand that traditional Korean foods may also be high in sodium, and they may not know about how to prepare them differently to meet dietary guidelines. Another cultural lifestyle difference may be reflected in Korean American study participants' low ranking of the item, "I put my feet up when I sit in a chair" (Jang, Toth, & Yoo, 2012, p. 251). The authors observed that Korean Americans, even if they have Western furniture, often find sitting on the floor more comfortable and may find the idea of putting their feet up when they sit in a chair as rude or offensive.

Finally, it is important to consider the role of social determinants of health in shaping self-care practices. If a person has medical insurance, they are much more likely to have access to medically prescribed forms of self-care such as dietary and exercise regimens. For people with insurance and access to formal health care, a combination of culturally based self-care practices and medical approaches has resulted in positive outcomes (Becker et al., 2004). However, people without health care insurance often must rely more heavily on self-care practices learned within their families. This raises the issue of whether self-care is truly a choice or may be enforced as a result of social conditions (Becker et al., 2004; Edgeworth & Collins, 2006). Health care providers' support of self-care practices is essential in either case. Globally, much self-care teaching is designed and delivered by the dominant culture, thereby potentially missing critical cultural factors.

It is evident that self-care and related concepts are a fundamental focus and concern of health care worldwide. What does this mean for the nursing profession?

Self-Care and Nursing

Most current models of health have as their focus the improvement of self-care as a major outcome of addressing the social determinants of health. All of the initiatives addressed earlier are extremely important. However, none of them identifies a specific role for nurses. Helping people take care of themselves has always been a focus of nursing. This focus has been and continues to be formalized through developments linking the science of self-care and nursing sciences. In the 1950s and 1960s, articles and books exploring what nursing is, and how it can be defined, started appearing in the nursing literature (Henderson, 1966; Peplau, 1952). For example, Henderson (cited in Tomey & Alligood, 1998, p. 102) identified the function of nursing as assisting an individual in performing activities related to health "that he would perform unaided if he had the necessary strength, will or knowledge. And to do this in such a way as to help him gain independence as rapidly as possible." Publication of proposed theories of nursing soon followed. Among these were two publications that are foundational to our understanding of the meaning of self-care: *Nursing: Concepts of Practice* (Orem, 1971) and *Concept Formalization in Nursing: Process and Product* (Nursing Diagnostic Conference Group [NDCG], 1979). The 1979 publication describes the activity of a group of nursing practitioners and scholars studying cases in an effort to define nursing, identify the variables associated with nursing practice, and depict the outcomes of nurse–patient interaction. This activity resulted in formalization of the Self-Care Deficit Theory of Nursing. The theory has been in use and has undergone continued development by scholars and practitioners working together since that time. It is this theoretical perspective that is key to understanding the role of the nurse in the current health care system worldwide with its growing understanding of the importance of self-care.

Orem stated that self-care is that daily care required by individuals "to regulate their own functioning and development.... Requirements of persons for this day-to-day regulatory care will be affected by, among other factors, age, developmental stage, health state, environmental conditions, and effects of medical care" (Orem, 2001, p. 20). From this description, we can see that one's ability to perform self-care is affected by his or her health state. In other words, a particular health state may interfere with a person's ability to regulate his or her own functioning and development. On the other hand, a positive health state can function as a resource for performance of self-care. Orem (2001) further stated that self-care is a "learned, goal-oriented activity of individuals... behavior that exists in concrete life situations directed by persons to self or to the environment to regulate factors that affect their own development and functioning in the interests of life, health, or well-being" (Orem, 2001, pp. 490–491). At the same time that the health state conditions a person's ability to perform self-care activities, it is also true that a person's deliberate and purposeful self-care actions can contribute to both health state and well-being.

It was established in Chapter 1 that a structured body of knowledge is a characteristic of a discipline, and that a unique body of knowledge is required for qualification as a profession. These factors, in conjunction with the rapidly changing world of health and health care with the focus on self-care and related concepts, lead to the conclusion that self-care is the appropriate focus of the discipline of nursing. The following chapters develop these ideas.

LEARNING ACTIVITIES

1. Identify your own social determinants of health and analyze how these have influenced your current state of health.

2. Select one theory of health promotion and consider its applicability to an at-risk or vulnerable population such as people who are homeless or elderly people in a nursing home.

3. Critically analyze the statement that "self-care is the appropriate focus of the discipline of nursing." Do you agree with this statement? Provide rationale for why you agree or disagree.

4. Describe situations where there is objective good health yet the person is not experiencing a feeling of well-being. What about a person who expresses well-being but, in fact, is seriously ill? What does this tell you about these two concepts?

References

Alliance for Self-Care Research. (n.d.). Retrieved from http://www4.rgu.ac.uk/fhsc/research/page_text.cfm?pge=87338

Antonovsky, A. (1996). The salutogenic model as a theory to guide health promotion. *Health Promotion International, 11*(1), 11–18.

Bandura, A. (1989). Social cognitive theory. In R. Vasta (Ed.), *Annals of child development. Vol. 6. Six theories of child development* (pp. 1–60). Greenwich, CT: JAI Press.

Becker, G., Gates, R. J., & Newsom, E. (2004). Self-care among chronically ill African Americans: Culture, health disparities, and health insurance status. *American Journal of Public Health, 94*(12), 2066–2073.

Bloom, D. E., Cafiero, E. T., Jane-Llopis, E., Abrahams-Gessel, S., Bloom, L. R., Fathima, S.,... Weinstein, C. (2011). *The global economic burden of noncommunicable diseases.* Geneva: World Economic Forum.

Bodenheimer, T., Wagner, E. H., & Grumbach, K. (2002). Improving primary care for patients with chronic illness: The chronic care model (Part 2). *Journal of the American Medical Association, 288*(15), 1909–1914.

Bronfenbrenner, U. (1979). *The ecology of human development.* Cambridge, MA: Harvard University Press.

Buccheri, R. K., Trygstad, L. N., Buffum, M. D., Lyttle, K., & Dowling, G. (2010). Comprehensive evidence-based program teaching self-management of auditory hallucinations on inpatient psychiatric units. *Issues in Mental Health Nursing, 31*(3), 223–231. doi:10.3109/01612840903288568

Centers for Disease Control and Prevention. (2011). *Healthy People 2020.* Retrieved from http://www.cdc.gov/nchs/healthy_people/hp2020.htm

Copeland, M. E. (1997). *Wellness recovery action plan.* Drummerston, VT: Peach Press.

Dalum, H. S., Korsbek, L., Mikkelsen, J. H., Thomsen, K., Kistrup, K., Olander, M.,… Eploy, L. F. (2011). Illness management and recovery (IMR) in Danish community mental health centres. *Trials, 12*(1), 195. doi:10.1186/1745-6215-12-195

Deci, E. L., & Ryan, R. M. (1991). A motivational approach to self: Integration in personality. *Nebraska Symposium on Motivation: Perspectives on Motivation, 38,* 237–288.

Deerochanawong, C., & Ferrario, A. (2013). Diabetes management in Thailand: A literature review of the burden, cost, and outcomes. *Globalization and Health, 9*(1), 11. doi:10.1186/1744-8603-9-11

Department of Health. (2005). *Self-care—A real choice. Self-care support—A practical option.* London, UK: Author. Retrieved from http://personcentredcare.health.org.uk/resources/self-care-%E2%80%93-real-choice-self-care-support-%E2%80%93-practical-option

Dickson, V. V., McCarthy, M. M., Howe, A., Schipper, J., & Katz, S. M. (2013). Sociocultural influences on heart failure self-care among an ethnic minority Black population. *Journal of Cardiovascular Nursing, 28*(2), 111–118.

Druss, B. G., Zhao, L., von Esenwein, S. A., Bona, J. R., Fricks, L., Jenkins-Tucker, S.,… Lorig, K. (2010). The health and recovery peer (HARP) program: A peer-led intervention to improve medical self-management for persons with serious mental illness. *Schizophrenia Research, 118*(1), 264–270. doi:10.1016/j.schres.2010.01.026

Economist Intelligence Unit. (2012). Never too early: Tackling chronic disease to extend healthy life years. Retrieved from http://digitalresearch.eiu.com/extending-healthy-life-years/report

Edgeworth, R., & Collins, A. E. (2006). Self-care as a response to diarrhoea in rural Bangladesh: Empowered choice or enforced adoption? *Social Science and Medicine, 63,* 2686–2697.

Garcia, A. A., Brown, S. A., Horner, S. D., Zuniga, J., & Arheart, K. L. (2015). Home-based diabetes symptom self management education for Mexican Americans with type 2 diabetes. *Health Education Research, 30*(3), 484–496. doi:10.1093/her/cyv018

Halfon, N., & Hochstein, M. (2002). Life course health development: An integrated framework for developing health, policy, and research. *Milbank Quarterly, 80,* 433–479. doi:10.1111/1468-0009.00019

Hancock, T. (1986). Lalonde and beyond: Looking back at "a new perspective on the health of Canadians." *Health Promotion, 1*(1), 93–100. doi:10.1093/heapro/1.1.93

Henderson, V. (1966). *The nature of nursing: A definition and its implications for practice, research, and education.* New York, NY: Macmillan.

Hsiao, C.-P., Moore, I. M., Insel, K. C., & Merkle, C. J. (2014). Symptom self-management strategies in patients with non-metastatic prostate cancer. *Journal of Clinical Nursing, 23*(3–4), 440–449. doi:10.1111/jocn.12178

International Self-Care Foundation (n.d.). Retrieved from http://isfglobal.org/what-is-self-care/a-brief-history-of-self-care

Jang, Y. S., Toth, J., & Yoo, H. (2012). Similarities and differences of self-care behaviors between Korean Americans and Caucasian Americans with heart failure. *Journal of Transcultural Nursing, 23*(3), 246–254.

Kennedy, M. G., Schepp, K. G., & O'Connor, F. W. (2000). Symptom self-management and relapse in schizophrenia. *Archives of Psychiatric Nursing, 14*(6), 266–275. doi:10.1053/apnu.2000.19089

King, I. M. (1981). *A theory for nursing: Symptoms, concepts, process.* New York, NY: John Wiley & Sons.

Leenerts, M. H., Teel, C. S., & Pendleton, M. K. (2002). Building a model of self-care for health promotion in aging. *Journal of Nursing Scholarship, 34*(4), 355–361.

Leininger, M. (1976). *Health-care dimensions: Transcultural health-care issues and conditions.* Philadelphia, PA: F. A. Davis.

Lorig, K. R., Sobel, D., Ritter, P. L., Hobbs, M., & Laurent, D. (2001). Effect of a self-management program on patients with chronic disease. *Effective Clinical Practice, 4,* 256–262.

Lucock, M., Gillard, S., Adams, K., Simons, L., White, R., & Edwards, C. (2011). Self-care in mental health services: A narrative review. *Health and Social Care in the Community, 19*(6), 602–616. doi:10.1111/j1365-2524.2011.01014.x

Mansyur, C. L., Rustveld, L. O., Nash, S. G., & Jibaja-Weiss, M. L. (2015). Social factors and barriers to self-care adherence in Hispanic men and women with diabetes. *Patient Education and Counseling, 98,* 805–810.

McCormack, D. (2003). An examination of the self-care concept uncovers a new direction for healthcare reform. *Nursing Leadership, 16*(4), 48–65. doi:10.12927/cjnl.2003.16342. doi: 10.1007/s11205-010-9757

Medicare.gov. (n.d.). Your Medicare coverage. Retrieved from https://www.medicare.gov/coverage/diabetes-self-mgmt-training.html

Millennium Development Goals. (2000). Retrieved from http://www.un.org/millenniumgoals

Millennium Development Goals Report. (2015). Retrieved from http://www.un.org/millenniumgoals/2015_MDG_Report/pdf/MDG%25202015%2520Summary%2520web

Nightingale, F. (1859). *Notes on nursing, what it is and what it is not.* Project Gutenberg. Retrieved from http://www.gutenberg.org/files/17366/17366-h/17366-h.htm

Nursing Diagnostic Conference Group. (1979). *Concept formalization in nursing: Process and product* (2nd ed.). Boston, MA: Little Brown.

Orem, D. E. (1971). *Nursing: Concepts of practice.* New York, NY: McGraw-Hill.

Orem, D. E. (2001). *Nursing: Concepts of practice* (6th ed.). St. Louis, MO: Mosby.

Ory, M. G., Ahn, S., Jiang, L., Smith, M. L., Ritter, P. L., Whitelaw, N., & Lorig, K. (2013). Successes of a national study of the chronic disease self-management program: Meeting the triple aim of health care reform. *Medical Care, 1*(11), 992–998. doi:10.1097/MLR.0b013e3182a95dd1; Retrieved from http://patienteducation.stanford.edu/programs/cdsmp.html

Papavlassopulos, N., & Keppler, D. (2011). Life expectancy as an objective factor of a subjective well-being. *Social Indicators Research, 104*(3), 475–505. doi:10.1007/s11205-010-9757-6

Pender, N. J. (1982). *Health promotion in nursing practice.* New York, NY: Appleton-Century-Crofts.

Peplau, H. E. (1952). *Interpersonal relations in nursing.* New York, NY: G. P. Putnam. (Reprinted 1991. New York, NY: Springer).

Plow, M., Bethoux, F., McDaniel, C., McGlynn, M., & Marcus, B. (2014). Randomized controlled pilot study of customized pamphlets to promote physical activity and symptom self-management in women with multiple sclerosis. *Clinical Rehabilitation, 28*(2), 139–148. doi:10.1177/0269215513494229

Prochaska, J. O., & DiClemente, C. C. (1982). Trans-theoretical therapy—toward a more integrative model of change. *Psychotherapy: Therapy, Research and Practice, 19*(3), 276–288.

Raingruber, B. (2014). *Contemporary health promotion in nursing practice.* Burlington, MA: Jones & Bartlett Learning.

Richard, A. A., & Shea, K. (2011). Delineation of self-care and associated concepts. *Journal of Nursing Scholarship, 43*(3), 255–264. doi:10.1111/j.1547-5069.2011.01404.x

Rosenstock, I. M., Strecher, V. J., & Becker, M. H. (1988). Social learning theory and the health belief model. *Health Education Quarterly, 15*(2), 175–183.

Saylor, C. (2004). The circle of health: A health definition model. *Journal of Holistic Nursing, 22*(2), 98–115. doi:10.1177/0898010104264775

Schulman-Green, D., Jaser, S., Martin, F., Alonzo, A., Grey, M., McCorkle, R., . . . & Whittemore, R. (2012). Processes of self-management in chronic illness. *Journal of Nursing Scholarship, 44*(2), 136–144. doi:10.1111/j.1547-5069.2012.01444.x

Seed, M. S., & Torkelson, D. J. (2012). Recovery journey in acute psychiatric care: Using concepts from Orem's self-care deficit nursing theory. *Issues in Mental Health Nursing, 33*, 394–398. doi: 10.3109/01612840.2012.663064

Shambley-Ebron, D. Z., & Boyle, J. S. (2006). Self-care and mothering in African American women with HIV/AIDS. *Western Journal of Nursing Research, 28*(1), 42–60.

Singh, D., & Ham, C. (2006). *Improving care for people with long-term conditions: A review of UK and international frameworks.* University of Birmingham, Institute for Innovation and Improvement. Retrieved from http://www.birmingham.ac.uk/Documents/college-social-sciences/social-policy/HSMC/research/long-term-conditions.pdf

Soto, M. A. (2013). *Population health in the Affordable Care Act era.* Retrieved from http://www.academyhealth.org/files/AH2013pophealth.pdf

Speck, R. M., DeMichele, A., Farrar, J. T., Hennessy, S., Mao, J. J., Stineman, M. G., & Barg, F. K. (2012). Scope of symptoms and self-management strategies for chemotherapy-induced peripheral neuropathy in breast cancer patient. *Supportive Care in Cancer, 20*(10), 2433–2439. doi: 10.1007/s00520-011-1365-8

Stanhope, M., & Lancaster, J. (2012). *Public health nursing: Population-centered health care in the community* (8th ed.). St. Louis, MO: Mosby.

Suarez, Z. E. (1992). Use of self-care by Hispanics: Culture, access, or need? *Journal of Health and Social Policy, 4*(2), 32–44.

Tao, H., Songwathana, P., Isaramalai, S., & Wang, Q. (2014). Taking good care of myself: A qualitative study on self-care behavior among Chinese persons with a permanent colostomy. *Nursing and Health Sciences, 16*, 483–489. doi:10.1111/nhs.12166

Tomey, A. M., & Alligood, M. R. (1998). *Nursing theorists and their work.* St. Louis, MO: Mosby. Retrieved from http://www.stritch.edu/Library/Doing-Research/Research-by-Subject/Health-Sciences-Nursing-Theorists/Virginia-Avernal-Henderson—Definition-of-Nursing

Topol, E. (2012). *The creative destruction of medicine: How the digital revolution will create better health care.* New York, NY: Basic Books.

Topol, E. (2015). *The patient will see you now: The future of medicine is in your hands.* New York, NY: Basic Books.

Wagner, E. H. (1998). Chronic disease management: What will it take to improve care for chronic illness? *Effective Clinical Practice, 1,* 2–4.

Wilkinson, A., & Whitehead, L. (2009). Evolution of the concept of self-care and implications for nurses: A literature review. *International Journal of Nursing Studies, 46*(8), 1143–1147. doi:10.1016/j.jnurstu.2008.12.011

Williams, C. C., & Tufford, L. (2012). Professional competencies for promoting recovery in mental illness. *Psychiatry: Interpersonal and Biological Processes, 75*(2), 190–201.

World Health Organization. (1946, June). *Preamble to the World Health Organization as adopted by the International Health Conference,* New York; signed on 22 July 1946 by the representatives of 61 States (Official Records of the World Health Organization, no. 2, p. 100) and entered into force on 7 April 1948. Retrieved from www.who.int/about/definition/en/print.html

World Health Organization. (1983). *Health education in self-care: Possibilities and limitations. Report of a scientific consultation.* Geneva, Switzerland.

World Health Organization. (1986, November). *The Ottawa Charter for Health Promotion. First International Conference on Health Promotion,* Ottawa, Canada. Retrieved from http://www.who.int/healthpromotion/conferences/previous/ottawa/en

World Health Organization. (2016). *Social determinants of health.* Retrieved from www.who.int/social_determinants

World Health Organization. (n.d.). *Health promotion.* Retrieved from http://www.who.int/topics/health_promotion/en

World Health Organization and United Nations Children's Fund. (1978, September). *Primary health care.* Report presented at the International Conference on Primary Health Care, Alma Ata, USSR. Retrieved from http://www.unicef.org/about/history/files/Alma_Ata_conference_1978_report.pdf

CHAPTER 3

THINKING AND DOING NURSING

Reflection or contemplation is linked to knowledge acquisition.

—Asselin, 2011

In Chapter 1, nursing is described as a profession and a discipline. The essence of these two elements for nursing is found in what we as *nurses* do and what we think about. In this chapter, we examine how we as nurses think and do nursing. This frames the metaparadigm of nursing when the focus is on self-care.

OBJECTIVES

After reading this chapter, the learner will be able to:

1. Identify the proper object of nursing
2. Explain the importance of knowing and understanding the proper object of nursing
3. Define *concept*
4. Describe a *concept map*
5. Describe the relationship between concepts, models, and theories
6. Explain the three stages of learning through use of a model
7. Identify major distinguishing factors between Orem's, Max-Neef's, and Maslow's understanding of human needs or requirements
8. Describe the basic self-care requisites of human beings from Orem's theoretical perspective
9. Define *human agency*
10. Identify different types of human agency

39

11. Explain what is meant by self-care limitations and provide examples of how these might occur

12. Discuss the pros and cons of having a common language in nursing

KEY CONCEPTS   proper object of nursing • concept • concept map • model • theory • interprofessionalism • self-care requisites • human agency • self-care limitations

AN ANALOGY

If you are a highly organized person, you will have all your desk or kitchen items in their proper places based on an organizing principle that makes sense to you. As you acquire new things, you know where to place them. And if someone asks you to retrieve something, you know right where to go or you can direct them to the correct place and they can find it quickly.

However, if you are like many of us, you will have that center desk drawer or that drawer in the kitchen where you haphazardly toss things and will then rummage through the drawer when you need an item. You know it is there and eventually you probably find it. A friend wants to borrow something. You know you have it in the drawer; however, can you find it quickly? Can you tell her where to find it? And if she wants two or more things, you have to think about where they might be. Are they related to some item in another drawer? Might they be in the same drawer? Or are they probably not even in the kitchen?

After this, you go to the store and buy organizers for the drawers. You begin to think about how you might put items into categories by size, function, and frequency of use, whatever has meaning for you. You no longer have to remember what is in each drawer. You can quickly refer to the drawer to find the item. You begin to see relationships between things that you had not thought about earlier. The same idea works with your computer—if you do not put a paper you are working on in the correct folder with a meaningful label, you can waste a lot of time and energy searching for it. Sometimes even Siri cannot help you.

A similar thing occurs within our brains as we store and retrieve knowledge. We get a new piece of information and need to store it so it can be retrieved; as we do this, we make associations with other data or concepts already present. We use those associations to help us quickly retrieve the information at a later time. For example, during the previous week, I took care of Mrs. Smith, who had fractured her hip. She was in extreme pain, and the medication did not seem to help as much as it might have. I remember a similar situation during the previous month with Mrs. Jones. What did we do to help relieve her pain? Did we change her position? Did we apply cold or heat? Did we sit and talk with her to distract her? What other things have worked in the past? What do I have in my repertoire of pain management that might work? As we reflect on the situation, we seek knowledge and experiences that are associated with this situation. We can retrieve knowledge, because we know its structure and can creatively seek associations. A theoretical structure of knowledge associated with nursing facilitates the storage and retrieval of data and allows us to use those as informative of practice. We develop explicit and tacit knowledge to aid in this process. We develop ways of approaching problems in a structured but not rigid way. And in the process, we gain new insights into practice.

THE OBJECT AND PURPOSES OF NURSING

Thinking nursing begins with conceptualizing what nursing is. Why does a person need a nurse? What is the object of nursing?

As early as 1922, the importance of identifying the object of nursing so as to identify the place of nursing in society was raised. Harmer (1922) noted the importance of:

> identifying the object of nursing so that we may have a goal to strive for, a guiding purpose by which we measure what we are and what we do and a central controlling idea by which we see the bearing and relation of all our studies and experience and which serves to link them together so that we may remember and utilize them. For, if we have a definite object in view, we are naturally interested in whatever leads us toward it and in what we are interested we eagerly pay attention, deriving both pleasure and profit and learning, not without effort—for nursing demands our highest efforts—but with the effort which brings a glow of satisfaction for work well done.
>
> Nursing is rooted in the needs of humanity and is founded on the ideal of service. Its object is not only to cure the sick and heal the wounded but to bring health and ease, rest and comfort to mind and body, to shelter, nourish, and protect and to minister to all those who are helpless or handicapped, young, aged or immature. Its object is to prevent disease and to preserve health. (Harmer, 1922, p. 3)

The need for knowing the object has not changed. The clarity brought about by understanding the object of nursing not only gives us the basis for knowing our own focus, but also provides us with the way to develop nursing science for the good of the people we serve. It also provides the basis for being able to see the nurse's role in interprofessional perspectives on caring for others. This is especially important as the focus on *interprofessionalism* continues to grow. In the current health care environment, nurses are at risk of being relegated to the tasks that nurses do rather than the overall contribution that nurses can make to the health and well-being of people in their care.

Doing Nursing: The Subject of Nursing

It should be obvious that the subject of nursing is the human person. It is the person to whom and for whom we provide our services. It is necessary to be more specific as to what it is about the person that guides our actions, and provides that guiding purpose that permits us to relate our knowledge and experiences in a meaningful way. This is referred to as the *proper object*. The proper object is important in that it indicates the differences in scientific disciplines, the methods for investigating and exploring knowledge, and the conclusions anticipated (Young, Taylor, & Renpenning, 2001, p. 7).

What is it about a person that would require nursing action? When a person has an illness, such as the acute or chronic manifestation of chronic obstructive pulmonary disease (COPD)? When the ability to care for self in a way that will restore or maintain health and well-being is compromised? Nursing may be required when a person is unable to care for self in a way that will restore or maintain health and well-being.

Expressed Proper Object of Nursing

The proper object of nursing presented here was first expressed by Orem and colleagues beginning in the 1950s, and it was further developed through conceptual thinking about experiences research. It is accepted worldwide by many nurses as a basis for practice and education. The proper object has been described as "the inability of persons to provide continuously for themselves the amount and quality of required self-care because of situations of personal health" (Orem, 2001, p. 20). The ideas presented in the next section are essential for understanding the proper object of nursing. As you continue on into the nursing-specific content of this book, you will come to understand the importance of these concepts. Remember that there are many disciplines that study these elements, and that will give you insights into their meaning and utility in knowing and doing nursing. Our view of the human person governs how we view nursing. Various disciplines have different focuses that define them. Various nursing theorists place different focus on aspects of the human—the person—and his or her place in the family/community/world/universe. These perspectives will be further explored and integrated in later chapters.

The proper object of nursing was proposed after studying nursing situations in search of answers to the following questions: "Why do people need nursing or what human condition brings about a need for nursing? What is nursing? What is the structure of the entity . . . we refer to as nursing?" (Taylor & Renpenning, 2011, p. 11). The model/concept map that presents the conceptual structure of nursing as presented in this book is shown in Figure 3.1. It includes the essential concepts and identifies relationships between them. The underlying structure of these concepts and relationships has been further developed in the self-care deficit nursing theory, and it is helpful as we work toward a conceptual understanding of the object and process of nursing.

Another way to think about the object of nursing is to think about what legitimates your saying to someone, "I'm your nurse." Imagine walking up to someone on the street corner and saying, "Hi. I'm your nurse." What kind of reaction would you get? The first thing that legitimizes your telling this to someone is the legal contract you have by virtue of being licensed in the jurisdiction in which you are practicing. The second thing is the establishment of a contractual relationship through your place of employment or a direct contract with the patient wherein you agree to provide nursing care. And the basis for establishing such a relationship is that you have something specific to offer. How would you define that? This could be defined as knowing the proper object of nursing and being able to offer services directly related to that object. You need to practice within your profes-

FIGURE 3.1 The Conceptual Structure of Nursing

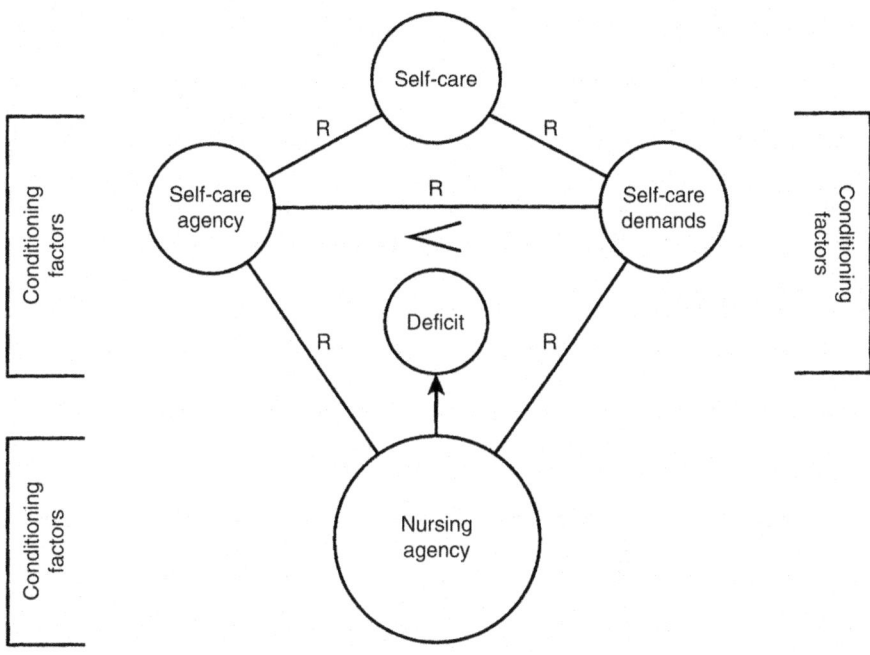

sional scope, which is congruent with the specific knowledge you have acquired through education, experience, and ongoing reflection.

THINKING NURSING

A journey into professional nursing is best made with a road map that helps you know your destination and the routes available to get you there.

> Conceptualizing nursing as a program with a purpose with identified responsibilities and tasks to achieve a defined end rather than as a collection of tasks can facilitate achieving the health-related outcomes of nursing practice. Nursing practice begins with a mental model of nursing and its goals. It asks the purpose of nursing in a particular situation and point in time. (Young et al., 2001, p. 37)

A discipline-specific nursing theoretical system provides the basis for conceptualizing nursing. The building blocks of a conceptual map of nursing begin with basic concepts and extend to the development of models and theories. The basic concepts and relationships between them come from the proper object of nursing.

Concepts, Models, and Theories

The object of nursing is understood as knowledge of the specific elements such as health or person. It is expressed through words, symbols, concepts, models, and theories. Concepts are the constituents of thoughts (Stanford Encyclopedia of Philosophy, 2006). A concept is a mental representation of an idea or entity that is expressed through the use of words. Words, semantics, and specific language are essential for communicating one's thoughts and observations. Words are important and convey meaning. Imagine how complicated life would be if every time you wanted to talk about a table you would have to describe it as a flat board, sometimes square or circular, with posts to support it, and with the number of posts varying with the size and shape of the board. Instead, the word *table* brings a picture to mind. A concept map is a way of representing relationships between ideas, images, or words in the same way that a sentence diagram represents the grammar of a sentence, a road map represents the locations of highways and towns, and a circuit diagram represents the workings of an electrical appliance. In a concept map, each word or phrase connects to another, and it links back to the original idea, word, or phrase. Development of a concept map may be a useful activity. It is a diagram that depicts suggested relationships between concepts. It is a graphical tool used to organize and structure knowledge. A concept map typically represents ideas and information as boxes or circles, which it connects with labeled arrows sometimes but not always in a downward-branching hierarchical structure.

The relationship between concepts can be articulated in linking phrases such as *causes, requires,* or *contributes to.* The technique for visualizing these relationships among different concepts is called *concept mapping.* The expression of relationships between concepts, in either words or symbols, is a way to further the development of theory and science. These relationships may be presented as a representational model wherein symbols are used (e.g., <=>, A + B = C). A model is a virtual or imagined system that bears varying degrees of relevant similarity to aspects of the real world it represents, for instance, a model airplane resembles the airplane we fly in (Young et al., 2001, p. 10). The conceptual structure is a model in the sense that it is what a theory represents (Figure 3.1). When we introduce a model, we use an identifying description, but the object itself is not exhaustively characterized by this description. Research then simply amounts to finding out more about the object thus identified. Models are vehicles for learning about the world. Significant parts of scientific investigation are carried out on models. By studying a model, we can discover features of and ascertain facts about the system that the model stands for; in brief, models allow for *surrogative reasoning* (Swoyer, 1991), that is, identifying or substituting individuals, primitive relations, and operations for building (compound) relations and propositions from these. These will then be easier to work with than the reality that they represent through a process of model-based reasoning.

Phenomena in the observed world are usually too complex to be understood by modeling all their parts and interactions; some form of simplification is necessary. Traditionally, scientists have simplified natural complexity by viewing individual items of observation in isolation from the complex set of relations that connect them with their environment and, ultimately, with the rest of the world. They have isolated the object of their investigations, and they are interested mainly in delimited inductive chains that could be readily mapped as linear—and perhaps circular—causality (that is, A affecting B, and B affecting C and possibly also A). Figure 3.1 shows a model of the conceptual structure of nursing. In looking at such elementary models, the essential components and relationships can be identified and learned from the simple to the complex, from the parts to the whole.

Models are useful in learning as well as in providing a basis for research and theorizing. Learning through using a model takes place in three stages: *denotation, demonstration,* and *interpretation* (Hughes, 1997). We begin by establishing a representative relationship (or *denotation*) between the model and the target. Then, we investigate the features of the model in order to demonstrate certain theoretical claims about its internal constitution or mechanism; that is, we learn about the model, *demonstration.* Finally, these findings have to be converted into claims about the target system: Hughes refers to this step as *interpretation.* Theories may be too complicated to handle. In such a case, a simplified model may be employed that allows for a solution. Models are tools that are used to find out about the causal relationships that hold between certain facts or processes, and it is these relationships that do the explanatory job (Stanford Encyclopedia of Philosophy, 2006). This leads to theorizing about the relationships. Multiple models of nursing practice have been developed.

Nursing practice in this book relies heavily on the model proposed by Orem related to self-care and the theories that comprise it. The totality of the conceptual system of Orem's theory of nursing is shown in Figure 3.2.

This simple model shows the relationship among the elements or constituent theories. One relationship that can be denoted is that in order to establish a nursing system there must be a definable need for self-care, called a *self-care deficit,* within the theory. Once the need for assistance with self-care has been identified, it would then be reasonable to develop ways of measuring elements of the self-care system. One might then see the relationship as follows: When the overall self-care need is greater than the person's ability to meet the need, a self-care deficit exists. These terms and relationships are explained in detail in the following chapters. Throughout this book, there will be representational models, concept maps, and theories that help in seeing relationships and understanding the theoretical ideas being presented that are foundational to nursing practice.

FIGURE 3.2   Constituent Theories: The Self-Care Deficit Theory of Nursing

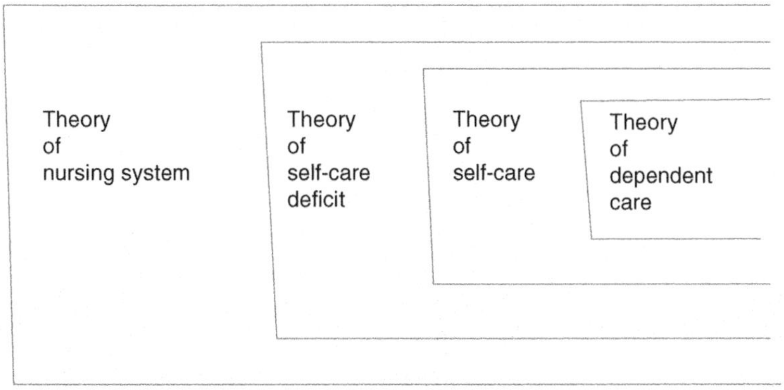

Theory of nursing system	Theory of self-care deficit	Theory of self-care	Theory of dependent care

Adapted from Orem (2001, p. 141).

THE HUMAN PERSON

The human person is a multidimensional unitary being, one who is interactive with the environment and who lives and survives by a series of interdependent relationships within the primary units of family, culture, and community. A *person* can be described as a unitary human being in the process of becoming, possessing free will (freedom of choice), self-examination, and other qualities. Human beings are experiencing beings, beings who attribute meaning based on their experiences (Banfield, 2001).

In nursing, we deal with the human being as a whole. When we speak of the thinking component, we refer to the object of nursing. When we do nursing, we use that knowledge or way of thinking in dealing with a subject—*Mrs. Smith. We use our understanding of many dimensions to come to know the person, recognizing that all dimensions are integrated into an irreducible one. I see the person standing in front of me, a material being. I acknowledge her physical being and use that to describe her physical appearance—tall, lean, sallow skin tone, dark hair, and so on.* But that is not the person Mrs. Smith is. She is a self, defined as the essential qualities that constitute a person's uniqueness or singularity, the essential being, the total or particular being of a person—the individual. The self is embodied with an "I," as known and perceived by the individual, and a "me," the referent used by the person to refer to the personality of the speaker or writer, or to something that may express it. In order to better know Mrs. Smith, I would need to ascertain her physio/bio dimensions, that is, her embodied self (organism) and her health state. I would also want information on how she thinks and feels, her cultural and social interactions, and so forth. Our ability to know a person is a function of what we can know about the various dimensions of that person, through science, literature, experience, and so forth. Our knowledge of Mrs. Smith is limited by what Mrs. Smith is willing to reveal to us and what we can see/learn from objective data and inferences. The self has biological, psychological, rational, and spiritual dimensions. The biological dimension includes organ systems, genetics, interior psychological structures, processes, and the nervous, endocrine, immune, cardiovascular, musculoskeletal, and reproductive systems. The psychological dimension includes how the person functions in "life situations that express their uniquely human qualities and personal development as they live and work [interrelate] with other persons in their community" (Orem & Vardiman, 1995, p. 165). This includes knowledge of the language, concepts, and social customs of the community. There is also a cultural view of self held by each person in accordance with his or her living system. The rational dimension means that the "person is able to symbolize, communicate, and interact with others" (Young et al., 2001, p. 74). It also defines the person as an agent with the capacity to deliberate and choose, make judgments, and take action. The actions can be directed at the self or to the environment. The person also has potentiality and the capacity for developing that potential. The spiritual dimension is an integrating force. This can be described as that which "quickens, animates, stirs, enlivens and gives life" (Johnson, 2014, p. 148).

The self is imperfect, that is, subject to limitations in knowledge, judgment and decision, and action. Through interactions with the person and those in relationship with her, our description of Mrs. Smith might broaden to include factors such as age, health state, mental status, family system, conditions of living, relationships, ability to communicate, and self-perceptions. Given this, we might further describe *Mrs. Smith as a 65-year-old divorced woman with one son who lives in the same city and has a supportive relationship with his mother. She recently retired from working as an administrative assistant in a small company. She lives and functions independently in the family home where she has lived for 35 years. She makes her own decisions about finances and other personal matters and has been doing so since her divorce 20 years ago. She participates in several group activities such as playing bridge with friends. She describes herself as spiritual but not religious. She speaks English, can read and write, though an idiopathic tremor makes writing difficult for her. She is confident that she will be able to manage any changes in her system of living as she ages.*

Basic Premises

Some premises underlying the view of human beings and nursing developed in this book include:

- Human beings require continuous deliberate inputs to themselves and their environments in order to remain alive and to function in accordance with natural human endowments.

- Human agency—the power to act deliberately—is exercised in the form of care of self and others, in identifying needs for self and others, and in making needed inputs.

- Mature human beings experience… limitations for action in care of self and others involving the making of life-sustaining and function-regulating inputs. Infants and children experience limitations in caring for self, which is congruent with their age and development.

- Human agency is exercised in discovering, developing, and transmitting to others ways and means to identify needs for self and others and to make inputs to self and others.

- Groups of human beings with structured relationships cluster tasks and allocate responsibilities for providing care to group members who experience limitations for making required deliberate inputs to self and others (Orem, 2001, p. 140).

HUMAN NEEDS AND SELF-CARE REQUISITES

Premise 1 reflects the needs of a person. These needs have been described by many scientists in various fields. Maslow proposed a hierarchy of interlocking needs, moving from the basic physiological needs to self-actualization. The intervening levels include safety, belongingness, and esteem. This was first offered as a theory of learning and motivation, though some nursing scholars use it as a model of basic human needs. Another iteration of fundamental human needs, presented by Max-Neef (Fisher, n.d.), is as follows: subsistence, protection, affection, understanding, participation, leisure, creation, identity, and freedom. Max-Neef extends the idea of needs by adding the concept of satisfiers. Although needs can be seen as universal, the way in which needs are met or satisfied changes with time and culture. He includes the resources, actions, and interactions that are necessary for meeting needs. For example, the fundamental need of subsistence (physical and mental health) requires resources of food, shelter, and work; actions needed include feeding, clothing, resting, and working in living environments and social settings.

The inclusion of actions is basic to the classification of needs. The focus is on the required inputs to the self and the environment as noted in Premise 1 of Orem's theory. These are basic requirements, referred to in Orem's theory as self-care requisites, and they include universal, developmental, and health-deviation requisites. An example of a universal requisite is the maintenance of sufficient intake of air. This approach includes the requirements for action to meet these needs or requisites. These requisites form the basis for self-care, expressing both the need and what the person needs to do or have done in order to maintain health and well-being, and are detailed in Chapters 5 through 7.

Reflecting on Mrs. Smith as we know her thus far, it would be possible to identify a number of her self-care requisites. Given her recent change from being employed to being retired, there are developmental requisites to be met. There is also a requisite to maintain a balance between solitude and social interaction and between rest and activity. The process of identifying the individual's requisites is presented in Chapter 6.

HUMAN AGENCY

This moves us to the characteristic of a person as an agent. Premise 2 of Orem's theory refers to the person's capacity for action (agency) taken on behalf of the self and others to meet these requirements for health and well-being. This is the basis from which we understand, make judgments, and take actions to care for self and others. The development of knowledge and skills occurs as self-care agency (SCA) is used and developed. *Some judgments we might make about Mrs. Smith are that her self-care agency is developed, operable (working), and adequate to meet existent requisites. These ideas are developed in Chapter 7. We can look at the life situation of Mrs. Smith to see whether she is taking appropriate action to meet her needs or demands. What actions is she taking to meet her transition from being employed to being retired? What is she doing to maintain balance between solitude and social interaction and between rest and activity? Are her actions appropriate, and are her demands being met?*

SELF-CARE LIMITATIONS

Our experiences and observations tell us that not all people are able to care for themselves at all times and under all circumstances. As expressed in Premise 3, people experience limitations for taking action. These limitations may occur in regard to limitations of knowing what to do and why, limitations in judgment and decision making, and limitations in taking or performing the appropriate action for care of self or others. There are many factors that determine the nature of these limitations. With a child, it may simply be his or her developmental stage; the younger the child, the greater will be the limitations. With an adult, it may be his or her state of health. A person with a broken arm will obviously have limitations in taking certain actions. As we reflect on Mrs. Smith, a possible limitation might be related to her idiopathic tremor. This could make it more difficult for her to perform actions requiring fine motor skills. See Chapter 7 for more content related to limitations.

Premise 4, in addition to Premise 2, also focuses on human agency (power or capacity for deliberate action) that is used to determine, develop, and communicate to others the needs for inputs to self and others. Human agency, the ability to "act with deliberate intentionality," allows human beings to "choose goals beyond biological survival and reproduction and act to achieve them" (Johnson, 2014, p. 261). Human beings consider principles of right and wrong in making choices. When used in determining needs and limitations for the self, human agency is called self-care agency (SCA). Human agency exercised in the care of others has different designations depending on who is doing the care. This book focuses on the care of self and on others who are dependent (dependent-care agency; Chapter 10). When care is given by a nurse, it is called *nursing agency*. Nursing agency is the power or capacity to act as a nurse in congruence with the proper object of nursing as earlier defined. The self is the operational unit in action and is both the source and locus of control for action. All agency is socially enabled and maintained through interactions with other similarly free, existential agents. One of the characteristics of human agency is the capacity for forecasting, predicting, or projecting into the future based on knowledge of both past and present. Much of what we do as nurses requires or is based on this kind of process. We see what is extant in the situation, relate that to our knowledge, and make judgments about what might happen to x if y occurs. We base our judgments about taking action on these predictions. We use the term *predicted outcomes* to express our projections. Health promotion activities are based on predictions of what a person or group needs to know or do about some event, designing a program or intervention to avoid the event or, should an event occur, how to respond. In some cases, such as parenting, this is referred to as *anticipatory guidance*. This is a form of surrogative reasoning.

RELATIONSHIPS AND CARE

The final premise of Orem's theory focuses on the propensity of humans toward organizations. Care begins in the family and extends from there to other sociocultural groups. Caregiving is an intentional, goal-directed response to a perceived health crisis, and it often consists of complex, interrelated, continuously refined, and negotiated behaviors that are carried out over time. Basic to the idea of organizing care are the concepts of interrelationships and care. Human development is dependent on relationships. Humans live and thrive through a series of interdependent relationships within the primary units of family, community, and culture (Taylor & Renpenning, 2011, p. 37). For humans, life begins with the person requiring assistance in meeting self-care requisites. This assistance, called *dependent care* within Orem's theory, is provided by members of the family or other designated social groups. Dependent care requires not only knowledge of the requisites of the dependent person but also the capability to make judgments and perform necessary actions. This dependent care is integrated with the caregiver's own self-care system. The characteristics and complexities of dependent care and care for others are described in Chapter 10.

THE LANGUAGE OF NURSING

How do we as nurses talk about what we do? For most nurses, the discussion reverts to the things that we do and the tasks that we perform. Orem (1988) as cited in Renpenning and Taylor (2003, p. 257) described her experiences with nurses in the

1950s: "I became aware of and somewhat overwhelmed by the inability of nurses to communicate nursing to their patients, to other nurses, to physicians, to hospital administrators, and to members of hospital boards of trustees."

Canam (2008) made a similar observation in response to concerns that nursing is largely invisible. In a study of clinical nurse specialists, she found that "nurses' silence is related to their understandings of the power dynamics operating within their practice environment" where the dominant language was technical, and caring discourse was not considered legitimate. She noted a number of advantages to a knowledge-based discourse of nursing practice: It has "the potential to improve working relations between doctors and nurses by decreasing the tension created by the binary thinking of technical knowledge as medicine's domain and relational knowledge as nursing's domain" (Canam, 2008, n.p.).

It has been the experience of many of those working from a self-care perspective and using the language of the theory that they are more confident in their knowledge; that is, they know how to do nursing, know how to express the outcomes of their actions, and can express to the management what they need in order to do their jobs effectively and efficiently as members of a care team where each one respects the others' contributions.

As a part of learning the language of nursing and using it to communicate with others, and with the advent of electronic health records (EHRs), some people express the desire for a standardized language for nursing. Given Canam's (2008) position that the dominant language and worldview in health care is that of medicine, standardized terminology tends to echo that worldview. As we move forward with the development of nursing science and other forms of nursing knowledge, nurses will benefit from a system that captures the essence and variability in the expression of nursing outcomes. At the present time, the American Nurses Association (ANA) has more than 10 approved languages (Rutherford, 2008). Dr. Norma Lang, a distinguished nursing leader, has asserted, "If we cannot name it, we cannot control it, practice it, teach it, finance it, or put it into public policy" (Clark & Lang, 1992, p. 109). Standardized language is an issue in practice that is related to nursing diagnosis and outcomes. These issues are addressed in Chapter 8.

One of the primary structured relationships of concern is that between the nurse and the patient. Nursing begins as an interpersonal relationship. The patient (receiver of services) may be an individual, family, group, or community. The variations in these relationships and the meaning for nursing are described in Chapters 10, 11, and 12.

LEARNING ACTIVITIES

1. How would you map your current view of nursing? What elements are part of that view? What relationships exist between the elements?
2. Consider the stress that you experience throughout the day. Construct a simple concept map representing the source(s) of your stress and actions that you take to manage it.

(continued)

LEARNING ACTIVITIES (*continued*)

3. Visualize an interdisciplinary or interprofessional team of health care and health care-related professionals similar to those you have worked with. Given what you have learned in this chapter, how would you describe the role that you would play within this team in provision of health care?
4. Write a paragraph analyzing the value of having a common language in nursing.

References

Asselin, M. E. (2011). Using reflection strategies to link course knowledge to clinical practice: The RN-to-BSN student experience. *Journal of Nursing Education, 50*(3), 125–133.

Banfield, B. E. (2001). A philosophical inquiry of Orem's self-care deficit nursing theory. In D. E. Orem (Ed.), *Nursing concepts of practice* (6th ed., p. xiii). St. Louis, MO: Mosby.

Canam, C. J. (2008). The link between nursing discourses and nurses' silence: Implications for a knowledge-based discourse for nursing practice. *Advances in Nursing Science, 31*(4), 296–307. doi:10.1097/01.ANS.0000341410.25048.d8

Clark, J., & Lang, N. (1992). Nursing's next advance: An internal classification for nursing practice. *International Nursing Review, 39*(4), 109–111, 128.

Fisher, K. (n.d.). *Max-Neef model of human-scale development.* Last revised 2012. Retrieved from http://www.rainforestinfo.org.au/background/maxneef.htm

Harmer, B. (1922). *Text-book of the principles and practice of nursing.* New York, NY: The Macmillan Co. Retrieved from http://www.archive.org/details/textbookofprinciharm or http://collections.nlm.nih.gov/bookviewer?PID=nlm:nlmuid-54130040R-bk

Hughes, R. I. G. (1997). Models and representation. *Philosophy of Science, 64*, S325–S336. Retrieved from http://plato.stanford.edu/entries/models-science

Johnson, E. A. (2014). *Ask the beasts: Darwin and the god of love.* New York, NY: Bloomsbury.

Orem, D. E. (2001). *Nursing: Concepts of practice* (6th ed.). St. Louis, MO: Mosby.

Orem, D. E., & Vardiman, E. M. (1995). Orem's nursing theory and positive mental health. *Nursing Science Quarterly, 8*(4), 165–173.

Renpenning, K., & Taylor, S. G. (2003). (Eds.). *Self-care theory in nursing: Selected papers of Dorothea Orem.* New York, NY: Springer Publishing Company.

Rutherford, M. A. (2008). Standardized nursing language: What does it mean for nursing practice. *Online Journal of Issues in Nursing, 13*(1). doi:10.3912/OJIN .Vol13No01PPT05

Stanford Encyclopedia of Philosophy. (2006). Last revised 2012. Retrieved from http:// plato.stanford.edu/entries/concepts

Swoyer, C. (1991). Structural representation and surrogative reasoning. *Synthese, 87*(3), 449–598. Retrieved from http://plato.stanford.edu/entries/models-science

Taylor, S. G., & Renpenning, K. (2011). *Self-care science, nursing theory, and evidence-based practice.* New York, NY: Springer Publishing Company.

Young, A., Taylor, S. G., & Renpenning, K. (2001). *Connections: Nursing research, theory and practice.* St. Louis, MO: Mosby.

CHAPTER 4

THE NURSING SYSTEM

In Chapter 1, nursing was described as both a discipline and a profession. In this chapter, we bring the two together as we describe how nursing is produced. Nursing is an action system and not simply something theoretical. A nursing system begins when a nurse engages with a client as the subject of the relationship. These actions are congruent with the purpose or object of nursing by an individual who is educationally prepared to take such actions in a knowing way. Nursing is not just a series of tasks performed on behalf of another person. Each of the individual actions is a part of a greater whole. Regardless of who has primary responsibility for the overall plan, all the involved people—client/patient, family, providers—should be a part of a plan that is designed for the good of the client. This overall plan is often referred to as a *care system*. When the proposed system is designed by a professional nurse with the object of helping clients regain or retain self-care, it is referred to as a nursing care plan. It becomes a nursing system as the designed system is put into action. The action system designed and used by an individual to maintain health and well-being is called a *self-care system*.

OBJECTIVES

After reading this chapter, the learner will be able to:

1. Define action systems
2. Distinguish between analytical/critical thinking and systems thinking
3. Identify properties of a system
4. Describe components of nursing agency
5. Discuss desirable characteristics of the nurse
6. Describe five methods of helping within the nursing system

7. Distinguish between the role of the patient and the role of the nurse within the methods of helping

8. Describe the dimensions of the nursing system

9. Examine factors related to patient disclosure within the nurse–patient relationship

10. Analyze the value and importance of caring in today's health care environment

KEY CONCEPTS action systems • nursing systems • nursing agency • methods of helping • dimensions of the nursing system

ACTION SYSTEMS

Action systems begin with problem identification, framing, and delineation. This is similar in many ways to the more traditional nursing process, and is discussed further in Chapters 8 and 9. For the nursing system, the problem will be identified and framed from the perspective of self-care. *As in Mrs. Smith's situation, the problem is related to her limited mobility postoperatively and her need to regain normalcy with regard to mobility through a series of actions, including learning to walk with assistive devices. In addition to that problem, she experiences difficulty in meeting her other requisites. How does her limited mobility influence her ability to meet her other needs for adequate food, hydration, and elimination? Is she able to sleep at night, or do pain and inability to get into a comfortable position interfere with her sleep? How does her limited mobility interfere with her social activities?*

There are often different interpretations of the problem because of the differing frames of reference used. The physician may see the problem as one related to a surgical site that needs to heal and may prevent further incidents by prescribing antibiotics, anticoagulants, and so forth. The nurse's focus will be on her limitations and abilities to meet her basic needs such as food and hydration. The alternative views of the problem are not necessarily competing but need to be coalesced into a meaningful plan of care for the patient.

When the purpose or mission of the system is described, then one can move on to designing a plan to deal with the problem, eventually implementing or executing the designed plan. Design, planning, execution, and production are interdependent and continuous activities. Depending on the fluidity of the situation, there may be simultaneous evaluation and adjustment of the plan. This is characteristic of most nursing systems.

Systems Theory

Before describing nursing systems, let us review what we know about systems. The idea of systems and a model of a general system is presented in Chapter 1. A common descriptor of a system is that the whole is greater than the sum of its parts. The word *system* connotes a complex (whole) of interacting components or elements together with the relationships between and among them that permit the identification of a boundary-maintaining entity or process with the following properties:

- Each element has an effect on the functioning of the whole.

- Each element is affected by at least one other element in the system.

- All possible subgroups of elements also have the first two properties. (Ackoff, 1981, pp. 15–16)

In addition, a system has structure, behavior, and interconnectivity. It contains parts that may be physical or conceptual. It exhibits processes that fulfill its function or purpose. The parts and processes are connected by structural and/or behavioral relationships. A subsystem is a set of elements, a system by itself, and a component of a larger system (Ackoff, 1981, pp. 15–16).

A system can have a physical reality or it may be conceptual. In nursing, we deal with both these aspects. The human person is a system with many subsystems, such as the digestive or cardiovascular subsystem. The relationship known as *family* is both a conceptual and a physical system. An organization is also such a system. Systems may also comprise actions. As noted earlier, systems are complex and adaptive, as shown in Figure 4.1.

The challenge to nurses in practice is to develop the ability to view situations as a whole and to engage in systems thinking. The central concepts in systems thinking are interconnections, feedback, and time delays. Systems thinking is about the relationship between the part and the whole. "Systems thinking is a discipline for seeing wholes. It is a framework for seeing interrelationships rather than things, for seeing patterns of change rather than static snapshots" (Senge, 2006, p. 53). Non-linear thinking is the heart of systems thinking. It emphasizes that it is not doing things right but doing the right thing that enables us to quickly reach our destination. In systems thinking, the fast is slow, which means that if you look for short cuts, it delays the process more. It is better to do the right thing wrong than the wrong thing right (Botla, 2009). Systems thinking is the process of understanding how things influence one another within a whole. It provides tools for understanding system structure, the system as a whole, and the dynamic behavior of a system. Contrary

FIGURE 4.1   Complex Adaptive System

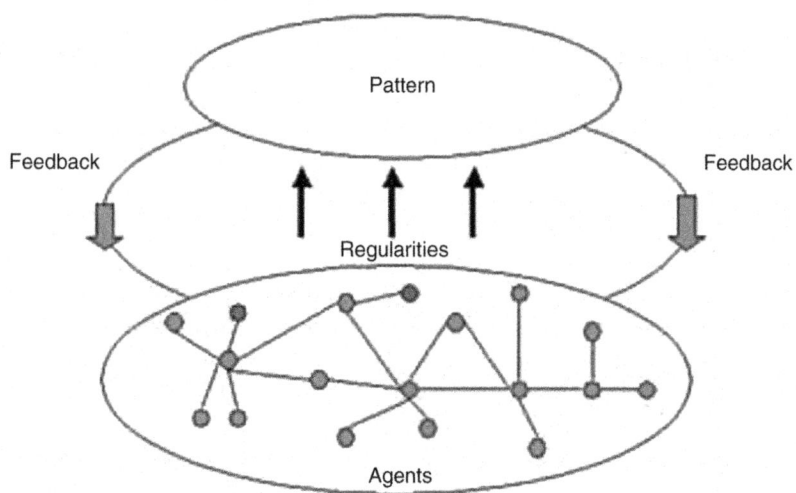

Used with permission from Peter Fryer and Jules Ruis.

to traditional analytical thinking, in systems thinking, the elements of the system are examined not only as distinct elements, but also as elements interacting with each other (Konkarikoski, Ritala, & Ihalainen, 2010). In contrast to critical thinking, systems thinking is interdisciplinary and may act as a bridge between the physical, natural, and social sciences (Cabrera, Colosi, & Lobdell, 2008). Systems thinking addresses parts, wholes, and the relationships among them; it is patterned and conceptual. An open system interacts with its environment and deals with concurrent information and energy. A human system is considered an open system, that is, one that exchanges information, matter, and/or energy between external and internal environments.

Furthermore, there are levels of systems or systems embedded within other systems, and these are often referred to as meta systems or subsystems. Meta systems or mega systems are large and comprise more than one describable system. A system may either comprise or include subsystems. The person doing a systems analysis determines the level of the system. For example, while thinking of Mrs. Smith from a systems perspective, we can consider her the central system of interest. When Mrs. Smith is the system, we can identify many subsystems, including anatomical, physiological, behavioral, and social subsystems. Once she interacts with another human system, the description may be of a mega system comprising two people with Mrs. Smith as the focal system. On the contrary, the dyad may be considered the system, in which case Mrs. Smith becomes a component or a subsystem. The plan of care could be viewed as a mega system comprising the client and medical, nursing, and physical therapy systems of care. The nursing system may have subsystems such as those that are designed to meet universal self-care requisites or developmental self-care requisites. A description of the properties of the system recognizes that each of the actions of the client, nurse, physician, and physical therapist has an effect on the whole; each element is affected by at least one other element. What Mrs. Smith and the physician do has an effect on the whole; similarly, what the nurse does has an effect on the whole plan of care. When the physician changes a prescription for anticoagulants, both the nurse and the client will need to make adjustments to their action systems.

Every real-world system contains a large number of components and is exposed to a large number of external forces and events. Self-care theory recognizes the complexity and dynamism of the components or elements of the theory when examining the conditioning effects of various factors such as those that exist between health state and self-care requisites (Figure 3.1). A change in a basic conditioning factor will affect the whole of self-care and other elements in the system. As Mrs. Smith's health state changed from that of a well woman to a woman recovering from surgery, her self-care system was transformed as did the elements of self-care demand and self-care agency.

Identification of the nursing system as a whole leads to questions about the parts—the elements or components—and their relationships to each other. The nursing system includes the patient variables of self-care agency and therapeutic self-care demand and the nurse variable of nursing agency. Essential to an understanding of the conceptual model is the underlying fact that the relationship is between people, basically between a nurse and a patient. Alternative nursing systems can and usually do include more than one nurse and variations in the constellation of clients (e.g., families or communities). These variations will be considered later.

NURSING SYSTEMS

The essence of the nursing system is that it is an action system that has social, interpersonal, and technological dimensions. The nursing system is an action system that comes into being with the establishment of a relationship between the person requiring nursing assistance and the nurse. This system is essentially an interpersonal system. It exists within a sociocultural context and, therefore, has both social and interpersonal dimensions. The technological dimension includes processes that are associated with establishing the relationship, data collection and analysis related to the client variables, and all the intervention strategies and procedures required. Nursing capabilities and actions are required relative to all three dimensions. In acute-care institutions today, there is often greater emphasis placed on the technological dimension than on the social and interpersonal ones. The seeming emphasis of nursing care on technical and biological factors related to the experience of health and illness at the expense of the critical importance of the nurse–client relationship is of current concern (D'Antonio, Beeber, Sills, & Naegle, 2014). However, as we learn more about the human person as a unified being, expand our understanding of the social determinants of health, and appreciate a more holistic approach to the delivery of health care services, there is a greater recognition of the need to attend to the social and interpersonal dimensions of nursing knowledge and capabilities.

Patient actions within nursing systems are focused on self-care and are expressed in the client self-care system. The self-care system is a function of the purposes or goals to be achieved, which are referred to as *self-care requisites* (discussed in Chapter 6), and the capabilities to act to achieve those goals (e.g., self-care agency, as discussed in Chapter 7). When a person's capabilities are not sufficient or appropriately developed to meet the goals, the person may need assistance from a nurse.

Nursing Agency

Agency is the power or capacity for action. When that action is directed toward the self, we call it *self-care agency*. The nurse demonstrates her power to act as a moral agent when making judgments about right or wrong actions. *Nursing agency* is the power or capacity to act in order to design and produce nursing systems for individuals, a dependent-care unit, groups or communities with limitations for engaging in the required self-care, dependent care, or care of families or other multi-person units (Orem, 2001). Some of the components that are specific to nursing agency are identified in Box 4.1.

Some characteristics of the nurse that reflect evidence of the preceding capabilities are listed in Table 4.1.

Nursing as Helping

The nursing system is a helping system. A helping system is an interactive system in which the actions of one person affect the actions or responses of the other. In situations where help is needed, there are two kinds of people: the person/ people who require help and the person/ people who provide help. These roles are, in part, related to societal and personal expectations and to ethical and cultural mores

---

BOX 4.1 Components of Nursing Agency

- Reliable knowledge of areas of nursing operation, including social, interpersonal, and technological
- Developed practical skills related to each of the three areas of nursing operation
- Sustained motivation and willingness to provide nursing
- Ability to unify action sequences toward achievement of desired results
- Consistency in performance of nursing actions
- Expertise to adjust actions associated with nursing operations because of current or emerging situations
- Ability to manage self in nursing practice situations

Adapted from Orem (2001).

TABLE 4.1 Desirable Nurse Characteristics

Social	Interpersonal	Technological
Is well informed about social and legal dimensions of nursing situations	Is well informed about psychosocial aspects of human functioning and factors that may help or interfere with interpersonal functions	Has mastery of techniques for diagnosis, prescription, and implementation of nursing actions related to meeting therapeutic self-care demands and for regulating development, exercise, and protection of self-care agency
Has knowledge of cultural differences and the importance of cultural influences	Has knowledge of conditions that are needed to develop helping relationships	Is experienced/becoming experienced in using techniques while performing technological aspects of nursing practice in nursing situations
Has social and communication skills that are necessary for interacting with a wide variety of people	Has interest in identifying and resolving human problems between people that cause pain and suffering	Can integrate methods of helping with technological operations toward production and management of nursing systems
Is respectful of self and others; courteous and considerate of others	Has interpersonal skills to work across the life span and with people who are ill, disabled, or debilitated	Is confident in nursing situations and able to mobilize for immediate and effective action to protect patient well-being

(continued)

TABLE 4.1 Desirable Nurse Characteristics *(continued)*		
Social	**Interpersonal**	**Technological**
Is responsible for provision of nursing within defined types of nursing situations	Can relate to patients and significant others in a way that conforms to conventions for human interactions	Seeks nursing practice experience, supervision, education, and training
Understands nursing as one of the health services provided for by society	Has communication skills, adjusted to specific needs, that are needed to form and maintain relationships for the production of nursing systems	Works toward formulation and testing of methods and techniques for technological operations of nursing practice
Understands the nature of professional and contractual relationships and is able to perform nursing practice within defined limits	Accepts people under nursing care and works with them in accordance with their self-care and dependent care roles	Endeavors to increase understanding of factors that condition patient variables, self-care agency, and therapeutic self-care demand, thus helping define requirements of nursing agency
	Identifies broader social and legal aspects of interpersonal situations	Identifies results obtained in nursing situations, compiles results over time, identifies associated factors, and compares results in various nursing situations
Adapted from Orem (2001).		

about appropriate behavior, as one person is being helped while another is a helper in health care situations. There are many kinds of helping systems besides nursing. Each system has its own goals and strategies to meet those goals. Not all helping systems are related to health; however, for our purposes, we will consider only those systems that are related to health. In recent health care literature, there is a great deal of emphasis on the partnership between professionals and patients: This is in contrast to the time when the professional was the authority and client records did not belong to the patient but to the health care system. Slowly, times are changing and we are getting past the situation where it was believed that only the doctor had knowledge and could share information; we are moving toward a more cooperative relationship.

The methods of helping that are described later are general. The specific selection of methods and correlated strategies are a function of the goal or purpose of helping. Nurses select the methods and strategies that correspond with the patients' needs and abilities to care for themselves.

THE METHODS OF HELPING

There are five primary categories of methods of helping. There may be more than one method of helping employed at any one time. In nursing, the methods of helping that are selected are a function of the characteristics of development, operability, and adequacy of the patient's self-care agency in relation to the nature of the self-care deficit. Helping requires interpersonal communication. It requires establishing a particular type of relationship with another person. If a person is unconscious, communication may occur only through touch and voice. If a person is able to participate in the helping relationship through decision making or doing, the responsibilities for the care actions are distributed between the person requiring the care and the helper or helpers. The moral and ethical dimensions and the influence of cultural beliefs are made evident not only in words but also in nonverbal communication. A helping relationship also has legal dimensions; these are based in the validity of the helper through laws, licensing, and education. An example of this is the Good Samaritan laws, which are enacted to encourage people to help while protecting helpers in certain situations such as automobile accidents.

Acting for or doing with another

This method may be employed when a person is unconscious. It may also be the method of choice in situations where the person is conscious but incompetent, or the person is unable to participate in making decisions. There are situations where the person should not be taking action, such as immediately after serious injury. Whenever this method is employed, the helper should respect the rights of the person being helped to know what is occurring and what to expect during the helping situation. Furthermore, to the extent possible, the person should be given an opportunity and encouraged to share likes, dislikes, and reactions. This method is probably the method of choice when specialized knowledge and techniques are required. It is not the method of choice when internal acts, such as controlling one's behavior, are required. *While Mrs. Smith is hospitalized she will need someone to do most things that require any physical action. She may be able to feed herself but would need someone to get the food to her. She may be able to decide she has a need for pain medication, but another person controls her access to the drugs.*

Guiding another

This method of helping may be appropriate when a person needs to choose one option over another or when he or she is able to pursue a course of action but only with direction and supervision. Communication between both parties is important. The patient must be able to perform required actions and be motivated to do so. The helper must provide appropriate suggestions, instructions, directions, supervision, and feedback. *When Mrs. Smith is able to walk with the use of an apparatus such as a walker, she may need guidance in deciding which is the most appropriate for her and how to manipulate the device.*

Supporting another

Support may be physical, psychological, or both. Supporting occurs when, for example, a person is helped by another to get through a painful procedure. Support may take the form of encouragement and assurance that the person being helped can do something, for instance, walking to the end of the hall. Again, communication is important, as the nurse must be sensitive to how much the person being helped is capable of doing. The person being helped must be able to communicate to the nurse when he or she can no longer continue to do what is required. *In the case of Mrs. Smith, she will also need physical support, probably in the form of a safety belt held by the assistant, until she regains strength and balance.*

Providing a developmental environment

Provision of a developmental environment may involve psychological and/or physical components. Respect for the individual is an essential component of this method of helping. The physical and psychological environments as well as social positions and roles are factors to be considered. This process begins in childhood, as adults help children to become independent and learn skills to master control over their environment. It continues throughout life. Attention to promotion of a developmental environment is particularly important when working with elderly, disabled, or challenged people so that well-intentioned caregivers do not take over decision making and/or activities that people are able to manage by themselves. This method of helping is often used in conjunction with teaching and other helping methods. This would also include play therapy equipment in the pediatric unit, equipment sized for children from toddlers to adolescents, and perhaps separate play areas for different ages.

Teaching another

When development of new knowledge and skills is required, teaching may be the method of helping. Teaching is more than just providing information and expecting a person to absorb and apply it. The nurse requires some understanding of learning theories and instructional strategies. In addition, use of this method begins with a clear understanding of the required behavior change, listening and exploration of the client's perception of the issue, current knowledge and understanding, and identification of cultural values that may be significant. It is important to understand what the patient knows, what the patient needs to know, and what he or she is willing and able to learn. The process may include designing learning experiences, utilizing group activity, input from a peer group, reference material, and so on. Behavior change in relation to self-care practices takes time; this change begins with establishment and achievement of little steps related to long-term goal achievement. In order to do this, the nurse must be aware of the clients' goals. In selecting a method of helping, it is also important to determine whether the required action has an internal or an external orientation. Actions such as learning, decision making, swallowing a liquid, and walking have an internal orientation; that is, "nobody can do it for you." Actions such as providing instruction, helping people select between various options, and helping someone walk have an external orientation. There are many teaching techniques that vary with the content to be learned, be it information or manual skills.

A summary of the methods of helping and associated nurse–patient roles is presented in Table 4.2.

There are many nursing intervention strategies that relate to the methods of helping. Many of those strategies are combinations of ways of helping. It is not uncommon that the nurse is teaching and supporting while doing for the patient. The interpersonal interactions while guiding a person to make a choice may also be supportive and instructive. The nurse may make a choice to do for the patient, even though the person is able to do for himself or herself. The intention here is to provide support, develop trust, or create a developmental environment. The

TABLE 4.2   Nurse and Patient Roles According to Method of Helping

Method of helping	Nurse's Role	Patient's Role
Doing or acting for/ with another	Acts in place of and for the patient	Receives care to meet therapeutic self-care demand and to compensate for self-care limitations Receives services that are relevant to resources and control of environment
Guiding and directing another	Provides information that is relevant to regulation of self-care agency or for meeting self-care requisites	Receives, processes, and uses information as a self-care agent or a regulator of a self-care agency
Providing physical support	Acts as a partner in performing self-care actions to help regulate a patient's self-care agency	Performs actions to meet self-care requisites or to regulate self-care agency in cooperation with a nurse
Providing emotional/ psychological support	Acts as a compassionate presence and an understanding listener who can enact other methods of helping as necessary	Confronts, resolves, and solves difficult problems and/or lives through difficult situations
Providing a developmental environment	Supplies and regulates environmental conditions and acts as a significant other in the patient's environment	Confronts living and caring for self in a way and in an environment that supports and promotes personal development
Teaching	Teaches: • Knowledge related to self-care requisites and therapeutic self-care demand • Methods and actions to meet self-care requisites • Methods of calculating therapeutic self-care demand • Methods of overcoming or compensating for self-care limitations • Methods of managing self-care	Acts as a learner who is engaged in knowledge and skills that are needed to provide continuous and effective self-care

Adapted from Orem (2001).

therapeutic self-care demands and self-care capabilities of the patient provide the basis for the selection of nursing intervention strategies.

The Dimensions of the Nursing System

The nursing system has been described as a three-dimensional system in which social, interpersonal, and technological components interact. Within each of these dimensions there are conditioning factors, some common and some unique to the particular dimension, that affect the choice of available actions. For example, socio-cultural values and beliefs vary among individuals and act as conditioning factors that influence the patient's action choices. With the introduction of the nurse as both person and nurse, the sociocultural values and beliefs of the nurse also influence the choice of technological options that the nurse considers in her interaction with the client. An extreme example of this is a situation in which the religious beliefs of the patient and/or nurse influence the options related to issues of birth control or right to life. Some cultural or religious values held by either the nurse or the patient may prevent a male nurse from caring for a female patient. A woman who is sexually abused may need a woman present to provide support and a developmental environment while being examined by a male provider.

Nursing actions are a result of and incorporate both art and science. Art includes a diverse range of human activities and the products of those activities. It involves the creation of objects or products in which the practical considerations of use are essential, for example, in a way that they usually are not in a painting. Art may refer to a process of using a creative skill or a product of the creative skill. Science can be creative, and art can be scientific. Both science and art are vital to a healthy, vibrant profession; both are equally important for innovation. The art expressed within the social and interpersonal dimensions also has a scientific base. Much of what we know about the social and interpersonal dimensions was developed in the related social sciences. Nursing looks to this knowledge from the perspective of seeking answers to nursing questions. This knowledge base is essential to nursing practice but it is important to ask, "What meaning does this theory or piece of information have for this nursing situation?" For example, what meaning does touch have in the religious preference of a particular patient and how does this affect nursing action? What meaning does personal space have in a particular situation?

In taking care of Mrs. Smith, the nurse demonstrates artful nursing in the manner in which she approaches her and positions her for maximum safety and comfort. The nurse is able to do this because of her knowledge and skill based in science.

The social and interpersonal dimensions also include conditioning factors such as the social environment in which a person lives, cultural values, family values, physical environment, access to human and economic resources, and so on. The following questions should be asked: Which of these factors is influencing the current situation? What expectations regarding the role of the health care provider and of the patient are of influence in the situation? How is this being manifested in the communications between the parties?

COMMUNICATION

The goal of communication is to convey meaning and information between people. Models of communication are changing as knowledge and technology are growing.

The earliest model was linear, that is, between two people or, more contemporaneously, from television or radio to a person, thus having no potential for feedback or clarification. Newer models take this into account. Now, the preferred models are interactive and transactional, allowing for feedback. The transactional model recognizes that communication is a simultaneous process. It also adds the environment, which embraces not only physical location but also personal experiences and cultural backgrounds. A transactional model of communication is shown in Figure 4.2.

In the early 1960s, a theory of goal attainment was developed by Imogene King. It describes a dynamic, interpersonal relationship in which a patient grows and develops while attaining certain life goals, and it uses a transactional model. Similar to the nursing system described in this chapter, the model has three interacting systems: personal, interpersonal, and social. Each of these systems has its own set of concepts. The concepts for the personal system are perception, self, growth and development, body image, space, and time. The concepts for the interpersonal system are interaction, communication, transaction, role, and stress. The concepts for the social system are organization, authority, power, status, and decision making. The goals to be attained are general to all helping professions.

The communications between the nurse and the patient are influenced by and a part of the social and interpersonal dimensions of the nursing system. Communication includes body language, language spoken, tone of voice, perception of position within a culture, cultural values, and vocabulary available to describe one's concerns, among others. With the availability of vast amounts of health-related information via the Internet, the health care provider is no longer viewed as the authority figure. Achieving health-related goals is a partnership between the person requiring assistance and the provider. Information available is filtered through a screen of culturally related beliefs, values, and choices made about suitable courses of action to be followed. There is a concern that nurses need to be more effective in dealing with people belonging to cultures other than their own. Dr. Madeleine Leininger was the creator of *Transcultural Nursing*. Transcultural nursing is a study of cultures that is undertaken to understand both similarities and differences in patient groups in which nurses practice according to the patient's cultural considerations. It begins with a culturalogical assessment, which takes the patient's cultural

FIGURE 4.2 Transactional Model

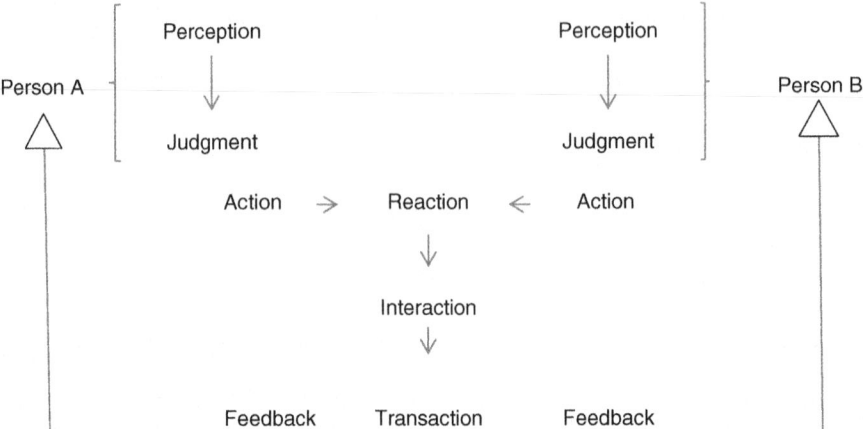

background into consideration in assessing the patient and his or her health. Once the assessment is complete, the nurse should use the culturalogical assessment to design a nursing system that also takes the patient's cultural background into consideration (Nursing Theory, 2015).

Sociocultural beliefs and values are also influential in the nurse–patient relationship. The nurse and the patient hailing from the same sociocultural background may be more comfortable with each other and find it easier to communicate. In addition, the common understanding about situations may mean less misunderstanding between the nurse and the patient.

One aspect of communication is determining the veracity of the information provided by the patient. This introduces the idea of disclosure. Under what circumstances do patients share all of the information related to the health situation that is of concern? Under what circumstances do they withhold information? What kind of information do they withhold? Why? What characteristics of nurse, patient, and/or nurse–patient relationship influence sharing and/or withholding information?

A man with Parkinson's disease visited his neurologist, who happened to be a colleague and friend, during a routine visit to assess the progress of his disease. The neurologist asked the man whether he could get out of bed on his own, to which the man replied, "Oh, yes. No problem." The man's wife disclosed that he was unable to get out of bed on his own and that he needed help to get up to void three or four times a night. Without verifying the patient's information, the physician would have made inaccurate changes to the care plan. Was this man withholding information or was his perception of the situation different from that of his wife? Perhaps his cultural beliefs as to the role of a wife influenced his view of the situation. Or perhaps he was reticent to reveal his vulnerability to the neurologist, who was a colleague and friend.

CARING

Caring has traditionally been regarded as an essential component of nursing action, as presented in Chapter 1. Caring is context specific and is characterized by expert nursing practice, interpersonal sensitivity, and initiation of close interpersonal relationships.

A nurse described her response to finding a patient who was crying: "I went to her, held her hand, and stayed with her until she settled. To this day, she thanks me for caring about her that day." Contrast this with what would happen if the person crying had been a Buddhist priest and the nurse tried to comfort him by expressing that she cared by reaching out to touch him. The caring, culturally sensitive nurse would know that this approach would not be acceptable.

There is much written in the nursing literature about caring and the carative process, notably the work by Jean Watson, in which 10 carative factors are identified as the core of nursing. Although Watson still considers these carative factors as relevant, her thinking has evolved to include a clinical caritas or a caring process with a more explicit spiritual focus. This caring process has meaning for other professions as well as for nursing. See Box 4.2 for Watson's Caritas™ Processes (Watson Caring Science Institute, 2015).

These caritas processes can provide direction and context for the development of meaningful and therapeutic nurse–patient relationships, along with other theoretical perspectives such as those provided by Peplau (1952). Peplau's work on the

---

BOX 4.2 Watson's 10 Caritas™ Processes

- Embrace altruistic values and practice loving kindness with self and others
- Instill faith and hope and honor others
- Be sensitive to self and others by nurturing individual beliefs and practices
- Develop helping–trusting–caring relationships
- Promote and accept positive and negative feelings as you authentically listen to another's story
- Use creative scientific problem-solving methods for carrying out decision making
- Share teaching and learning that address individual needs and comprehension styles
- Create a healing environment that respects human dignity for the physical and spiritual self
- Assist with basic physical, emotional, and spiritual human needs
- Be open to mystery and allow miracles to enter

Source: Watson Caring Science Institute (2015). Reprinted by permission of Jean Watson, PhD, RN, AHN-BC, FAAN, Distinguished Professor and Dean Emerita, University of Colorado College of Nursing.

---

transformative power of interpersonal relationships in nursing is seminal. D'Antonio et al. (2014) contend that Peplau's ideas have a renewed place in today's health care environment with its emphasis on patient-centered care. These authors do not suggest that Peplau's original work be transported to the 21st century; rather, they advocate returning to her focus on the power of interpersonal relationships to heal and to "move all nurses away from reductionist foci on diseases and treatments and toward more inclusive formulations about the experiences of illness in individuals, families and the health systems in which they find their expression" (p. 312). Caring, like communication, is not a concept that is associated exclusively with nursing, although it is a central component.

There are other aspects of social and interpersonal dimensions to be considered within each of the clinical specialty areas of nursing. Family and social interpersonal relationships are important in establishing an effective system for the client. To the extent that relationships are good, the family can be supportive and facilitative of care. When there are tensions within the family, the opposite may be true. It has been found that families and social relationships can be a source of both support and tension simultaneously, and this possibility should be assessed (Pickens, 2003).

PATIENT-CENTERED CARE

Patient-centered care is both a philosophy and a program. "Providing care that is patient centered indicates a true collaboration exists between provider and patient.

Instead of telling the patient what he or she should do, the emphasis is to engage the patient in making decisions about care, and provide support, so he or she can achieve the goals of care" (Silver, Keefer, & Rosenfeld, 2011, p. 447). *Culturally sensitive health care* has been defined by the U.S. Office of Minority Health (cited in Tucker, Marsiske, Rice, Nielson, & Herman, 2011, p. 2) as care that reflects "the ability to be appropriately responsive to the attitudes, feelings, or circumstances of groups of people that share a common and distinctive racial, national, religious, linguistic, or cultural heritage." Patient-centered care is ideally culturally sensitive care that has been shown to positively influence health behaviors and outcomes.

Person-centered care requires the development of all three dimensions of a nursing system. It is a value that is frequently expressed in relation to the social and interpersonal dimensions of the health care delivery system both generally and definitely in reference to nursing. What does that mean? How is this value operationalized in nursing? Operationalization of patient-centered care begins with a particular kind of critical thinking that "involves two skills: the skill of self-examination, and the skill of using a style of reasoning that does not begin with the specifics of evidence, but rather, with the general goals of nursing" (Lazenby, 2013, e12).

Critical thinking begins with being clear about what one cares about and the outcome that is desired, which is derived from the object of nursing. This involves a certain amount of self-examination in determining how one's actions as nurses fit with the general goals of nursing, which is an example of "thinking nursing" (Chapter 3). This begins with thinking about the broad goals of nursing—maintenance of health and well-being, and promotion of development. These goals become further defined by the particular view held by the nurse about the object of nursing, that is, the inability of a person to provide the quantity and quality of self-care required. Nursing theory and nursing science provide a road map for further exploration of this domain, leading to:

- Identifying and naming the variables of concern to nursing—the self-care system, self-care agency, therapeutic self-care demand, nursing agency, and nursing system
- Establishing the relationships between and among the variables of concern and the role of nursing in relation to those variables, that is, meeting the therapeutic self-care demand by protecting self-care agency, facilitating development of self-care agency, and/or acting on behalf of the person or people

In every nursing situation, nurses must ask themselves two questions: What action is required to achieve these goals? How do my actions fit with these goals? These goals are very different from the tasks of changing a dressing or giving medications.

Answering these questions requires nurses to think holistically by using systems thinking, which necessarily includes all components of the system, including the patient's perspective as well as that of nursing. The result is cultivating a way of thinking that recognizes that each person's predicament is unique to him or her. The right nursing act as defined by evidence or established standards may not be that which is needed by for the individual (Lazenby, 2013, e13). Thinking holistically or using systems thinking requires that nurses consider the following three dimensions of the nursing system: social, interpersonal, and technological.

Patient-centered care, therefore, is the way in which a nursing system should be designed and produced. Lazenby describes a reasoning process that moves from the general goals of nursing to the specifics of a particular situation in consultation with patients and families, in order to determine which particular acts will accomplish the goals particularized to the situation. Using inclusive sympathy, as described by Lazenby, leads nurses "to cultivate in themselves the ability to imagine the actual lives and predicaments of those for whom they care and how these actual lives and predicaments may dictate different care" (p. e13).

It is exam time. Mary has flu-like symptoms and goes to the health clinic for advice. The nurse practitioner (NP) confirms that Mary does, in fact, have flu and advises Mary to limit contact with others, include more sleep and rest in her daily routine, increase her fluid intake, including more fruit juices, and return for a follow-up visit if she does not feel any better. On a follow-up visit, Mary is feeling no better. This time, using inclusive sympathy, the nurse spends more time with Mary and finds out that Mary lives at home and is responsible for caring for a parent who has significant disabilities associated with arthritis. In addition to being responsible for all of the grocery shopping and meal preparation, Mary frequently has interrupted sleep, as she worries about her responsibilities at both home and school. This encounter incorporates all three dimensions of the nursing system: In addition to assessment strategies used to diagnose flu, the nurse uses interview techniques and looks for alternative methods for helping Mary deal with her complex issue.

There are both personal and institutional person-centered care features. Unless the institution within which care is being given maintains a system that promotes individual person-centered care, it will be difficult to maintain that value. This issue is further considered when the organization and delivery of care to groups is discussed. The U.S. Centers for Medicare and Medicaid (CMS) is promoting patient-centered medical homes (PCMH) "as a way to improve care. The concept of PCMH combines the tenets of primary care (first contact, comprehensive, and coordinated care) with systematic improvement of the health of the practice's patient population (via use of electronic information systems, disease management, continuous quality improvement, and so on)" (Bao, Casalino, & Pincus, 2013; 2012, n.p.). Or "for professionals it involves less doing for and more doing with" (Warren, 2012, p. 233). The ways of thinking and doing nursing presented in this book are patient centered and encourage a consideration of cultural differences. The development of cultural competency and/or sensitivity is left up to the individual nurse.

CONCLUSION

Never doubt that a small group of thoughtful, committed citizens can change the world. Indeed, it is the only thing that ever has.

—Margaret Mead

So what does this all mean to you as you transition to professional nursing roles? First, it would suggest that you cultivate or develop ways of thinking that are patient centered within a specific nursing focus. From the perspective of change and evolution, these may be countercultural to the existing emphases in health care. The discussion of how nursing evolved lends credence to Mead's statement. There are areas of knowledge that contribute to nursing knowledge and to our understanding of the multiple roles and responsibilities that come with being a nurse. Part II of this book presents you with ways of using a conceptual model of nursing.

LEARNING ACTIVITIES

1. You are the nurse caring for Mr. Jones, who lives in a small town in a rural part of the Midwestern United States with his wife and three children. His elderly parents live nearby, and he has two brothers and one sister who also live in the same town with their families. He is a member of the Lutheran Church and of the local Kiwanis club. Identify the systems, subsystems, and meta systems or mega systems included in this scenario.

2. Describe the steps that would be necessary to develop a teaching plan for a 47-year-old Hispanic woman who has recently been diagnosed with type 2 diabetes. What other methods of helping would be appropriate to incorporate into her overall plan of care?

3. Consider the questions related to disclosure in this chapter and respond to each of them: Under what circumstances do patients share all of the information related to the health situation that is of concern? Under what circumstances do you think they might withhold information? What kind of information might they withhold? Why? What characteristics of nurse, patient, and/or nurse–patient relationship may influence sharing and/or withholding information? (For an overview of the concept of disclosure, see Saiki & Lobo, 2011.)

4. Answer the following questions about caring: What are the characteristics of expert nursing practice that are important to the caring process? How specifically does a nurse develop a trusting relationship with a patient or a client? What characterizes interpersonal sensitivity? How is caring expressed in close interpersonal relationships that nurses may have with patients? How is caring expressed in relationships with family members of patients? What are the antecedents to caring in reference to patients? Nurse? Environment?

References

Ackoff, R. L. (1981). *Creating the corporate future: Plan or be planned for.* New York, NY: Wiley.

Bao, Y., Casalino, L. P., & Pincus, H. A. (2013; 2012). Behavioral health and health care reform models: Patient-centered medical home, health home, and accountable care organization. *Journal of Behavioral Health Services & Research, 40*(1), 121–132. doi:10.1007/s11414-012-9306-y

Botla, L. (2009). Systems thinking: The Gandhian way. *Journal of Human Values, 15*(1), 77–90. doi:10.1177/097168580901500106

Cabrera, D., Colosi, L., & Lobdell, C. (2008). Systems thinking. *Evaluation and Program Planning, 31*(3), 299–310. doi:10.1016/j.evalprogplan.2007.12.001

D'Antonio, P., Beeber, L., Sills, G., & Naegle, M. (2014). The future in the past: Hildegard Peplau and interpersonal relations in nursing. *Nursing Inquiry, 21*(4), 311–317. doi:10.1111/nin.12056

Konkarikoski, K., Ritala, R., & Ihalainen, H. (2010). Practical systems thinking. *Journal of Physics: Conference Series, 238*(1), 012007. doi:10.1088/1742-6596/238/1/012007

Lazenby, M. (2013). On the humanities of nursing. *Nursing Outlook, 61*(1), e9–e14. doi:10.1016/j.outlook.2012.06.018

Mead, M. (n. d.). Retrieved from www.brainyquote.com/quotes/quotes/m/margaretme 101283.html

Nursing Theory. (2015). Retrieved from http://nursing-theory.org/nursing-theorists/Madeline-Leininger.php

Orem, D. E. (2001). *Nursing: Concepts of practice* (6th ed.). St. Louis, MO: Mosby.

Peplau, H. E. (1952). *Interpersonal relations in nursing*. New York, NY: G. P. Putman. [Reprinted 1991]. New York, NY: Springer.

Pickens, J. M. (2003). Formal and informal social networks of women with serious mental illness. *Issues in Mental Health Nursing, 24*(2), 109–127. doi:10.1080/016128 40305296

Saiki, L. S., & Lobo, M. L. (2011). Disclosure: A concept analysis. *Journal of Advanced Nursing, 67*(12), 2713–2722. doi:10.1111/j.1365-2648.2011.05741.x

Senge, P. M. (2006). *The fifth discipline: The art and practice of the learning organization* (Rev. and updated.). New York, NY: Doubleday/Currency.

Silver, G., Keefer, J. M., & Rosenfeld, P. (2011). Assisting patients to age in place: An innovative pilot program utilizing the patient centered care model (PCCM) in home care. *Home Health Care Management & Practice, 23*(6), 446–453. doi:10.1177/1084822311411657

Tucker, C. M., Marsiske, M., Rice, K. G., Nielson, J. J., & Herman, K. (2011). Patient-centered culturally sensitive health care: Model testing and refinement. *Health Psychology, 30*(3), 342–350. doi:10.1037/a0022967

Warren, N. (2012). Involving patient and family advisors in the patient and family-centered care model. *Medsurg Nursing, 21*(4), 233–239.

Watson Caring Science Institute. (2015). Ten Caritas™ processes. Retrieved from http://watsoncaringscience.org/about-us/caring-science-definitions-processes-theory/global-translations-10-caritas-processes/

PART II
THE PRACTICE OF NURSING

In Part I, the object of nursing was identified as the inability of a person to maintain life and health and to promote development. In order to make use of this as the basis for providing nursing care, the elements of a self-care system are examined.

Nursing is produced through a series of complex thinking and actions to which we refer as *practice operations*—a term that is more reflective of nursing activity than the nursing process. A practice operation is a mental process or one of a practical nature that is necessary in some form of work or production. The practice operations associated with nursing that will be explored in the section include:

- Diagnosis and prescription
- Design and planning
- Production and control

The elements of an individual's health-related self-care system provide the subject matter for nursing. Health-related self-care involves engaging in purposeful activities that are associated with maintaining life, health, continuing personal development, and well-being. Self-care is viewed as a complex adaptive system of actions. In looking at the system of self-care, the essential components are as follows: What is to be done and why? What are my abilities to meet these requirements? What actions will I choose to take care of myself? What is it about me and my environment that leads me to the decision to act or to carry out the actions?

We can look at the answers to these questions in a common-sense way. Mrs. Smith would ask herself: "Given my current state of knowledge and my action capabilities, I know that I cannot get exercise by running or walking. Therefore, I will do chair exercises as my therapist showed me." But to evaluate that decision from a nursing perspective, it is helpful to have and use a more structured, scientific approach. The development of nursing sciences correlative with a self-care focus is based within a conceptual model as shown in Figure 1.2. As the questions become more complex, using an established structure is helpful (Figure II.1).

FIGURE II.1 A Schematic Representation of the Elements of Concern in Nursing Practice

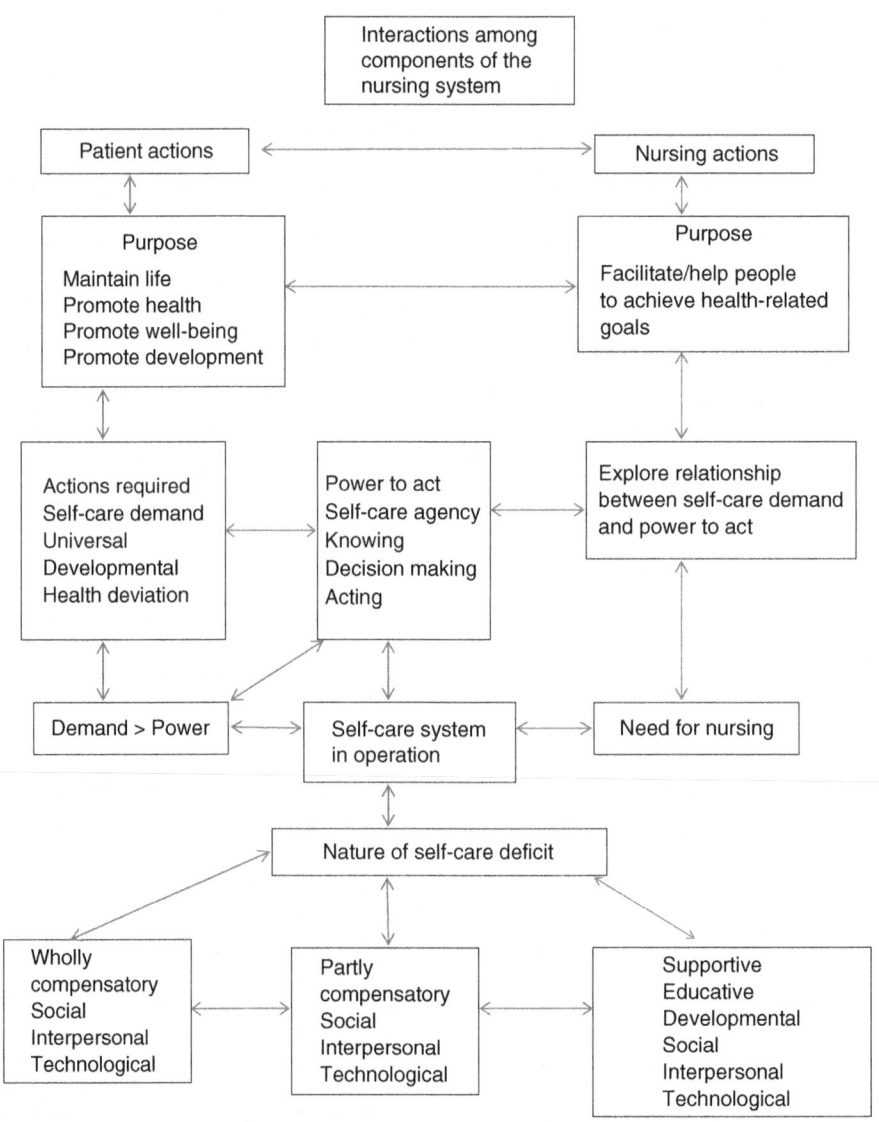

The need for self-care, referred to as *self-care requisites,* provides the structure for examining what the person needs to do or have done to maintain health, develop as a person, and recover from illness or injury. As individual requirements or demands are identified, we begin to see connections and relationships between and among them. We begin to see what factors in the environment condition these requisites. Mrs. Smith has a requisite to maintain an adequate intake of food. What does that mean to an elderly woman recovering from surgery after a fall? What should be the distribution of nutritional elements, such as protein, calcium, vitamins, fiber, and so on? Information to answer those questions can be found in a number of sciences. Some of this can be found in already established standards.

From there we can examine the person's agency to care for self in regard to taking action to meet these requisites. The specific elements that form the structure and content of a self-care approach to nursing provide the analytic lens for designing and providing nursing care. Structuring of this model began in the 1950s with work done by Orem (Renpenning & Taylor, 2003). Continuing development has been done by many nursing scholars, clinicians, and researchers worldwide who find it a helpful way to view practice and to conduct research in nursing. Figure II.I is a schematic representation of the elements of concern in nursing practice.

Reference

Renpenning, K. M., & Taylor, S. G. (Eds.). (2003). *Self-care theory in nursing: Selected Papers of Dorothea Orem.* New York, NY: Springer Publishing Company.

CHAPTER 5

CONDITIONING FACTORS AND HEALTH-RELATED SELF-CARE

This chapter begins the discussion linking the science of self-care, nursing sciences, and nursing practice through the theory of self-care. To this point, self-care was discussed as a general idea. In order to use these concepts for a patient, they need to be made specific to the individual person in a particular point in time who is affected by specific circumstances. How an 80-year-old Caucasian woman takes care of herself is obviously different from the way a 21-year-old African American man takes care of himself. How do we explain or describe these differences in a meaningful way? In this chapter, the focus is on the factors that condition or influence the requirements for self-care. These conditioning factors represent a point of articulation of nursing sciences with other sciences that inform health-related situations. They are also associated with the social determinants of health described in Chapter 2. The individual has very little control over the social determinants that exert a predominant influence over the choices available to people as they lead their everyday lives. The role of nursing is to help people make wise choices, understand options available, help them develop related skills to act, and/ or provide assistance when they are unable to act on their own behalf.

OBJECTIVES

After reading this chapter, the learner will be able to:

1. Identify factors that condition the action component of the self-care system
2. Provide some examples of the relationship between conditioning factors and self-care system actions

KEY CONCEPTS   basic conditioning factors • personal sociocultural factors • family system factors • health care and health care system factors • resources • conditions and patterns of living • development and developmental care system factors • health state and health care system factors

BASIC CONDITIONING FACTORS

Courses of action to accomplish the required self-care are many and varied. The courses of actions required, the courses available, and the courses chosen by an individual are influenced by the conditioning factors that are present at a particular time and in a particular place. These factors have been collectively named *basic conditioning factors* (BCF). A diagram illustrating these factors and their interrelationships is presented in Figure 5.1.

Nurses access the body of nursing knowledge and knowledge from related disciplines to facilitate an understanding of the influence of these factors on self-care. In the following discussion, the kind of data pertinent to each conditioning factor is presented. Since time, place, circumstances, and influence of other conditioning factors are of varying importance in each patient situation, the degree to which specific conditioning factors are of influence will vary. Consequently, it may not be necessary or expedient to collect detailed information for each conditioning factor. Rather, in the process of interacting with the patient, the specific conditioning factors that are currently influencing the situation should be addressed and their relationship to other components of the self-care system can then be established. As a nurse with a developing body of knowledge about specific populations of interest, it is possible and preferred to establish models that elicit the essential information. A cautionary note as we move from the data-gathering process to using

FIGURE 5.1   Basic Conditioning Factors

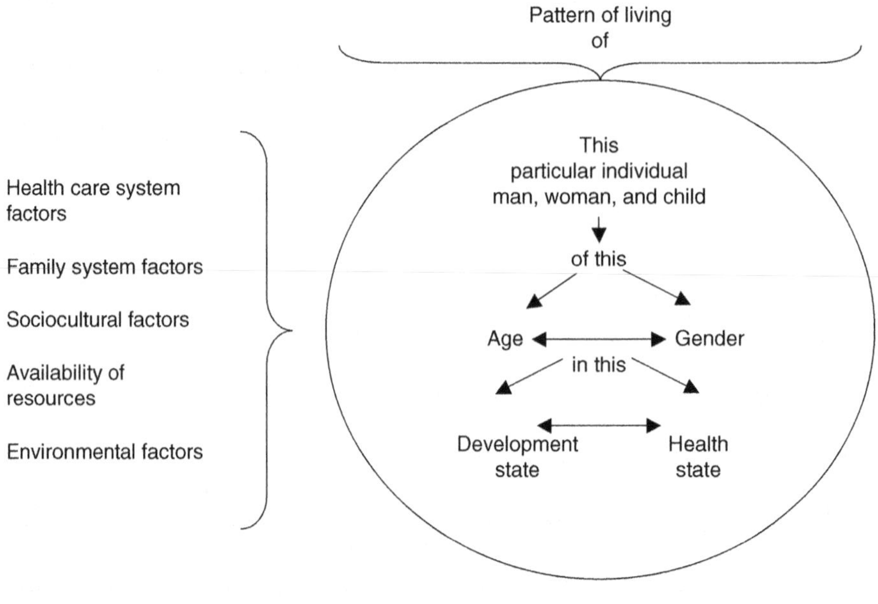

that information with our patients: Be wary of assumptions and personal biases; as you proceed, take time to validate your conclusions.

Gender

While reading research studies and analyzing information in relation to the best practices, it is important to note the gender of the population being studied, as gender differences have been demonstrated in the expression of disease conditions and in medication effectiveness. The traditional gender-related research addressed two genders: male and female. Little research has been done with populations representing other definitions of *gender*. An example of findings from gender-related research shows, for example, that women may have some different signs when having a heart attack than do men.

In reference to Mrs. Smith, some health conditions are more predominant in one gender. Postmenopausal women are likely to have osteopenia or osteoporosis. X-rays revealed that Mrs. Smith had osteoporosis, a factor conditioning her demands for prevention of hazards and probably was a problem in her current health situation.

More recent studies suggest that gender be viewed more broadly to consider, for example, individuals who are transgendered. In studies developed from an intersectionality perspective, it is suggested that the influence of gender be considered even more broadly, not as a fixed category but rather as changeable and contingent in nature (Hankivsky, 2012).

Health State and Health Care System Factors

HEALTH STATE

Health state factors include the person's description of why he or she is seeking assistance; the medical diagnosis, if there is one; the perception of another (family or friend) as to why the person requires nursing assistance; the reason for referral to nursing; and so on. The diagnostic activities, findings, and treatment plans of the various members of the health team (including findings of a physical assessment) should be considered. Most importantly, the nurse should try to begin to understand what all of this means from the perspective of the self-care system of the patient and his or her family, if applicable. What are the pertinent components of the current self-care system? What changes may be required in self-care practices? What new knowledge, skills, and abilities may be required? Is there evidence of motivation to change, if required? What factors appear to impede implementing suggested changes? Again considering Mrs. Smith: *What is Mrs. Smith's state of health? At this time, her health state is that of a person with a fractured hip and with osteoporosis. While in the hospital awaiting surgery, she receives analgesia and is on bedrest until the surgery can be performed. Her son is with her, and all understand her need for nursing to meet her self-care. She is beginning to understand that she will need assistance not just during the hospitalization but also in the rehabilitation phase of recovery. A significant percentage of individuals who sustain a hip fracture have increased mortality for up to one year. Often, the individuals who survive hip fracture do not return to their pre-fracture functional status or living arrangements.*

PATIENT PERCEPTION OF HOW HEALTH STATE IS AFFECTING SELF-CARE PRACTICES

Important questions to be explored about patient perception of health state and how self-care practices are affected are addressed in Box 5.1.

OTHER HEALTH CARE WORKERS AND AGENCIES INVOLVED

It is important for nurses to know about the diagnoses and treatment plans of other health care workers as they consider the efficacy of the self-care practices. This information should be considered in the assessment process and in developing the plan of care. It may affect the way in which self-care requisites are met, helps determine capabilities and dispositions that the patient requires in a particular situation, and influences the nurse's action. It is essential information that influences both patient action and nurse action. The more health care providers are involved in a patient situation, the more knowledge and skill the person requires to sort out conflicting information regarding health care management. What is the role of nursing in clarifying health care information? *In the initial stage of treatment for Mrs. Smith, the surgeon's plan of action is dominant and nursing judgments are made to meet Mrs. Smith's demands within that framework. In the rehabilitation phase, the physiotherapist will be important. After surgery, she will spend probably three days in the acute-care setting, after which she will be discharged to either home or a rehabilitation facility.*

PAST HEALTH STATE, INCLUDING EXPERIENCES WITH THE HEALTH CARE SYSTEM

Experience is a great teacher! The experiences that a person has had with the health care system may have been either positive or negative and may strongly influence his or her perception of the current situation. Perceptions and feelings about past and current experiences should be explored.

Research related to adherence with medication regimes, diet, and other instructions has shown that the patient often does not follow the directions of health

---

BOX 5.1   Patient Perception of How Health State Affects Self-Care Practices

- What are your major concerns? How are you managing?
- What things do you have to do differently?
- What do you know you should do but choose not to do?
- Are you able to manage to do all the things you need to do in your daily schedule?
- What kind of help do you need?
- Who is available to help you and who helps?
- How does having the particular health issue, including treatment, affect your overall view of both life and self?

care providers. Decision-making and information-processing theories have been incorporated into studies in attempts to understand the reasons for nonadherence. From the perspective of the theory of self-care, lack of adherence to a prescribed course of action may be related to any one of the components associated with the power to produce self-care, which is the topic of Chapter 7. *Mrs. Smith's prior experiences within the health care system are limited. She was hospitalized for the birth of her child but has had no acute illness. She has experienced the usual seasonal illnesses. As the nurse–patient relationship develops, more information about many of the BCF can be acquired through interaction with her or perhaps with her son.*

HEALTH CARE SYSTEM

The health care system includes all aspects of the provision of health care from providers to bureaucrats who manage the system, insurers, pharmaceutical companies, medical device manufacturers, and so on. In some places, the system is organized at a national level, as it is in Germany and Great Britain; or, as in Canada, where it is funded at the national level, and policies are primarily established at the provincial level, whereas services are provided through a combination of private and public facilities at the local level. In other places, such as the United States, the system is not organized and is a combination of private and public facilities or services. In the developed world today, we take for granted that some health care services are available. There is also a belief that some degree of health care is a human right. Little thought is given to the nature of these services and of how one accesses them unless they become a political issue, or one requires them and then encounters difficulties in obtaining services or becomes concerned with the quality of service. Some questions to consider in relation to the health care system include the following: Is access to health care services a right in society, as is education, or is it the responsibility of the individual? How does the answer to this question impact the health of the individual? How does location of services influence access? How does access to transportation influence utilization of services?

In an integrative review of issues related to accessing health services by chronically ill Canadians, Spenceley (2005) found the construct of symmetry (like to like—person requiring health care in relation to provider) to be useful in making sense of the data. Factors that promoted symmetry, such as common cultural background of patient and provider, facilitated access. Asymmetry in power, status, and knowledge (attributes of the provider) resulted in the patient experiencing feelings such as fear, uncertainty, lack of confidence, and perception that his or her knowledge was neither relevant nor valued. In some instances, although the power of the physician was acknowledged as reassuring, services of other providers were not as credible. Prior negative experiences with insensitive or judgmental providers produced feelings of mistrust, shame, and embarrassment in the patient. Such experiences caused people to avoid services. Gender or sexual identity, generational similarity or difference were factors that served to either facilitate or interfere with symmetry in the relationship. Providing medical information in an understandable form was a facilitator. Barriers to access had origins in asymmetry between identity and beliefs and between provider and patient, including marginalized groups and strongly held cultural beliefs about health and disease. Cultural views held by Asian and Aboriginal populations frequently resulted in patients relying on traditional healing methods. Other factors affecting access and utilization of services included transportation; hours of availability; flexibility of scheduling; choice of service options; culturally appropriate services, including interpreters; and explanations regarding preparation and procedures. The procedural requirements of the system may also act as barriers to access, such as the requirement for referrals, insurance limitations, and lack of communication between various providers.

How the health care system will condition Mrs. Smith's demands and how access to services to help her meet those demands vary greatly by the political/social/cultural system within which she resides. If she lives in the United States, she would be eligible for Medicare and with a supplemental insurance policy, most, if not all, of her hospital costs could be met. The benefits available to her are dependent on the specific insurance program in which she is enrolled. Within the Canadian system, Mrs. Smith would have fewer concerns as to follow-up care and payment. In both systems, a social service person would most likely be the one to make the arrangements for follow-up care. The nurse would want to be involved, as some of the decisions as to type of care or specifics of care relate to the nursing care needed.

Conditions and Patterns of Living

The environment, conditions of living, and everyday patterns and activities influence the choices available to people and the choices they will make in relation to self-care activities. It is important to explore with regard to the person how the conditions and patterns of living interfere with or facilitate self-care.

For example, how does the homeless person you have seen sleeping on a park bench manage personal hygiene, access drinking water, and stay warm and dry? Environmental factors are concerned with the surroundings where the person works and/or lives. Is the location itself hazardous? Is there clean air, adequate sanitation, and clean water supply? Are environmental changes possible? If not, what adjustments can be made in the self-care system?

Environmental factors conditioning Mrs. Smith's demand at this time are a function of being in the hospital and her health state. She is not able nor allowed to manipulate her environment. Her home is in an urban area, with bedrooms on the second floor. The entry has three steps and no hand rail.

CONDITIONS OF LIVING

The purpose of collecting data about the conditions of living is to determine how they influence or interfere with the actions that a person must take to care for himself or herself or his or her capability to do so. In an extreme example, Allison and Renpenning (1999) describe the exploration of health-related issues in a low income community with many transient people. One of their findings was that many individuals were constantly on the move, thus living in one place for less than a month. The accommodation they did have was primarily in temporary shelters or in run-down repurposed hotel rooms, most of which had shared bathrooms in a central location. If people have no access to a kitchen, how do they meet their nutritional needs? If they live in temporary shelters, how do they maintain a balance between rest and activity? Do people choose to live on the streets rather than in temporary shelters with many other residents so they can have some privacy? Areas to be explored regarding conditions of living are included in Box 5.2.

BOX 5.2   Questions Related to Conditions of Living

- With whom does the patient live?
- Could that individual or those individuals assist with components of the self-care requirements?
- Is the residence adequate?
- Do accommodations need to be made to facilitate the required self-care?
- Are the available resources adequate (time, money, social support, access to transportation, etc.)?

PATTERNS OF DAILY LIVING

Daily activities, other activities in which the person regularly takes part, and the responsibilities the person has will influence how he or she feels about the situation and the actions he or she will be willing to take. Are there variations in lifestyle that may be considered different from the norms in society? If so, how do these affect the actions a person takes or will be willing to take in health-related matters? The influence of lifestyle on capability to act also needs to be identified and considered in developing the plan of action. For example, if a person follows a strict vegetarian diet, this will influence the choices he or she makes, which may or may not be consistent with nutritional requirements. *Mrs. Smith leads a comfortable life. She has a pension, social security, and some investments that are for her retirement. Her monthly resources are adequate to meet her needs with some left to add to savings. She is trying to establish good health practices, although her usual pattern of eating included fast food or frozen prepared meals. She does not drink alcohol or smoke.*

Family System Factors

Self-care is learned within the family. The capacity of the person to act and the self-care actions usually performed are closely linked to experiences within the family and other family influences, including the family value system. It is important for the nurse to identify ways in which family system factors may influence or interfere with the actions that patients should or would be willing to take and also influence their capabilities to act. The role of nursing in relation to family will be explored in more detail in subsequent chapters. In this chapter, the family is considered as conditioning the development and exercise of the self-care system.

CHARACTERISTICS OF FAMILY MEMBERSHIP

How does the patient describe his or her family, including family membership? Development of a genogram, a diagram of family membership and relationships, is a useful way of describing the composition of a family. *Mrs. Smith views herself and her son as her family. She has no other close relatives. Both her father and mother died of heart disease at the age of 70 and 75, respectively.*

BOX 5.3 Assessment of Problem-Solving Skills of the Family

How do family members:

- Identify problems?
- Identify sources of problems?
- Communicate the nature of problems to appropriate people?
- Identify and select alternative courses of action, and act on selected courses of action?

PERCEPTION OF FAMILY MEMBERS REGARDING THE PATIENT'S HEALTH STATE AND GENERAL PATTERN OF FUNCTIONING

Altered health state of any member of the family will affect the family system and how that system functions. Therefore, it is important to explore the understanding and belief systems of family members in relation to the patient's health state and the changes that the family thinks should be made. The changes that the family is willing or not willing to make are of concern in designing the nursing system. How do family members perceive that the patient's health state is affecting family functioning? Has it been or will it be necessary to alter who does what in the family? Are outside resources being utilized or should they be? If outside resources are being utilized, are there problems in incorporating these resources into family functioning? What changes in self-care practices of family members are or may be required to accommodate the changes in the patient's health state?

PROBLEM-SOLVING SKILLS OF THE FAMILY

The problem-solving skills of family members and how the family members individually and collectively habitually solve problems affect the self-care systems of all family members. It is important to explore the extent and characteristic ways in which family members identify and approach problem solving. Important considerations related to problem-solving skills of the family are addressed in Box 5.3.

Mrs. Smith's son, John, who helps her at home, has had little personal experience with illness or injury. He works as an information system technician and has good problem-solving ability related to his work.

INTERPERSONAL AND TASK FUNCTIONING OF THE FAMILY

Effective families act as a unit to accomplish certain family functions that are associated with self-care—feeding, sheltering, socializing, teaching, promoting development, and so on. Accomplishment of these tasks requires that members of the family accept responsibility to execute these tasks and have certain capabilities to do so. Acting as a unit requires skills in communications, perception of other members as people, empathy, and understanding that all family members require the help of others. Areas of exploration regarding interpersonal skills and task functioning of the family are included in Box 5.4.

BOX 5.4 Assessment of Family Interpersonal Skills and Task Functioning

To what extent can family members:

- Convey clear and direct messages between members?
- Describe how members are feeling about the situation?
- Anticipate and recognize needs of members?
- Meet self-care demands of dependent members?
- Mobilize resources and provide comfort when members are distressed?
- Respect individuality and independence of family members?
- Attend to family management tasks?

Content related to dependent and family care is addressed in more detail in Chapters 10 and 11.

Personal–Sociocultural Factors

Self-care behaviors are learned, and self-care capabilities are developed within a sociocultural context. The nurse collects data that assist in understanding the person's behavior, actions he or she may be motivated or not motivated to take, and potential for developing self-care capabilities from this frame of reference.

SOCIAL, CULTURAL, AND RELIGIOUS NORMS AND PRACTICES

Social, cultural, and religious norms and practices may have a strong influence on self-care practices and the development, operability, and adequacy of self-care capabilities. If a patient is a member of a distinctive social, cultural, or religious group, are his or her beliefs and practices closely aligned with those of that group?

Listed in Box 5.5 are some questions that might be helpful in determining cultural factors that may be influencing the person's perception and understanding of his or her current health state.

Additional questions that may be explored include:

- Is this condition good or bad?
- What have you been doing for this problem/condition in the past?
- What are you presently doing and what do you plan to do in the future to manage the situation?
- How should a person who has this condition act? How should one who has this condition/problem be treated by family members?

LANGUAGES SPOKEN AND UNDERSTOOD

If English is not the first language of the patient and of his or her family members, it is important to identify that even though people speak English there may be a

> **BOX 5.5   Assessment of Cultural Factors That May Influence Perception/Understanding of Health State**
>
> - What do you think has caused your problem?
> - Why do you think it started when it did?
> - What does your sickness do to you? How does it work?
> - How severe is your sickness? How long do you think it will last?
> - What kind of treatment do you think you should receive?
> - What are the most important results you hope to get from this treatment?
> - What are the chief problems your sickness has caused you?
> - What do you fear about your sickness?
>
> Adapted from Tripp-Reimer, Brink, and Saunders (1994).

difference of interpretation of information exchanged between patients, family members, and health care providers. This difference may be related to understanding the language or to cultural differences. Do the people involved have a language/vocabulary to accurately describe symptoms and health concerns? Is the nurse asking questions and interpreting answers from the cultural perspective of the patient? A patient was admitted to an emergency service in an inner-city hospital saying, "I ain't seen nothin' for three months." An ophthalmology resident was called to see the patient. In discussion with her, he discovered he was the wrong specialist in the case. She was pregnant and was referring to her menstrual periods, not her eyesight (personal communication, 2010).

Educational System Factors

Educational factors influence the development of abilities to care for self. These include previous education, attitudes toward education, and success and failure with mastering written material, learning styles, and so on. Does the person regularly access the Internet and does he or she question the reliability of information gained? What other sources does the person rely on for health-related information—friends, family members, magazines, local health store personnel?

Mrs. Smith is a high school graduate. She learned her skills on the job. She is an avid reader.

Resources

Resources available include monetary, personal, and societal resources. The adequacy of financial resources, the availability of family and community resources, and the willingness of the patient to enlist the aid of a support system may be important information for the nurse to have. When looking at resources, it is important to also look at the availability of sufficient time to accomplish self-care.

Since she retired, time is not an issue. Mrs. Smith was considering finding part-time or seasonal work to supplement her retirement funds. This plan will likely be altered due to her current health condition.

Developmental State and Developmental System Factors

Age is important and so is developmental state, which may or may not be appropriate to the stated age. The patient's view of the future may have significance. Also, developmental state may influence choices and capabilities to manage patterns and conditions of living, social conditions, and health state.

Developmental factors that may facilitate or interfere with self-management are included in Box 5.6.

Mrs. Smith's self-care demands and capabilities are conditioned first and foremost by her health state and health system factors. Her mobility and comfort are conditioned by her injury and medication received to relieve her pain. Her son's presence could have a positive or negative effect on her depending on their relationship and his ability to control his responses to her injury. If he is unable to control his response to her injury and impending surgery, Mrs. Smith may be directing her energy and attention to solacing him rather than working on understanding and accepting her own health situation. At this time, he is feeling anger and helplessness.

BOX 5.6 Developmental Factors That May Influence Self-Management

Cognitive Development

- Attention span, reasoning, learning capability, perception, memory, decision-making capability, language development

Physical Development Appropriate for Age

- Motor abilities, gross and fine movement, coordination

Psychosocial Development

- Emotional, self-concept, socialization, play/vocational, moral, religious, sexuality, relationship with family/significant other

---

LEARNING ACTIVITY

Read the following articles and consider the relationships between BCF and self-care practices illustrated in each.

Arvidsson, S., Bergman, S., Arvidsson, B., Fridlund, B., & Tops, A. B. (2011). Experiences of health-promoting self-care in people living with rheumatic diseases. *Journal of Advanced Nursing 67*(6), 1264–1272. doi:10.1111/j.1365-2648 .2010.05585.x

(*continued*)

LEARNING ACTIVITY (*continued*)

Collins, P. (1989). Learning from the outside within: The sociological signifi-cance of Black feminist thought. *Social Problems, 33*(6), S14–S32.

Davidson, P. M., Daly, J., Leung, D., Ang, E., Paull, G., DiGiacomo, M., & Thompson, D. R. (2011). Health-seeking beliefs of cardiovascular patients: A qualitative study. *International Journal of Nursing Studies, 48*(11), 1367–1375. doi:10.1016/j.ijnurstu.2011.02.021

Finnstrom, B., & Soderhamn, O. (2006). Conceptions of pain among Somali women. *Journal of Advanced Nursing, 54*(4), 418–425.

Pickens, J. M. (2003). Formal and informal social networks of women with seri-ous mental illness. *Issues in Mental Health Nursing, 24*(2), 109–127. doi:10.1080/01612840305296

Tomstad, S. T., Söderhamn, U., Espnes, G. A., & Söderhamn, O. (2012). Living alone, receiving help, helplessness, and inactivity are strongly related to risk of undernutrition among older home-dwelling people. *International Journal of General Medicine, 5*, 231–240.

References

Allison, S., & Renpenning, K. (1999). *Nursing administration in the 21st century: A self-care theory approach.* Thousand Oaks, CA: Sage Publications.

Hankivsky, O. (2012). Women's health, men's heath, and gender and health: Implications of intersectionality. *Social Science and Medicine, 74*, 1712–1720. doi:10.1016/j.soc med.2011.11.029

Spenceley, S. M. (2005). Access to health services by Canadians who are chronically ill. *Western Journal of Nursing Research, 27*, 465–486. doi:10.1177/019394590427238411

Tripp-Reimer, T., Brink, P., & Saunders, J. (1994). Cultural assessment: Content and process. *Nursing Outlook, 42*(2), 76–82.

CHAPTER 6

THE "WHY" OF SELF-CARE

Determining the Self-Care Demand

As a nurse, the basic content presented in this chapter will be familiar to you. The difference is how content is organized and how it is used to answer nursing questions when the focus of nursing is on determining the adequacy of the self-care system. Self-care is carried out through a series of actions. An action system has purpose and structure. The purposes are there, because we are human—eating, drinking, loving—and the actions we need to take vary with our current health state. In this chapter, a structure that recognizes all those things that we have to do is identified. This structured list is then used to collect and organize patient information. Once we know the details of the patient information, we can draw on our knowledge of physiology, anatomy, pathology, and human behavior to determine the actions required to achieve more than treating the immediate medical problem; this will also help the patient develop the knowledge and skills required to look after himself or herself in the long term. Construction of this action system requires that the nurse address the interpersonal, sociocultural, and technological factors that are at play in the situation. This requires employing a systems perspective in the collection and analysis of the data. The structure that is outlined presents an articulation point between nursing knowledge and knowledge developed in related disciplines, thus helping to answer nursing questions.

OBJECTIVES

After reading this chapter, the learner will be able to:

1. Utilize the framework of self-care requisites to collect and organize patient data
2. Identify which conditioning factors are of concern in particular situations

3. Identify the self-care requisites that are the most likely affected by the conditioning factors present

4. Illustrate what is meant by conditioning effect of the self-care requisites

5. Determine the purposes for action in relation to self-care requisites of concern in a particular situation

6. Construct an appropriate action system to meet the requirements for self-care in a particular situation

KEY CONCEPTS   self-care as action • universal self-care requisites • developmental self-care • health deviation self-care • therapeutic self-care demand

THE SELF-CARE DEMAND

The requirement for self-care is a characteristic of being human. It is the way in which health is maintained. This requirement or demand is made up of a collection of purposes and actions related to maintaining life. The term *demand* is used to emphasize the fact that it is imperative that these purposes be attended to. These purposes and associated actions have been named *self-care requisites*. You may be familiar with the expression "meeting basic human needs." The self-care requisite associated with meeting the need for air is stated as "maintain a sufficient intake of air." This statement provides direction for action. First, the question that must be answered is: What is sufficient for this person at this point in time? "Sufficient" is different for a sedentary person as opposed to a person running a marathon. The second question to be answered relates to the method of intake. Is there an unobstructed airway, a supply of oxygenated air that is free of pollutants? Just as the concept of a tabletop does not produce a picture of a table in your mind, so the concept of need by itself does not fully represent the purpose to be achieved or the associated action system, and thus does not provide direction for action.

From the analysis of nursing cases, nursing scholars (Allison, 2007; Denyes, Orem, & Bekel, 2001; Nursing Development Conference Group, 1979; Orem, 2001) have identified a structure and processes that are useful to nursing in determining the kind and quality of self-care required in particular situations. Three general categories of purposes to be achieved in relation to self-care are identified. These are universal requisites, which apply to all people across the life span; developmental requisites, which are related to growth and development across the life span; and health deviation requisites, which are associated with variations in health state. These requisites are summarized in Table 6.1.

These general statements are not specific enough to provide direction for practice. They have to be made more specific to the individual situation to be useful. This is accomplished by exploring the relationship between conditioning factors and individual requisites. This makes it possible to prescribe, in concert with the patient, a suitable course of action. For example, if a person wishes to lose weight, the requisite "Maintain a sufficient intake of food" may be expressed more specifically for a woman as the ability to "maintain a daily caloric intake of no more than 1,200 calories." The general requisite is stated in relation to a particular individual

TABLE 6.1   Self-Care Requisites

Universal Self-Care Requisites	Developmental Self-Care Requisites	Health Deviation Self-Care Requisites
Maintenance of sufficient intakes of air, water, and food	Provision of conditions that promote development	Seek and secure appropriate medical assistance.
Provision of care associated with elimination	Provision of conditions that facilitate engagement in self-development	Be aware of and attend to effects of pathological conditions, including effects on development.
Maintenance of a balance between activity and rest	Provision of conditions and promotion of behaviors to prevent occurrences of conditions that interfere with development	Effectively carry out prescribed diagnostic, therapeutic, and rehabilitative measures.
Maintenance of a balance between solitude and social interaction	Provision of conditions and experiences to lessen or overcome existent harmful effects on development	Be aware of and attend to discomfort or harmful effects associated with prescribed care measures, including effects on development.
Prevention of hazards to life, functioning, and well-being		Modify self-concept, thus accepting oneself as being in a particular health state and requiring health care.
Promotion of normalcy		Learn to live with effects of pathological conditions and effects of diagnostic and treatment measures, while adjusting lifestyle to promote continued personal development.

Adapted from Orem (2001).

or situation. The action system related to this particularized requisite would include following a designated meal plan, preparing specific food, and so forth. In the case of a person with type 2 diabetes, maintaining a sufficient intake of food may be made more specific by stating it as "maintain a daily intake of a 1,500 calorie diet composed of 'x,y,z' to keep the hemoglobin A1C within a specified range." The action system would then be developed to meet the demands of that specific person.

Universal Self-Care Requisites

Eight universal self-care requisites are proposed. These apply to all people over the life span and are stated as purposes to be achieved through action.

MAINTAIN AN ADEQUATE INTAKE OF AIR

The purpose to be achieved in meeting this requisite is to "prevent interference with the natural process of breathing to ensure inspirations of air sufficient to maintain pulmonary ventilation with air that has a partial oxygen pressure consistent with air at sea level or below 12,000 feet" (Orem, 2001, p. 239). We know these parameters from the sciences of physiology, physics, and medicine. Again, remember that for most people, this requisite is met automatically through the process of respiration. But there are times when the person needs to pay attention to this. Taking specific action to meet this requisite would be significant for patients who have respiratory diseases such as chronic obstructive lung disease, asthma, and pneumonia. Problems related to the cardiovascular system and the neurological system may also affect the functioning of the respiratory system. Some conditioning factors associated with meeting or not meeting this requisite may include infections, structural abnormalities, obstructions, lack of oxygen-carrying capacity of the blood, hemorrhage, and even extreme stress. Environmental factors include decreased oxygen availability at higher elevations, poor air quality associated with dust and pollens, presence of noxious gases, and similar irritants and contaminants.

When considering whether this requisite is being met, the following evidence would be important:

- No signs of dyspnea at rest or with moderate exertion
- Rapid recovery of a normal respiratory rate after exertion
- Oximeter readings within normal limits
- Blood gas levels within normal range

Indicators that this requisite is not being met may include:

- Shortness of breath, rapid and/or irregular respirations, cyanosis
- Rapid pulse, blood oxygen levels of less than 90% saturation
- Fatigue on mild exertion
- Cyanosis

Some areas to consider as the data are collected include:

- What is sufficient for this person at this point in time under the current circumstances?
- Are physical structures that are associated with the respiratory system intact?
- Are the cardiovascular and respiratory systems and other involved body systems functioning normally? These data are obtained through a physical assessment, laboratory findings, reports of other disciplines, and other health state data.
- What hazards are present that might interfere with meeting each of these requisites? Is it possible for the individual to control or eliminate these hazards? Is community action required?

- Can normal functioning and development be promoted as these requisites are being met? For example, consider the implications of requiring oxygen continuously or periodically.

- What changes may a person have to make in self-care practices to meet this requisite?

Mrs. Smith's requisite for maintaining an adequate intake of air is conditioned by the fact that she is on bedrest and has received medications that may depress respiration. Monitoring shows that her respirations are normal and it is determined that the demand is being met.

MAINTAIN AN ADEQUATE INTAKE OF FOOD

Again, the question arises: What is adequate? Again, the answer lies in understanding what is to be regulated and the purpose to be achieved. Unlike breathing or respirations, this requisite must be attended to on a regular (daily) basis. The purpose of this requisite is to maintain a total intake of appropriate foods that are sufficient to supply the metabolic need of people, with consideration of their energy demands, environmental conditions, physiological state, age, and gender. Conditioning factors that are particularly significant in relation to meeting this requisite include:

- Health state with particular requirements for modification of diet

- Age

- Conditions of living

- Adequate resources for procuring food, including financial resources, access to transportation, food preparation area, and knowledge about appropriate foods

- Activity level

Some indicators that this requisite is being met would include:

- Body mass index within normal range

- A balanced diet

- Regular intake of food

Some indicators that this requisite is not being met would include:

- Being overweight or underweight as per recommended norms

- Lack of access to appropriate foods and/or food when needed or desired

- Lack of knowledge about what is appropriate food

- Lack of appropriate storage of facilities for foods

- Lack of appetite or lack of willingness to eat

Some conditioning factors affecting meeting this requisite include the following broad general interferences:

- Access to food, including resources, availability, storage facilities, and so on

- Structural or functional abnormalities in the digestive tract that interfere with digestive processes

- Inability to communicate needs, likes and dislikes, sensory deprivation, sensory overload, anxiety, confusion, and coma
- Self-concept that interferes with realistic assessment of requirement for food—bulimia, anorexia nervosa, acceptability of food available as influenced by culture, religion, familiarity, appearance, taste, odor, texture, and so on
- Perception of social acceptability during eating process

Questions to be asked of the data collected in reference to this requisite include:

1. What is sufficient for this person at this point in time under the current circumstances? The answer to this question is, in part, found by determining the height and weight ratio or body mass index, age, gender, requirements associated with particular health state and environmental conditions, and other conditioning.

2. Are the body systems involved functioning normally (e.g., in relation to digestion, elimination, cognitive reasoning, communication)? These data are again obtained through observation, questioning, physical assessment, laboratory findings, reports of other disciplines and family members, and data related to health state.

3. What hazards are present that might interfere with meeting this requisite (e.g., lack of adequate storage facilities; unsafe, inadequate, or inappropriate food supply)? Can these hazards be eliminated or controlled by the individual? By family action? By community action?

4. Can normal functioning and development be promoted during the course of meeting this requisite? For example, consider the implications of expecting a teenager to change a diet from one of potato chips, burgers, and sodas to a more balanced diet.

"Nutrition also includes cultural and social aspects, and meals are considered to symbolize care, friendship, love, security and concern" (Tomstad, Söderhamn, Espnes, & Söderhamn, 2012, p. 232). For people who have lost a partner, living, cooking, and eating may appear to have lost their meaning. This may account for older people living alone being at risk for undernutrition. Availability of some nutritional screening tools is reported in the literature.

Until her injury, Mrs. Smith's requirements for intake of food were adequate to meet her basic energy needs. Her diet was insufficient in factors affecting calcium intake and utilization as manifest by the osteoporosis. Her diet will now be supplemented with high energy protein preparations containing minerals and vitamins.

MAINTAIN AN ADEQUATE INTAKE OF WATER

An adequate intake of water is required to keep concentrations of water constant in the blood plasma, tissue, and intracellular fluids and in balance considering output.

Much research and development activity in the biomedical, pharmaceutical, and related fields has been devoted to understanding the impact of meeting or not meeting this requisite, as well as to developing technologies to meet it. The sciences of nutrition, exercise physiology, and sports medicine contribute to this area. There are also personal factors to consider when evaluating adequacy of intake.

Indicators of the state to which this requisite is being met include changes in body weight, physical evidence of dehydration, physical evidence of excess fluid intake or retention, disturbance in body chemistry detected through visual and chemical analysis of body fluids, and cognitive changes such as confusion and disorientation.

Mrs. Smith's fluid requirements are increased after the surgery. She was NPO (nothing by mouth) before the surgery. Until she is able to retain fluids postsurgery, intravenous (IV) fluids will be used to maintain intake and output. As soon as she is able to tolerate liquids, her intake will be switched to oral fluids.

Indicators that this requisite is not being met include:

- Physical signs of dehydration or overhydration (polydipsia)

- Cognitive signs of dehydration or overhydration such as confusion or disorientation

- Evidence of disturbance in acid–base balance or electrolytes

Processes involved in ensuring this requisite is met include:

- Ensuring the availability of a safe water supply

- Knowing and maintaining awareness of the quantity of the required intake

- Drinking appropriate fluids

- Determining the adequacy of the intake

- Limiting fluid intake if needed

PROVISION OF CARE ASSOCIATED WITH ELIMINATION

The body accomplishes elimination of wastes through the lungs, the skin, the urinary tract, and the digestive tract. The elimination processes are interactive with the products and processes that are associated with intake. They begin at the cellular level and end at the visible level where there may be evidence of external structures being affected by the elimination processes. In addition, the requisite is concerned with proper disposal of the waste products within the person's immediate environment.

Indicators that this requisite is being met would include:

- Normal color, odor, and consistency of excrements—urine, stool, sputum, perspiration

- Frequency of elimination of urine and stool being within normal limits

- Safe disposal of waste products

Questions to be asked of the data associated with this requisite include:

- Is the individual pattern of elimination within normal limits?

- Has there been a recent change in elimination patterns?

- What are the factors conditioning or affecting the situation?

Processes associated with meeting this requisite include:

- Acquiring knowledge about normal functioning and attaching meaning to signs of abnormalities associated with elimination processes

- Acquiring knowledge about adequate disposal of excrements and hazards associated with inadequate disposal

- Protection of physical structures associated with elimination to prevent obstructions that interfere with elimination functions

- Provision of equipment, facilities, and community services that ensure sanitary disposal of excrements

Until Mrs. Smith is mobile, her elimination is problematic. The use of indwelling catheters is not recommended. She will/should have an output of urine that is compatible with her intake. Her bladder needs to be emptied regularly to prevent retention or incontinence, both of which are hazardous. Once she receives solid food, she should have a bowel movement within 2 days.

MAINTAIN A BALANCE BETWEEN REST AND ACTIVITY

Although both rest and activity are essential for health, it is important that these occur within the total system of living. Too much of one or the other or both is not healthy. Allison (2007) further developed this requisite, identifying two subrequisites that provide more specific direction. She suggests that the purposes to be achieved include:

(a) To maintain a level of physical activity in accord with capabilities and the current standards established for health and well-being, and

(b) To obtain a sufficient amount of rest and relaxation to maintain the required and desired level of activity (p. 69).

In the following discussion, these two subrequisites are discussed as well as the balance maintained between activity and rest.

Activity

Activity has been identified as a contributing factor in improving health and well-being, specifically affecting weight management, blood pressure, bone density, decreased mortality from heart and other chronic diseases, and reduced risk of some cancers. Allison (2007) also suggests that the processes involved in engaging in the required amount of activity include:

- Knowing the quality and quantity of activity required for physical parameters (e.g., age, sex, weight, health state, physique, intensity of activity)

- Determining whether daily activities provide a sufficient amount of exercise

- Determining what additional activity is necessary if activities of daily living do not provide a sufficient amount of exercise

- Engaging in exercise and/or planned activity on a regular basis

Rest

Rest is essential so that human beings conserve and restore physical, mental, and emotional energy. The concept of rest not only embodies inactivity but may also involve activities that are engaged in to provide relief from stresses. However, rest may also have negative connotations, as has been demonstrated in studies that have described the effects of immobilization on healthy people and studies associated with the space program that have demonstrated the effects of weightlessness on bone density, muscle mass, and circulation.

Allison (2007) also suggests the processes involved in meeting the requirement for rest, including:

- Recognizing the conditioning and deconditioning effects of factors such as age, gender, weight, health state, physique, and emotional stress
- Engaging in activities that are restful to the individual
- Recognizing and acting to mitigate harmful effects of excess rest or activity
- Responding to body cues, and pacing activities to prevent energy depletion

The purpose of balancing rest and activity is to achieve and sustain a state of physical and psychological equilibrium that supports optimum physical, mental, cognitive, and emotional functioning. The result of maintaining a balance between rest and activity is a state of equilibrium in which there is efficient use of energy and resources, as activities are pursued that promote a sense of accomplishment and satisfaction. A balance between rest and activity is essential to maintaining normal body rhythms, such as heart functioning. It protects the body from the damaging effects of excesses of activity or excesses of rest. Processes associated with maintaining a balance between activity and rest include the following (Allison, p. 73):

- Awareness of the quantitative and qualitative standards for activity and rest
- Awareness of current needs, body cues, level of performance, and recommended standards for activity and rest
- Implementation of reliable measures that are appropriate in relation to age, gender, level of development, health status, capabilities, and limitations

The questions to be asked as data collection proceeds include:

- What constitutes a balance between rest and activity for this person at this time and under current conditions?
- How do the current patterns compare with previous patterns?
- What kinds of rest and activity may be hazardous for this person? For example, if the person is confined to bed, the lack of mobility may be hazardous. On the other hand, if recovering from the placement of an extensive skin graft, activity may be hazardous.
- What action should be taken to meet this requisite?

In the immediate postoperative period, Mrs. Smith requires an increase in rest. As she moves to the rehabilitation phase of her recovery, she will continue to have needs for recuperative rest and also for an increase in the amount of activity.

MAINTAIN A BALANCE BETWEEN SOLITUDE AND SOCIAL INTERACTION

Maintenance of a balance between solitude and social interaction has been shown to affect the physical and mental aspects of health and well-being. Human beings live in a world with other humans. Solitude and social interaction are components of daily life. Theories that help to understand the dimensions of this requisite are found in the social sciences.

Baumeister and Leary (1995) evaluated empirical literature and found support for the hypothesis that humans need to form and maintain strong, stable interpersonal relationships. They hypothesized that humans have a need for frequent, affectively pleasant interactions and that these "must take place in the context of a temporarily stable and enduring framework of affective concern for each other's welfare" (p. 497). Conversely, a lack of belongingness may cause a variety of ill effects. The authors suggested that this interpersonal motive is the cause of much human behavior, emotion, and thought. Social isolation has been found to be a risk for morbidity and mortality. A review of the literature by Hawkley, Burleson, Bernson, and Cacioppo (2003) found evidence that living alone, small social networks, less frequent social interactions, and smaller households increased the risk for all-cause mortality. They describe studies that identified that variations in specific physiological indicators, namely total peripheral resistance and cardiac output, were demonstrated in lonely and non-lonely people in a sample of college-age students. This finding may have an impact on health status in later life. More recently, in a study involving data from more than 5,000 patients, Shankar and McMunn (2011) found that both social isolation and loneliness were associated with a greater risk of being inactive, smoking, and reporting multiple health-risk behaviors. Their findings led them to suggest that social isolation may also affect health through processes that are associated with development of cardiovascular disease.

Harris (1989, personal communication) studied the behavior related to maintaining a balance between rest and activity in a population of men with schizophrenia who lived in an institution. He identified 18 behaviors related to solitude, which, on further analysis, clustered around distancing and organizing, and 10 behaviors related to interaction, which clustered around managing situations. He concluded that people with the serious mental illness managed their environments through self-care behaviors that were directed at maintaining a balance between solitude and social interaction. In another example of similar action, a mother with an autistic child described how her son met this requisite when they were travelling by lying on the floor in the space between the bed and the wall with his iPad.

Social interaction may be experienced in a variety of ways, including through work, for instance, through paid, domestic, and volunteer activities. The complexity of work appears to be associated with improvement in mental flexibility, and associated with status and self-esteem. Participation in physical and nonphysical leisure activities may play a part in self-concept, reducing depression, controlling anxiety, enhancing self-esteem, and facilitating social interaction. They also contribute to feelings of an increase in general psychological well-being and life satisfaction and may contribute to improving cognitive functioning.

There is a body of research that has explored leisure as a means to transcend negative life events. Conclusions in this literature point to leisure as contributing to physical, social, emotional, and cognitive health. This occurs through prevention, coping, and transcendence strategies. This, in turn, leads to consideration of leisure counseling as a therapy. Consideration of leisure counseling as a therapeutic action leads to consideration of the role of society and community policies and programs and their relation to the overall health of individuals. Barriers to maintaining a balance between work and leisure appear to be more societal and global rather than individual (Haworth & Lewis, 2005). This is a further example of social determinants of health.

Some conditioning factors that are associated with maintaining a balance between solitude and social interaction include the following:

- Personal, family, societal, and cultural values and perceptions about work, leisure, use of time, and the interrelationships among these variables
- Family responsibilities
- Availability of resources
- Available social programs facilitating leisure activities

Some factors that may interfere with meeting this requisite include:

- Personality, temperament, anxiety about being with others (social phobia), and concerns about physical attributes
- Feeling a need to be in constant contact with another
- Sensory impairments and inadequate communication skills
- Life situation that requires continuous contact and interaction with others during waking hours
- Continuous involvement in provision of care for another
- Conditions of living
- Availability of social contacts and interactions

Maintenance of a balance between rest and activity and a balance between solitude and social interaction are closely related, and some of the processes are the same. The following are proposed as processes to be considered in maintaining a balance between solitude and social interaction:

- Acquiring knowledge about the influence of solitude and social interaction and the balance between them in maintaining health and promoting well-being
- Making judgments about what to do in planning and establishing effective daily routines to facilitate and maintain a balance between solitude and social interaction
- Having knowledge of and utilizing available resources to promote and ensure an adequate program for maintaining a balance between solitude and social interactions

As Mrs. Smith processes the meaning of her injury and future recovery, the nature of her social interactions will change. She will have needs for more purposive social interactions—people to help her with her mobility, and provide support as she works through the rehabilitation process and attempts to reestablish her independent living.

PREVENTION OF HAZARDS

The purposes to be achieved in reference to this requisite include promotion of human functioning and development. This requisite is intertwined with each of the other universal self-care requisites.

What hazards exist in the individual's environment (e.g., secondary smoke, use of drugs among peer group)?

- What will happen if a hazard is not eliminated or controlled?
- What individual values and actions may be causing hazardous conditions (e.g., living within a drug culture, following an extreme lifestyle)?
- What should the individual do to become aware of, prevent, or control hazards?
- Are there potential hazards in the home (e.g., stairs, scatter rugs)?

PROMOTION OF NORMALCY: PROMOTION OF HUMAN FUNCTIONING AND DEVELOPMENT WITHIN SOCIAL GROUPS IN ACCORD WITH HUMAN POTENTIAL, KNOWN HUMAN LIMITATIONS, AND THE HUMAN DESIRE TO BE NORMAL

The purposes to be achieved by meeting this requisite include developing and maintaining a realistic self-concept and acting to promote one's own development. It is also concerned with the action a person may take to achieve a personal or group norm but one that may be hazardous to well-being or health, such as teenagers smoking marijuana because it is the group norm. In defining *normalcy*, the boundaries that have been identified include three reference points:

1. The social group of the person
2. Human potential and known human limitations
3. Human desire to be normal

These reference points would imply that consideration must be given to the personal perception of what is normal and the person's desires regarding normalcy. Orem (2001) states, "*Normalcy* is used in the sense of that which is in accord with the genetic and constitutional characteristics and talents of individuals" (p. 225). This would infer that the frame of reference for normalcy is the individual within a sociocultural context. There are no absolute scales to measure normalcy. In working with this requisite, it is particularly important to listen to the patient. As one person being interviewed by a nurse said, "I've known myself for forty years. I know me better than you ever could."

Promotion of normalcy includes consideration of physiological, cognitive, and psychological human functioning. Which of these areas are significant in the current situation? What are the purposes to be achieved in relation to each of these areas? How do the action systems available for meeting each component of this requisite interact with each other? Whenever there is a requirement for modifying self-concept as in learning to live with a variation in health, a chronic illness, or an injury with lasting consequences, attention should be paid to this requisite.

Whenever there is a need to attend to promotion of normalcy, promotion of development should also be explored. Studies related to the experience of living with a health deviation, mental or physiological, provide some insight into the importance of normalcy in daily living and into what it means (Pickens, 1999). There is frequent reference on the part of the patient and the family for normalcy, a desire to return to normal, a desire to be normal, and a desire for things to be as they were before "x."

Achievement of a sense of normalcy when there is a change in conditioning factors appears to take place over time as people learn a new way of life, incorporating new actions into daily living along with a new perception of self, and possibly incorporating new roles into their daily lives. Some examples from studies reported in the literature provide us with a glimpse of the way in which people perceive normalcy and attempt to promote normalcy in their lives. In their study, Harris and Williams (1991) report that homeless men expressed that normalcy meant getting money, keeping clean, and having clean clothes. People dealing with spinal cord injuries described normalcy as getting to the point when they could focus on their abilities rather than on their limitations, considering themselves or a person in a wheelchair as normal as anyone else, and finding a purpose in life (DeSanto-Madeya, 2006).

Behavior and expressions of satisfaction or dissatisfaction with one's life may be indicators of the extent to which this requisite is or is not being met. Questions to consider in data collection include:

- How does the person see himself or herself (data related to self-concept)? Is this view realistic?

- Is the need for health care identified and is appropriate care obtained?

- Is action taken to promote health?

- How does the patient define normalcy, quality of life, and related factors?

- How does the patient's perception of normalcy influence other self-care requisites?

- How does meeting of other self-care requisites interrelate with promotion of normalcy?

When health deviation self-care requisites are discussed later in this chapter, you will note that there are two requisites that are closely associated with the promotion of normalcy. Whenever promotion of normalcy is a concern, attention must be paid to modifying self-concept and learning to live with the effects of pathological conditions and treatment measures in a lifestyle that promotes continued personal development. Conversely, when these two requisites are the focus of concern, the promotion of normalcy must also be considered. These two requisites vary from promotion of normalcy in that they are of concern when there is some altered health state in addition to the requirement for promotion of normalcy, which is universal and pertains to all people. There is also an overlap between promotion of normalcy and the developmental self-care requisites. In many situations, development is the prime concern, and specific actions are required to promote development. However, it is important to realize that the actions taken to meet universal self-care requisites will influence the meeting of developmental self-care requisites and that the reverse is also true.

From the perspective of the individual, promotion of normalcy includes:

- Developing and maintaining a realistic self-concept
  - Knowing and accepting the reality of structure and functioning
  - Recognizing that the environment is important
  - Recognizing the relationship between self-concept and goal achievement
- Fostering certain specific human developments
  - Making choices that promote all aspects of human development and that stimulate interest in and give meaning to life
  - Expression of individual interests and talents, promotion of sense of personal worth and responsibility
  - Avoiding situations that interfere with exercise of self-control and self-direction
  - Periodic self-assessment and awareness of effects of one's behavior on self and others
- Promoting integrity of structure and functioning
  - Care of body (e.g., ensuring adequate nutrition, controlling conditions to maintain body temperature)
  - Interference—lack of feeling, interest in, or respect for others
- Attending to deviations from structural and functional norms
  - Collect factual information about what is normal regarding physical structure, functioning, and behavior patterns and identify manifestations of deviation.
  - Be aware of the significance of what has been mentioned earlier.

Mrs. Smith needs to change her perception of normalcy, at least during the rehabilitation phase of recovery. She may or may not need to modify her self-concept after the recovery period, since she had previously planned to get a part-time job to supplement her retirement income.

DEVELOPMENTAL SELF-CARE REQUISITES

Development is viewed from the broadest perspective, including growth and development of the physical structure of people: psychological, social, emotional, moral, and behavioral development. Detailed assessments in any one of these areas are usually done by specialists in the particular area. For example, the pediatrician and nurses in well-baby clinics are concerned with physical, cognitive, and behavioral development of infants and toddlers, as all these areas are interrelated. Many benchmarks of progress have become established norms for these age groups. Children are evaluated against these norms and if deviations are found, they may be referred for more detailed assessments. Development in all areas continues throughout the life span. In mature individuals, it tends to occur in response to the whole situation that the individual is experiencing, including the changes in physiological functioning and social interaction that are associated with the aging process. Research related to developmental processes in adults is very limited.

Varying theoretical schools and theories have developed within the social sciences to explain and to facilitate an understanding of the processes of development. Advances in the neurosciences are providing information about the interrelationships among cognitive development and decline, the chemistry of the brain and associated pathology, and behavior.

An understanding of the relationship between self-care and development from the perspective of the interests and concerns of nursing entails exploring the articulation between nursing sciences and the sciences in which studying particular kinds of development is the focus of concern. The articulation between nursing science and developmental science takes place as nurses explore the related scientific literature to answer nursing questions. For the purposes of nursing practice, development is viewed from two perspectives. One perspective is as a basic conditioning factor that influences the actions to be taken to meet self-care requisites and the capability to act. The other perspective is as a self-care requisite with the requirement to promote development throughout the life span and/or to take action to overcome factors that interfere with promotion of development.

Some examples of nursing questions as suggested by the self-care deficit nursing theory include the following: How is development promoted across the life span? What parenting behaviors facilitate/interfere with promotion of development? What is the relationship between culture and promotion of development? How do various illnesses and/or health states impact developmental processes? What is the relationship between the promotion of normalcy and the developmental self-care requisites?

Three categories or sets of developmental self-care requisites have been suggested (Orem, 2001). These are provision of conditions that promote development, engagement in self-development, and prevention of or overcoming effects of human conditions and life situations that can adversely affect development.

Provision of Conditions That Promote Development

The independent person can or should be able to maintain his or environment in such a way that it leads to a positive, healthy life. There are some agreed-upon stages of development with associated tasks that promote development. Conditions that may interfere with normal development include poverty, abusive family relationships, limited mobility, chronic illness, and unfortunately, in our current society, social conflict and war.

In periods of social dependency such as infancy, childhood, or declining age, these self-care requisites are met by actions of a dependent-care agent—a parent, a guardian, or an adult child of an aging parent. *Social dependency* is defined as "a condition that exists when persons require assistance from other members of society. It occurs within the context of a particular social unit. The provision of assistance and the nature of the assistance provided are a function of the general culture and culture of the specific groups" (Taylor & Renpenning, 2011, p. 108). A dependent-care agent may be a parent or another family member. He or she is a mature or maturing individual who accepts responsibility to know and to meet components of the therapeutic self-care demand of people who are socially dependent on them. They also assume responsibility for regulating development and exercise of self-care agency for the person who is dependent. Some specific conditions that may need to be provided to meet this requisite that are adapted from Orem (2001, pp. 251–252) include the following:

- Provision and maintenance of an adequate supply of water, food, and conditions that are essential for ongoing physical development

- Provision and maintenance of physical, environmental, and social conditions that ensure feelings of comfort, safety, closeness to another human, and a sense of being cared for

- Provision and maintenance of conditions that prevent both sensory deprivation and sensory overload

- Provision and maintenance of conditions that prevent and sustain affective and cognitional development

- Provision of experiences and conditions to facilitate development of skills for life in society, including intellectual, perceptual, interpersonal, and social skills

- Provision of experiences to foster awareness of self and of being a person with the world of family and community

- Regulation of the physical, biological, and social environment to mitigate development of states of fear, anger, or anxiety

Mrs. Smith is successfully transitioned through adult developmental stages. As she returns home, she probably will need to engage in some other activities that help her move forward, given her recent retirement and injury.

Engagement in Self-Development

As part of knowing and meeting his or her own therapeutic self-care demand, the mature and maturing person acts to promote his or her own self-development. This includes, but is not limited to, the following:

- Develop insights about self, one's perception of others, relationships to others, and attitudes toward them.

- Accept feelings and emotions leading to insights about self and others and about relationships to others, to objects, and to life situations.

- Through development of talents and interests, prepare for engaging in and maintaining productive work in society.

- Engage in clarification of goals and values in situations that demand involvement.

- Assume responsibility in life situations in accord with one's role and with one's developing self-ideal.

- Value positive emotions, including desire to know, variations of human love, joy of making and doing, laughter, religious emotions, and happiness.

- Seek to understand impact of negative emotions and action impulse, including feelings of guilt, states of guilt, and unconscious conflict.

According to Orem and Vardiman (1995), it is important to promote positive mental health through a deliberate effort to function:

- Within a reality frame of reference
- To bring about and maintain order in daily living
- With integrity and self-awareness
- As a person in a community
- With an increasing understanding of one's own humanity

Interference with Development

Throughout life, there are events, conditions, and problems that interfere with development. As part of knowing the therapeutic self-care demand, it is necessary to recognize the circumstances under which these conditions may occur and strategies for mitigating the impact they may have on development. For example, consider the effect that an accident resulting in paraplegia may have on the process of development of an adolescent. The experience of independence will be limited, relationship to a peer group will be altered, normal adolescent social experiences may be limited, schooling may be interfered with, and future employment may be affected. What is the impact on a child of having to follow a restrictive diet composed of what he or she does not like? The goals of situational developmental self-care requisites include:

- Provision of conditions and promoting the behaviors that will prevent the occurrence of deleterious effects on development
- Provision of conditions and experiences to mitigate or overcome existent deleterious effects on development

Some situations that are readily recognized as affecting development include deteriorating health or disability, terminal illness, and impending death. Changes of residence can be significant for adults as well as for children. Living conditions may interfere with development. Loss of relatives, friends, associates, possessions, or occupational security may also impact development. The interactive effect between the universal self-care requisites and the developmental requisites has been previously discussed. It is important to again stress the interaction between promotion of normalcy and development. Mathew has been in daycare since he was a year old. He is now 3 years old. His mother has just had a new baby and since she has a parental leave from her job, Mathew does not go to daycare. What is the impact of this on Mathew?

As Mrs. Smith works to regain her independence, she also needs to recognize her developmental and safety needs. Are there hazards, such as throw rugs, in the house? Is she realistic in accepting her limitations and the need to work for recovery?

HEALTH DEVIATION SELF-CARE REQUISITES

Health deviation self-care requisites have their origins in the health states of individuals and in the health care systems factors that are present. Health deviation self-care requisites address situations when there is a health state that deviates from the normal or when a person is undergoing health-related diagnosis or treatment. Illnesses, disabilities, and diagnostic tests influence/condition actions that are required to meet universal and developmental self-care requisites and to manage the existing health state. Much of nursing is focused on this area. Assisting the patient to meet these requisites requires a high level of skill on the part of the nurse, particularly in light of the shortened inpatient stays and complicated health care systems that the patient has to navigate.

Seek and Secure Appropriate Medical Assistance

The modern health care system is complicated. Access may be limited due to costs, insurance requirements, availability of services, transportation, and lack of knowledge about who to contact and how. The nature of the assistance required will, in part, determine the appropriate health care provider. Throughout history, healers, medicine men, shamans, and so on, have been present in many cultures and in some, they are the dominant health care providers. In Western cultures, such services are referred to as alternate health care. For the most part in the developed world, it is becoming more common that the beliefs associated with these alternate health practices are respected while simultaneously encouraging acceptance of treatment that is more scientifically based.

Exploration about a person's feelings, understanding, and experiences in reference to the health care system and health care providers is important. It is not uncommon for these personal factors to be the reason that treatment plans are not followed and do not succeed.

Mrs. Smith recognized her need for assistance after her fall. By calling 911, she sought appropriate assistance. She might have called her son to help but he would neither be able to transport her nor be able to provide pain relief.

Be Aware of and Attend to the Effects and Results of Pathological Conditions and States, Including Effects on Development

This requisite points to the need to identify the articulations and interrelationships among the universal, developmental, and health deviation self-care requisites. The effects of illnesses and disabilities on the universal self-care requisites tend to be quite obvious. For instance, if one has the flu, there is a decreased appetite, fluid intake may be diminished, and the person has little energy to engage in social interaction. Less obvious are the effects of altered health states on development. But consider the effects of living with an asthmatic condition on development of a child. Consider how a car accident resulting in lower-body paralysis can affect development of a 16-year-old. The concepts of awareness and attention are not well understood in the nursing literature. Until a patient internalizes and accepts that he or she has a situation that needs attending to, there is a high likelihood that he or she will be nonadherent with our expectations for self-care.

The following areas should be explored in relation to this requisite.

- Which self-care requisites will be affected by the current health state and how?

- Does the person have the knowledge and understanding to identify which self-care requisites will be affected and how they will be affected?

- What changes are required in self-care behaviors?

- Does the person have the knowledge, skill, and abilities to make these changes?

- Taking into account the person's capabilities, what adjustments should be made in prescribing the desired action system?

Mrs. Smith attended to her condition by agreeing to have hip surgery. After surgery and postoperative recovery, she will have to attend to rehabilitation. Depending on how that progresses, she will have to make adjustments to her diet and need to modify her activity and rest.

Effectively Carry Out Medically Prescribed Diagnostic, Therapeutic, and Rehabilitative Measures

This requisite addresses the collection and analysis of data to determine the changes required in the self-care system that are specific to the diagnosis and treatment of the current health state. These changes require assessment that focuses not only on the changes in action but also on consideration of the person's intention or motivation to act and the kinds of capabilities required to carry out the proposed actions. An example of how complex the meeting of this requisite can be and the nature of the cognitive skills required in management of one condition is described by Backscheider (1974). Since the article was published, many of the details regarding the diabetic condition and its management have changed; whereas the complexity of that management has not. The everyday activities involved in managing a regimen for diabetes include blood testing, monitoring how one feels, eating the appropriate diet, incorporating exercise, and taking medication regularly. The specific capabilities required to successfully execute this regime included, among others, the capability to discriminate and to classify clusters of events as being necessary to recognize symptoms along the hypoglycemia–normal–hyperglycemia continuum. Memory and learning are capabilities that are associated with food selection and taking medication. Attention span underlies the ability to learn and follow through on details of the diabetic regime. The meaning of and meeting this requisite can be complicated. There is a tendency to label people who do not follow advice as noncompliant. The practice of nursing from the perspective of self-care deficit nursing theory provides another framework for explaining such behavior, which is in accord with the current usage of the term *nonadherence*, that is, *there is a reason behind all behavior*. And it is the job of the nurse to determine what the underlying reasons might be.

Mrs. Smith will need to make adjustments in many aspects of her daily life, at least until her rehabilitation is completed. One of these will be to manage the osteoporosis medication and monitor its effects. For a time, Mrs. Smith will need assistive devices such as a walker or a cane. If she should refuse or be reluctant to use a walker, it would be important to determine why that might be. Time will tell whether she has other mobility issues.

Be Aware of and Attend to or Regulate the Discomforting or Deleterious Effects of Treatment Measures Performed or Prescribed by a Health Care Professional, Including Effect on Development

It is not uncommon for people to not follow a treatment regime, because the side effects of a treatment are more debilitating or perceived to be worse than the condition being treated. Meeting this requisite includes knowing that there may be side effects that are associated with the diagnosis or treatment, what these are, and strategies for dealing with them. Having access to this information is a major component of meeting the requisite. With the current access to information via the Internet, it is even more important to help people to filter through the information available with reference to potential side effects. Having some knowledge of the processes associated with development underlies being able to address the impact of the treatment itself or the actions associated with meeting the requisite on development.

Modify Self-Concept (and Self-Image) Accepting Oneself as Being in a Particular State of Health and Learn to Live in a Lifestyle that Promotes Continued Personal Development

These two requisites will be considered together. Both of these requisites articulate with promotion of normalcy, particularly when long-term management of a health state is required. Some examples of findings reported in the literature are helpful in understanding these requisites. The first example describes the trajectory of learning to live with a serious mental illness, the second describes women living with chronic pain, and the third is about people who have lived with a spinal cord injury for some time.

Pickens (1999) identified that people with serious mental illness in the population studied expressed the desire for normalcy as having normal things, undergoing normal experiences, doing meaningful activities, and being well and safe. They also expressed normalcy as not harming self or another, and as not using drugs. Gender-related normalcy meant being free from physical or sexual abuse. Expressions related to normalcy were also related to age and developmental issues: Older people were concerned with a place to live, whereas younger people were more concerned with acquisition of material goods.

DeSanto-Madeya (2006) explored the meaning of living with spinal cord injury five to ten years after the injury occurred. Reading this article provides much food for thought about the role that health care providers can play in promotion of normalcy and in overcoming the interference with development and day-to-day enjoyment of life in the presence of a chronic disability. This study identified seven themes: "looking for understanding, stumbling along an unlit path, viewing self through a stained glass window, challenging the bonds of love, moving forward . . . and reaching normalcy" (p. 265). The findings portrayed that living with spinal cord injury involved continuing challenges to deal with unfamiliar equipment, complications, terminology, changing responsibilities, and lack of freedom for the whole family. Only when the existence of the permanence of the injury and associated changes and challenges were accepted as the new normal were members of the family able to move on. The families expressed frustration with the lack of understanding and support from health care providers.

Skuladottir and Halldorsdottir (2011) report in their study that women living with chronic pain described the experience as affecting feelings of well-being, daily activities, and emotions. These women acted to control the pain rather than having the pain control them by reorganizing their lives, pacing activities, taking pain medication, and being aware of triggers that affected pain levels. The people in this study described how they managed the misunderstanding and disbelief associated with living with chronic pain by concealing their suffering so as to appear normal. The presence of pain changed their self-image and to cope with this they tried to behave as strong people. Participation in family life and social activities appeared to help them to achieve a sense of normalcy. Findings of this sort emphasize the links among the requisites related to solitude and social interaction, rest and activity, as well as normalcy and promotion of development.

These requisites require Mrs. Smith to contemplate her current situation and draw some conclusions as to what kind of changes she might need or want to make.

THE THERAPEUTIC SELF-CARE DEMAND

Considering All Aspects of the Current Health Situation, What Actions Are Required to Maintain Life and to Promote Health, Well-Being, and Development?

The term *therapeutic self-care demand* is used to refer to the totality of all of the care measures required to meet the self-care requisites identified as important in the situation. Again, back to the example of the word *table*, standing for that flat board with four legs, the therapeutic self-care demand is an expression that represents all of the purposes and related actions associated with self-care over a specific period. It is complex and, because of its complexity, it takes time to fully appreciate the utility in providing direction for nursing action. However, it is one of the most useful conceptual organizers in that it not only provides direction for collecting and analyzing data but also provides direction for nursing practice and for organizing nursing knowledge. Just as the term *appendicitis* is useful as an organizer of information in medicine, bringing together a collection of symptoms and treatments, so the term *therapeutic self-care demand* is useful as a means of categorizing information of concern to nursing.

Thinking this way takes time. In some ways, attaching meaning to this term is like learning a new language. The chief nursing officer in a health care setting where self-care deficit nursing theory had been found to be useful to frontline nurses wanted to eliminate the term *therapeutic self-care demand*, saying it was too foreign to most nurses, not common to other disciplines, and not necessary. The nurses in practice disagreed, saying that the term was the most useful to them, as it gave them a full picture of the situation. It represented a whole complex of knowledge and activities required in a particular patient situation, providing specific direction for their practice. As we focus more holistically on the patient, a construct such as therapeutic self-care demand becomes even more relevant. If we are to view the patient as a whole, we need to be able to see how the parts fit together into a whole, where the whole is greater than the sum of the parts. Later, as we present the concept of nursing process operations, this will be brought into focus.

Conceptualization of the therapeutic self-care demand as a whole is difficult. It might be considered as analogous to baking a cake. The cake is made up of flour, sugar, eggs, seasonings, and so on. The final product is very different than the constituents. Expression of the therapeutic self-care demand must be preceded by careful consideration of the self-care requisites that are affected by the conditioning factors in the particular situation and simultaneous consideration of the relationships among all of the significant requisites. It involves agreement being reached with the patient about priorities, what should be done, and when. In sharing this with the patient, the goal is to have the person ultimately able to calculate his or her own therapeutic self-care demand. People with chronic illnesses, although they do not name the product, implement the results of calculating their own therapeutic self-care demand through their self-care practice.

A Clinical Example: The Therapeutic Self-Care Demand for Patients With Heart Failure

Heart disease is one of the leading causes of morbidity and mortality in North America. As a result, there have been many studies done that contribute to our understanding of the changes in self-care practices that are required to successfully manage living with heart failure. Although the studies have not been framed from a self-care theory perspective, the findings constitute some common elements of therapeutic self-care demand for a person with heart failure. The requisites of concern, the related action systems, and some associated conditioning factors are indicated.

The components of the demand listed next are based on findings from Riegel et al. (2009). These findings have been used by the American Heart Association (AHA) to develop practice guidelines. Lainscack et al. (2011) suggest that there is not sufficient research evidence to support some of the clinical practice guidelines identified by Riegel and colleagues, and adopted by the AHA, but the work to date represents a useful beginning.

The following outline of components of therapeutic self-care demand cannot be considered an exhaustive description, but it is presented to help the reader to understand the components, complexity, and utility of the construct therapeutic self-care demand. It illustrates the process of identifying or particularizing the self-care requisites for a particular disease entity, heart failure. There is a judgmental factor at play in calculating the self-care demand. Once again, we are faced with recognizing that there is an art as well as a science in the provision of nursing. The expression of the therapeutic self-care demand in individual situations can only be accomplished through a careful examination of interrelationships in consultation with the person/people involved to determine the desired course of action for the particular situation. The following outline is limited to the demand component of the self-care system. This list of actions is reflective of guidance from the theory of self-care. The theory of self-care proposes that self-care is purposeful, and that the purposes are achieved through an action system, the self-care system. The specific capabilities that are required for action and make up the other half of the self-care system are discussed in Chapter 7.

The Self-Care Demand for People Living With Heart Failure

- Maintain a sufficient intake of food and water.
    - Adjust the intake of food and water to accommodate physiological changes associated with heart failure.
    - In keeping with current known standards, limit daily sodium intake to less than 2.3 g/d or as prescribed by the health care provider.
    - In keeping with current known standards, limit fluid intake to less than 2 liters per day.
    - Monitor weight daily.
    - Recognize and correctly interpret changes in weight.
    - Adjust fluid intake and diuretic dosage as prescribed to accommodate physiological changes.
    - Restrict alcohol consumption.
- Maintain a balance between rest and activity, solitude and social interaction.
    - Engage in exercise programs to increase anaerobic threshold, peak oxygen uptake, and coronary flow reserve.
    - Establish and adhere to a regular exercise program.
    - Prevent/alleviate depressions that are often associated with heart failure.
    - Adhere to an exercise regime.
    - Include social interaction in self-care activities.
    - Recognize and seek treatment for anxiety and/or depression.
- Prevent hazards.
    - Prevent infection and inflammatory response.
    - Engage in regular hand washing.
    - Attend to maintaining dental health.
    - Maintain immunizations.
    - Avoid recreational drugs.
    - Stop smoking.
    - Avoid secondhand smoke.
- All health deviation self-care requisites are of concern.
    - Take prescribed medications.
    - Obtain initial and refill prescriptions; be aware of why the prescribed medication regime is not being followed and discuss with the health care provider.

- Discuss taking of nonprescription drugs with the health care provider to determine possible interactions.
- Incorporate taking medications into daily activities.
- Adjust medication schedule regarding travel, appointments, changes in health state, and so forth.
- Monitor self to detect variations in health state.
- Know how to monitor.
- Know what to monitor.
- Establish and follow routine for monitoring.
- Respond appropriately to variations in monitoring data.
- Differentiate symptoms that are associated with comorbidities.
- Recognize meaning of changes identified, for example, edema, dyspnea, chest pain, and dizziness.
- Evaluate change.
- Decide on course of action.
- Take action.
- Evaluate response to action taken.
- Accept self as having heart failure and needing to take specific action to manage health state.
- Contact health care providers.
- Keep appointments.
- Recognize when symptom management is beyond individual's knowledge and/or capabilities.

LEARNING ACTIVITIES

1. Keep a diary of your food intake for 3 days, including everything you eat—meals, snacks, candies, drinks. Download a set of national food guidelines and compare your diet over the preceding 3 days to the recommended intake. What changes should be made in your diet? What factors are influencing your choice to make or not make the required choices?

2. Describe specific ways in which the community in which you live has taken steps to promote normalcy for people with physical disabilities, for those who are developmentally disabled, and for those who are academically challenged.

3. Consider a case situation familiar to you. Identify the self-care requisites and conditioning factors that were significant in that situation. What changes in self-care practices did that person have to make?

References

Allison, S. E. (2007). Self-care requirements for activity and rest: An Orem nursing focus. *Nursing Science quarterly, 20*(1), 68–76. doi:10.1177/0894318406296297

Backscheider, J. (1974). Self-care requirements, self-care capabilities and nursing systems. *American Journal of Public Health, 64*(12), 1138–1146.

Baumeister, R. F., & Leary, M. R. (1995). The need to belong: Desire for interpersonal attachments as a fundamental human motivation. *Psychology Bulletin, 117*(3), 497–452.

Denyes, M., Orem, D. E., & Bekel, G. (2001). Self-care: A foundational science. *Nursing Science Quarterly, 14*(1), 48–54.

DeSanto-Medaya, S. (2006). The meaning of living with spinal cord injury 5 to 10 years after the injury. *Western Journal of Nursing Research, 28*, 265–289. doi:10.1177/0193945905283178

Harris, J. L., & Williams, L. K. (1991). Universal self-care requisites as identified by homeless elderly men. *Journal of Gerontological Nursing, 17*(6), 39–43.

Hawkley, L. C., Burleson, M. H., Bernson, G. G., & Cacioppo, J. T. (2003). Loneliness in everyday life: Cardiovascular activity, psychosocial context and everyday life. *Journal of Personality and Social Psychology, 85*(1), 105–120. dx.doi.org/10.1037/0022-3514.85.1.105

Haworth, J., & Lewis, S. (2005). Work, leisure and well-being. *British Journal of Guidance and Counselling, 33*(1), 67–79. doi:10.1080/03069880412331335902

Lainscack, M., Blue, L., Clark, A., Dahlstrom, U., Dickstein., K., Elman, I., . . . Jaarsma, T. (2011). Self-care management of heart failure: Practical recommendations from the Patient Care Committee Heart Failure Association of the European Society of Cardiology. *European Journal of Heart Failure, 13*(2), 115–126. doi:10.1093/eujhf/hfq219

Nursing Development Conference Group. (1979). *Concept formalization in nursing: Process and product* (2nd ed.). Boston, MA: Little, Brown.

Orem, D. E. (2001). *Nursing: Concepts of practice* (6th ed.). St. Louis, MO: Mosby.

Orem, D. E., & Vardiman, E. M. (1995). Orem's nursing theory and positive mental health: Practical considerations. *Nursing Science Quarterly, 9*(4), 165–173.

Pickens, J. M. (1999). Living with serious mental illness: The desire for normalcy. *Nursing Science Quarterly, 12*, 233–239. doi:10.1177/08943189922107007

Riegel, B., Moser, D. K., Anker, S. D., Appel, L. J., Dunbar, S. B., Grady, K. L., . . . Whellan, D. J. (2009). State of the science: Promoting self-care in persons with heart failure: A scientific statement from the American Heart Association. *Circulation, 120*, 1141–1163. doi:10.1161/CIRCULATIONAHA.109.192628

Shankar, A., & McMunn, A. (2011). Loneliness, social isolation and behavioral and biological health indicators in older adults. *Health Psychology, 30*(4), 377–385. doi:10.1037/a0022826

Skuladottir, H., & Halldorsdottir, S. (2011). The quest for well-being: Self-identified needs of women in chronic pain. *Scandinavian Journal of Caring Sciences, 25*, 81–89. doi:10.1111/j.1471-6712.2010.00793.x

Taylor, S. G., & Renpenning, K. (2011). *Self-care science, nursing theory and evidence based practice*. New York, NY: Springer.

Tomstad, S. T., Söderhamn, U., Espnes, G. A., & Söderhamn, O. (2012). Living alone, receiving help, helplessness, and inactivity are strongly related to risk of undernutrition among older home-dwelling people. *International Journal of General Medicine, 5*, 231–240.

CHAPTER 7

THE "HOW" OF SELF-CARE

Self-Care Agency

One of the most exciting developments to take place in nursing has been the contribution of nurse scholars in putting forth a structure for exploring the capability and the power to engage in self-care/self-care agency. This structure and the related elements will be discussed in this chapter. The structure of self-care agency provides direction for articulation of nursing knowledge with knowledge from other disciplines to help answer nursing questions and to help nurses better understand why and how people make the choices they do in regard to self-care or self-management. Through case analysis, research, and theoretical advances in nursing and related disciplines, we are gradually developing an understanding of the elements that are associated with the power to engage in self-care. This understanding is foundational to evidence-based nursing practice.

OBJECTIVES

After reading this chapter, the learner will be able to:

1. Describe the development of the capability to engage in self-care (self-care agency) over the life span
2. Explore components of the structure of self-care agency in nursing practice
3. Make decisions about the degree of development of self-care agency and its impact on production of self-care
4. Identify factors that facilitate development of self-care agency
5. Identify factors that facilitate or interfere with the exercise of self-care agency

6. Appreciate the value of nursing theories in bringing a nursing perspective to knowledge developed in related disciplines

KEY CONCEPTS   self-care agency • self-care limitations • self-care operations • power components for self-care • foundational capabilities and dispositions

OVERVIEW OF THE CAPABILITY FOR ENGAGING IN SELF-CARE

The accomplishment of self-care involves a complex set of abilities. This "basketful" of capabilities has come to be known as *self-care agency* (Chapter 4). *Self-care agency* is defined as "the complex acquired ability of mature and maturing persons to know and to meet their continuing requirements for deliberate, purposive action to regulate their own human functioning and development" (Orem, 2001, p. 522). This multifaceted theoretical construct or term represents a number of physical and cognitive capabilities. It cannot be measured as a whole. However, we can examine self-care practices and through that exploration gain an understanding of the capabilities required to accomplish self-care, how these capabilities develop over the life span, and how factors facilitate or interfere with their development.

There are many ways to view self-care—ranging from the perspective of being responsible for self to the view reflected in this book, that is, as a characteristic or function of being human. As previously stated, self-care is required to maintain life and health and to promote development. The combination of knowledge, skills, abilities, and motivation to engage in self-care is learned over time within a sociocultural environment. It begins in childhood and continues throughout one's life. Development of health-related self-care agency is intertwined with the daily practices that become habitual, often with little or no recognition that these practices may be health related.

Self-care agency is developed as one learns from his or her family members and others in society to care for self. An essential part of this process involves encouragement to care for self, being allowed to do so, being assisted in acquiring the necessary knowledge and skill, and having the resources to do so. As this process takes place, a person gradually develops a concept of self as self-care agent (one who acts on his or her own behalf). Through this process, a person sees himself or herself as having some responsibility and capability for attending to health-related needs. Think of someone you know who has a chronic condition. What knowledge, skills, and abilities has that person developed in response to his or her health state? How long did it take that person to develop the required capabilities? What factors interfere with people you know who are taking required action in relation to their health?

The knowledge and capabilities required to accomplish self-care are a function of the goals of self-care and the associated actions. These, in turn, are a function of external conditioning factors such as society, culture, environment, available resources, and family practices. In addition to knowing the actions to be taken, the development of the capabilities to act is a function of the opportunity to acquire and to exercise those capabilities, including resources available and environmental factors. They are also a function of the physical, cognitive, and emotional characteristics of the person. For the most part, unless there is a problem, we learn to take care of ourselves without giving much thought to what is required or the associated capabilities. A good example of this is learning to care for one's skin. Within North American culture, an adult bathes the baby, and then the child learns to wash hands when directed to, gradually takes over the whole bath, and in time takes over decision making about when and how to wash himself or herself. These self-care practices become habitual and we do not think of the associated capabilities as developing over time or as being related to particular conditions of living, sociocultural orientations, or availability of resources. But think how different these practices are in any one of the following situations: when the child is developmentally challenged, the bathroom is a shared one down the hall, there is no access to running water, lifestyle is nomadic, the family lives in a refugee camp, temperatures are below freezing for months on end, or being a member of a religious subculture that advocates strict gender roles. The capabilities developed to meet the requirements for self-care in each of the foregoing examples will have some features in common and some will be specific to the situation. Understanding the capability required to engage in self-care begins with exploration of self-care practices.

As nursing scholars studied patient situations, they began to recognize the importance of self-care in relation to health and well-being, identifying specific things that people did to maintain health. In analyzing those situations in more detail, they came to understand that there were two interrelated components to self-care—the requirement for action to maintain health and promote well-being (the therapeutic self-care demand discussed in Chapter 6) and the capabilities or power to act. This power came to be known as *self-care agency* and reflected that a person is acting on his or her own behalf or as an agent in relation to self-care (Nursing Development Conference Group [NDCG], 1979). This power to act is made up of knowledge, ability to think, ability to move body parts, skills, and motivation, and it is influenced by genetics, environment, energy levels, and so on.

Not everyone acts appropriately in relation to self-care. Why? Answering this question requires an in-depth exploration of the components of self-care agency. What exactly goes into the decision-making process? What are the influencing or conditioning factors? Answering this question has been and continues to be accomplished by studying cases to determine the capabilities that are required in specific situations followed by exploring nursing literature and that of related disciplines to learn more about how these capabilities are developed and activated. Through this kind of activity, nurses have and are continuing to build a knowledge base about the elements that make up self-care agency and the relationships among the elements. This understanding is developed within the sciences of both self-care and self-care agency, with contributions from practicing nurses and scholars, and also with contributions from many other disciplines, particularly the social sciences. One such contribution comes from the field of action science.

ACTION THEORY AND UNDERSTANDING SELF-CARE AGENCY

Knowledge in various fields is interrelated. Nursing theories and nursing knowledge do not stand alone. Developments in the field of action science have been foundational to the developing understanding of self-care agency. An action system is a series of actions or operations performed at a particular point in time to accomplish a specific purpose (Argyris & Schön, 1978). The self-care system is an action system. The operations associated with producing self-care involve knowing, decision making, and acting. Each of these operations requires that the person have the capabilities and dispositions that are specific to that operation.

Self-Care Operations, Related Capabilities, and Limitations

Knowing and decision making are cognitive processes requiring an intact and functioning cognitive system. These processes are influenced by cognitive development; perception; understanding of the situation, culture, and value system; available resources, including educational background; conditions of living; developmental state; sensorimotor state; environmental factors; previous experiences; and other conditioning factors.

Decision making involves reflection about which course of action to follow, projecting the possible outcomes of following one action or another, and making a decision either to follow a specific action or not to engage in any action. Carrying out this operation involves cognitive capabilities to enable comparison, differentiation, evaluation, and determination of preferred courses of action. It involves being able to anticipate and understand consequences of action. Moral and ethical judgments may be involved. Again, culture, personal values and preferences, family influences, available resources, and so forth will also influence the course(s) of action chosen. In making choices, individuals consider, "Is it beneficial for me? Can I do it" (Orem, 2001, p. 271). The completion of this operation results in a conclusion that one course of action is preferable to another or that none should be pursued, and a decision is made to follow through accordingly.

Limitations for decision making may be knowledge related, that is, there may be a lack of knowledge about the situation, not having enough information to know what questions to ask, or not having enough background information to make an informed decision. Emotions may impede decision making. There may be cognitive limitations. There may be a lack of ability to project into the future and visualize the result of a particular course of action. Or there may be a lack of interest or motivation in determining what should and should not be done in relation to self-care.

The productive phase is the most complex. It involves preparing self and the environment, performing the productive operations within a specific period, and monitoring the conditions that can affect the performance of the actions and the results—desired or not. This phase also involves deciding whether or not to continue a course of action, temporarily suspend it, or discontinue it.

The capabilities associated with carrying out the plan of action may be cognitive as well as psychomotor. They include cognitive abilities to ready the self, psychomotor skills to prepare materials and the environment, and capabilities associated with acting in a certain way and within a specific period. Cognitive capabilities are required for monitoring effectiveness of a course of action and for modifying it. Being able to categorize like events and to attach meaning to events is a part of production. Cognition and motivation to continue, to alter, or to cease production of certain courses of action are the other capabilities that are associated with production operations.

Limitations associated with implementing courses of action may also be present. Examples include a lack of specific skills or resources related to accomplishing the required self-care. A lack of energy has been identified as a limiting factor in exercising self-care agency. There may be other priorities for action, lack of interest, motivation, and persistence to act. Culture plays a part in implementing self-care actions as do family values and family system functioning. External interferences such as family crises or obligations, role functioning, and social disasters are obvious interferences in the exercise of self-care agency. The productive operations, that is, the practical work of carrying out the planned course of action, are influenced by many of the same factors that condition processes that are associated with decision making. In addition, they are influenced by the ability to perform the required actions, level of energy, motivation, opportunity, and so on.

The following example illustrates these self-care operations.

If Mrs. Smith develops an infection that is amenable to antibiotics, the action required is to take the antibiotic. The action system to accomplish this includes that a person has the knowledge and understanding of the symptoms of an infection, recognizes these symptoms, knows he or she must visit a health care provider to get a prescription, visits a health care provider and gets a prescription, goes to a pharmacy to get the prescription filled, reads and understands the instructions for taking the medication, understands the signs and symptoms of undesirable side effects, integrates plans for taking the medication as directed, takes the medication, assesses the results of taking the medication, and reports to the health care provider if the antibiotic is not effective or there are undesirable side effects.

The foregoing action system seems simple enough. But each of these actions requires specific capabilities:

- Perceptual and cognitive capability to recognize the need for attention of the health care provider

- Motivation to seek assistance

- Knowledge and belief that the antibiotic is appropriate

- Knowledge of the location of the pharmacy and how to get there—motivation to go to the pharmacy

- Ability to read

- Ability to understand directions

- Ability and motivation to incorporate taking medication into daily self-care

- Ability to retain information about timing of medication

- Ability to monitor for effectiveness and for undesirable side effects

- Recognition of the need to seek assistance of the health care provider

Foundational Capabilities and Dispositions

As illustrated in the preceding discussion, each of the self-care operations has specific capabilities and dispositions or characteristics that are associated with them. These capabilities and dispositions are foundational to all types of knowing, decision making, and acting, as well as to all types of deliberate action. Exploration, theories, and knowledge development related to these elements take place in disciplines that are associated with social sciences as well as in nursing and other health care disciplines. Identification of these capabilities is detailed and precise work but it is valuable to nursing. This work provides a point of articulation between nursing and other disciplines whose research is helping answer nursing questions.

For example, Backscheider (1974), a nurse with a sociology background, catalogued specific actions that patients needed to take to manage their diabetic condition. She then identified the specific capabilities required to perform each of these actions. She categorized these into physical, mental, motivational, and orientating capabilities. This was followed by an analysis of the data from the perspective of work done by Piaget (Wadsworth, 1984) and Furth (1977) that was related to cognitive development. This listing (Table 7.1) is a useful addition to our understanding of areas to explore in relation to self-care agency.

Some examples of research that has been conducted related to foundational capabilities and dispositions include Anderson and Olnhausen (1999); Meyer (2002); and White, Peters, and Schim (2011).

The Power Components for Self-Care

The results of Backscheider's work (1974) were integrated into the work of the NDCG (1979) as they analyzed cases to gain an understanding of the power that was specific to performance of self-care: What capabilities are involved? How do they develop? What are the cognitive components? What part do emotions play? How do people make decisions to act? What interferes with taking action?

As the work of studying data about self-care agency progressed, the NDCG proposed a set of capabilities that articulated with self-care operations on one hand and with the foundational capabilities and dispositions on the other hand. They became known as the power components for self-care (Table 7.2).

The power components provide more specific direction for exploring capabilities and limitations related to the production of self-care in particular situations. For example, if a person knows what action is required but does not follow through with the action, referencing the power components may provide insight as to why they do not act, thus providing direction for nursing. The power components also provide direction for accessing related literature and help nurses to use the knowledge gleaned for nursing purposes.

In reviewing the power components, you will note that many of these are concerned with some aspect of cognition. Continuing developments in the neurosciences and social sciences are key to helping us understand more about these power components. There is a great deal of variation in the extent to which the individual power components have been studied, and their underlying substructure has been explored. In the following discussion, illustrations of the utility of the power components are drawn from nursing studies and links to knowledge developed in related disciplines are introduced. This is not meant to be an exhaustive exploration of individual power components.

TABLE 7.1   Foundational Capabilities and Dispositions

Conditioning Factors and States
Genetic and constitutional factors
   Arousal state
   Social organization
   Culture
   Experience

Capabilities and Dispositions
Selected basic capabilities
   Sensation
      Proprioception
      Exteroception
   Learning
   Exercise or work
   Regulation of the position and movement of the body and its parts
   Attention
   Perception
   Memory
   Central regulation of motivational and emotional processes

Knowing and doing capabilities
   Rational agency
   Operational knowing
   Learned skills
      Reading, counting, and writing
      Verbal, perceptual, and manual
   Reasoning
   Self-consistency in knowing and doing

Dispositions affecting goals sought
   Self-understanding, self-awareness, and self-image
   Self-value, self-acceptance, and self-concern
   Acceptance of bodily functions
   Willingness to meet needs of self
   Future directedness

Significant orientative capabilities and dispositions
   Orientations to time, health, other people, events, and objects
   Priority system of value hierarchy
      Moral, economic, aesthetic, material, and social
   Interests and concerns
   Habits
   Ability to work with the body and its parts
   Ability to manage self and personal affairs

TABLE 7.2   Power Components for Self-Care

1. Ability to maintain attention and exercise requisite vigilance with respect to: (a) self as self-care agent and (b) internal and external conditions and factors that are significant for self-care
2. Controlled use of available physical energy that is sufficient for the initiation and continuation of self-care operations
3. Ability to control the position of the body and its parts in the execution of the movements that are required for the initiation and completion of self-care operations
4. Ability to reason within a self-care frame of reference
5. Motivation (i.e., goal orientations for self-care that are in accord with its characteristics and its meaning for life, health, and well-being)
6. Ability to make decisions about care of self and to operationalize these decisions
7. Ability to acquire technical knowledge about self-care from authoritative sources, to retain it, and to operationalize it
8. A repertoire of cognitive, perceptual, manipulative, communication, and interpersonal skills adapted to the performance of self-care operations
9. Ability to order discrete self-care actions or action systems into relationships with prior and subsequent actions
10. Ability to consistently perform self-care operations, integrating them with relevant aspects of personal, family, and community living

Source: NDCG (1979). Copyright Johns Hopkins University.

EXPLORING THE POWER COMPONENTS FOR SELF-CARE

1. Ability to maintain attention and exercise requisite vigilance with respect to (a) self as self-care agent and (b) internal and external conditions and factors that are significant for self-care.

This first power component addresses the importance of attention and vigilance.

Attention is the behavioral and cognitive process of selectively concentrating on a discrete aspect of information while ignoring other perceivable information. "Attention is a multidimensional term that refers to at least three different cognitive processes—concentration or effortful awareness, selectivity of perception, or the ability to coordinate two or more skills at the same time" (Moran, 2012, p. 39).

When we concentrate on something, we exert purposeful energy. Personal experience will tell you that it is possible to attend to more than one thing at a time or to attend to only certain things in a situation. As nurses, you do this many times every day. It is a skill that can be developed. A lack of ability to attend may manifest itself as an attention deficit disorder. *Vigilance* is commonly understood as the process of paying continuous and close attention. Nursing studies related to vigilance have addressed vigilance being demonstrated by family members in relation to relatives in intensive care and to children in inpatient settings. Researchers have described vigilance as a "strategy" used by individuals to cope with uncertainty

(Suffet & Lifshitz, 1991), and as a process for preserving self (Morse & O'Brien, 1995). Factors that interfere with the exercise of vigilance include, but are not limited to, health state, role responsibilities, energy levels, and neurochemical factors.

Meyer (2002) explored the process of vigilance in women who had migraine headaches and developed a substantive theory of vigilance from the analysis of her findings. The presence of a migraine interferes with daily functioning of the person. Through vigilance, conceptualized as the "art of watching out," the women studied were able to better manage daily functioning. Vigilance began with the women having a name for their condition—a diagnosis—and accepting the label. This was followed by "making the connections," which involved recognizing the patterns, that is, associating internal sensations with the onset of migraine headache. This process also involved learning about forms of treatment to become familiar with options available to them. Watching out emerged from the data as the core phenomenon associated with vigilance. Four subcategories were associated: assigning meaning to "what is," calculating the risk, staying ready, and monitoring the results. Deciding what to do preceeded any action. The decision-making process consisted of "determining the actions to be taken, selecting the actions to be avoided, and optimizing benefits over risks" (p. 1230).

Data related to exploring this power component include the observed level of consciousness. Is the person oriented to time, place, and person? Are there problems related to short-term memory? Do they express concerns about short-term memory? Does the attention span appear to be within normal limits? Are the responses to questions consistent and congruent? Do they recognize responsibility for their actions?

2. Controlled use of available physical energy that is sufficient for the initiation and continuation of self-care operations.

Maintaining a balance between rest and activity has been identified as a universal self-care requisite. This power component addresses the ability to manage energy expenditure to meet that component of the therapeutic self-care demand and other components. For example, in studies related to medication-taking behavior in people with heart failure, inconsistent taking of medication was associated with inadequate amounts of sleep and lack of energy. Adequate sleep has been linked with pursuing and persisting with an exercise program. Community health nurses visiting new mothers continuously find the new mother lacking in sleep and neglecting her own needs in favor of those of the new babe. Have you ever thought of how much energy it takes to do grocery shopping and to prepare meals? Perhaps this is why seniors living alone at home resort to "tea and toast" meals.

Underlying this controlled use of available physical energy are variables such as personal and cultural values, role responsibilities, role models, health state, availability of resources, and even available transportation, among other factors.

Areas to be explored include evidence of increased pulse or respiratory rate during activity. Another area is the expression of being tired, lethargic, and not having enough energy to do what a person wants to do or for accomplishing daily activities. Are there environmental or personal factors that interfere with adequate sleep or eating appropriate foods, such as weight, mental state, health state, changes in role responsibilities, excessive demands of other family members, or job situation? Should the person be limiting activities for some reason, and is he or she doing so?

3. Ability to control the position of the body and its part in the execution of the movements that are required for the initiation and completion of self-care operations.

This power component involves sensorimotor capabilities. In addition to muscle function, strength, pain, energy level, weight, and so forth may be inhibiting factors. This is probably one of the more obvious power components. The importance of this ability is evident in infancy and again as one ages.

Data collection includes observation of gross and fine motor skills. It also includes disclosure about limitations in movement, presence of pain, and verbalization about inability to perform daily tasks or job-related skills because of physical limitations.

4. Ability to reason within a self-care frame of reference.

Reasoning within a self-care frame of reference is a cognitive capability; thus, the state of cognitive development influences reasoning ability. It takes place within a personal and sociocultural frame of reference. The knowledge base from which the person is working is significant. This is strongly influenced by culture, family experiences, and so on. Not only is knowledge of what is required necessary but also self-concept, self-efficacy, and self-valuing may be involved in the reasoning process along with motivation.

In some cultures, particularly many Asian cultures, the importance is on the group and not on the individual. Davidson et al. (2011) studied health-seeking beliefs, a component of reasoning within a self-care frame of reference, of people of Chinese origin living in Australia who were recently discharged from the hospital after having been admitted for an acute cardiac event. They found cultural beliefs to be profoundly important in understanding the reasoning of some members of this population in relation to self-care. This included the emphasis on collectivism, the importance of family and tradition, and the need to integrate traditional beliefs with beliefs of Western medicine. The beliefs that the heart is the main organ of the body, and that the heart is central to emotion, meant that having heart disease resulted in a disruption of equilibrium and harmony in life balance. These beliefs required accessing traditional therapies to restore balance. This reflects the cultural component of understanding what is meant by reasoning within a self-care frame of reference.

Being aware of food choices and making decisions about what to eat is another example of reasoning within a self-care frame of reference. This comes into play throughout life—making decisions in relation to school lunches, losing weight, and alcohol consumption. Culture, religious teachings, family experiences, and availability of resources will impact the reasoning process. In a study of older home-dwelling individuals at risk for undernutrition, Tomstad, Söderhamn, Espnes, and Söderhamn (2012) found that when there was a change from living with another person, eating alone appeared to have an impact on an individual's pleasure in preparing meals and on appetite.

Ability to reason includes being able to perform inductive reasoning, that is, using specific facts to arrive at a general conclusion. In addition, one must be able to perform deductive reasoning or to use general principles to arrive at specific conclusions. Is the person able to identify cause–effect relationships? Does he or she associate needs and self-care actions? Is there evidence of moral and ethical judgment, a sense of differentiating between right and wrong? Does the person appear to value self-care? How is the person managing his or her current health state?

5. Motivation (i.e., goal orientations for self-care that are in accord with its characteristics and its meaning for life, health, and well-being).

Multiple theories have been developed in the social sciences in an attempt to understand motivation. Piaget's cognitive theory was an integral component in the studies done by Backscheider to help understand self-care behavior in the patients in the diabetic outpatient clinic. Social cognitive theory represented by Bandura (1997) has been widely used by nurses in research studies and to guide construction of education programs that are associated with health promotion. These cognitive theories along with learning theories have been helpful in developing educational programs that are related to specific health states.

Studies in neuroscience have led researchers to an understanding that the ability to persist with a course of action is, in part, controlled by certain structures of the brain and chemicals produced by those structures. Research in mental health is beginning to link the lack of ability to persist in an activity exhibited by people with schizophrenia to this chemical control.

Motivation has been described as both internal and external (Ryan & Deci, 2000). Conditions that promote internal motivation to accomplish tasks are those that are more personal to the individual, are linked to everyday life, and support autonomy through the opportunity to make choices (Medalia & Saperstein, 2011). An approach that uses this understanding of the value of intrinsic motivation is motivational interviewing (MI), which has been defined by its originators as "a directive, client-centered counseling style for eliciting behavior change by helping clients to explore and resolve ambivalence" (Rollnick & Miller, 1995, p. 325). When exercising this approach, the health care provider uses genuine and accurate empathy and reflective listening to help provide a supportive environment. The provider develops discrepancy between the person's health goals and his or her current behavior, acknowledges and honors the person's resistance rather than arguing for change, and supports self-efficacy. These methods demonstrate a way of being with the patient to help identify and support his or her own reasons for resolving ambivalence and ultimately making behavioral change (Miller & Rollnick, 2014). Although defined as being directive, this method is never authoritative, and does not involve giving advice or telling the patient what to do, since this usually results in further resistance to change (Miller & Rose, 2009). Rather, the approach is collaborative, supportive, and patient centered, since it values patient autonomy and recognizes that ultimately it is the person who will change or not. Even though MI was initially developed for use in counseling with people who have substance use disorders, it has been adapted for use in brief consultations within a variety of health care settings (Anstiss, 2009; Britt, Hudson, & Blampied, 2004; Mason, 2008). Since the intention of MI in health settings is always focused on increasing a patient's readiness to make health-related change, this approach is often used in conjunction with the Transtheoretical Model of Change, which views change as a process rather than as a discrete event, and it includes stages of precontemplation, contemplation, preparation, action, and maintenance (Prochaska & DiClemente, 1983).

Data related to this power component would include expression about the value that people place on health and health-related self-care, including priorities that facilitate or interfere with self-care, and how they manage those priorities. Do they persevere in working to accomplish health-related goals?

6. Ability to make decisions about care of self and to operationalize these decisions.

Decision making was discussed earlier as one of the operations associated with self-care. Operationalization of decisions may be both cognitive and psychomotor. As with motivation, advances in psychology and the neurosciences highlight the complexity of trying to understand the cognitive aspect of decision making. It appears to involve, at a minimum, anatomical structures, neurochemical systems, and past experiences. It may appear to be rational or irrational depending, in part, on the perspective of the person making or observing the decision-making process. It can be based on information and values within the conscious awareness of the decision maker. In this case, the basis for the decision making is explicit. Or decision making may be tacit, in which case the person is not explicitly aware of why particular choices are being made. The role of intuition in decision making has been studied, as well as what has been termed *naturalistic decision making*. Data include determining whether the person has a desire to change self-care routines and has a plan to do so or would like help in developing a plan. Do they engage in activities to prevent illnesses, have regular health-related checkups, and so forth?

7. Ability to acquire technical knowledge about self-care from authoritative sources, to retain it and operationalize it.

This ability is very complex, beginning with the ability to hear, see, or both, and then to process the information that is gathered through the senses. Older people watching television programs often complain that the dialogue moves too quickly for them to follow comfortably. This may be associated with changes in hearing, change in speed with which the brain processes data, or both. People with Parkinson's disease have trouble reading because of the slowing of the eye movements associated with dopamine transmission, which makes tracking and processing the written words difficult. They also may have trouble following audio–visual material. Then, there is the requirement to access information from authoritative sources. There may be limited access to appropriate information. Differentiating between reliable sources, advertising, hearsay, "old-wives" tales, cultural beliefs, and so on, can be difficult. Both processing and retaining information require intact cognitive functioning as well as reliable short-term and long-term memory. Understanding and operationalizing the knowledge goes back to the previous discussion about the processes of deliberate action.

Are authoritative sources accessed? Are cultural beliefs and informal sources valued over scientifically based information? Does the person have the skills and cognitive capacity to seek out appropriate information, to retain it, and to operationalize it? When they are required to change their lifestyle, can they explain the benefits of doing so?

8. A repertoire of cognitive, perceptual, manipulative, communication, and interpersonal skills adapted to the performance of self-care operations.

Is there evidence of ability to acquire knowledge? Is the cognitive system intact? Does the person take advantage of memory aids to augment cognition? Are the sensory systems intact? Is the person able to sustain effective interpersonal relationships?

To understand the complexity of this power component, list all of the self-care activities in which you engage in one 24-hour period. For each of these activities, identify the cognitive, perceptual, manipulative, communication, and interpersonal skills required to successfully act.

9. Ability to order discrete self-care actions or action systems into relationships with prior and subsequent actions.

This may be a problem for people with attention deficit disorder. Another example of this ability in action is the routine that one follows when getting ready for the day—washing, brushing teeth, and dressing appropriately for the weather. Think of a person who has diabetes. How would having that condition alter his or her morning activities? Now imagine a person who oversleeps. What new capabilities or coping skills are required to adjust the usual morning activities?

Does the person demonstrate the ability or describe being able to construct a systematic action system related to self-care? Does he or she have goals related to health and a systematic approach to accomplishing these goals? On the flip side, is the person obsessed with following a routine or is he or she unable or unwilling to do so?

10. Ability to consistently perform self-care operations, integrating them with relevant aspects of personal, family, and community living.

We live in a social world. Each person has a variety of role responsibilities for which he or she feels accountable. Often, these responsibilities may interfere with or be perceived to interfere with performance of self-care operations. When new self-care activities are required as a result of changing health state, new action systems may need to be developed. It is not uncommon for people to neglect various aspects of self-care as a result of any one or more of the foregoing situations. Self-esteem, self-concept, energy levels, and other factors may play a part in exercising this ability. Being unable to order an action sequence may interfere with integrating self-care into one's daily activities and responsibilities. Again, this may be especially true of children or adults who have attention deficit disorder.

THE STRUCTURE OF SELF-CARE AGENCY

Self-care agency has been described as a theoretical construct. It cannot be seen or measured as an entity. But the results of activating self-care agency can be evaluated—engagement in adequate or inadequate self-care practices. Then, the question follows: What differences in capabilities exist when self-care is adequate or inadequate? It is these capabilities that are the focus of concern in the diagnostic process. The structure of self-care agency outlined in Figure 7.1 provides an organizing framework for the diagnostic process associated with self-care agency. It references the therapeutic self-care demand and the components of self-care agency that are essential if the demand is to be met; these components have been discussed in the previous section.

Three clusters of capability have been identified as being useful to nursing practice (Taylor & Renpenning, 2011, p. 64). The first, level 1, is the most general—the operations of knowing, decision making, and acting. Does the person know what to do? Is he or she making appropriate decisions to act? Is he or she acting appropriately?

The second cluster, level 2, is a set of capabilities that are specific to self-care. These have been named the *power components* for self-care (Table 7.2). For example, two of the power components are the ability to attend to self as self-care agent and controlled use of available physical energy. An example of these being an area of concern is during an initial postpartum home visit. Attention is paid to whether or

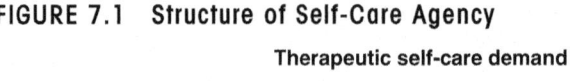

FIGURE 7.1   Structure of Self-Care Agency

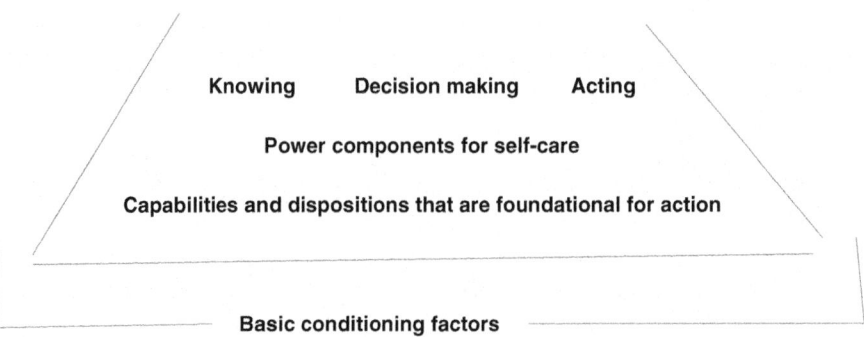

not the mother has an adequate diet and is getting sufficient rest. These are areas of concern, as they may affect having an adequate supply of breast milk.

In addition, basic conditioning factors also influence the capabilities to act.

The next cluster, level 3, is made up of capabilities and dispositions that are foundational to all forms of deliberate action (Table 7.1). They underlie each of the self-care operations. Information about these capabilities and dispositions provides more specific insight into why a person is or is not performing any one of the following: knowing, decision making, or acting. Examples include perception, memory, self-image, awareness, and learned skills such as reading and counting. Much of the knowledge related to this cluster has been developed in disciplines other than nursing but is accessed to answer nursing questions.

Underlying and influencing all of what has been mentioned earlier are the basic conditioning factors.

The diagnostic process can begin at any of the levels identified in the structure. For example, in the intensive care unit (ICU), the nurse may begin with determining whether the patient is conscious (a basic conditioning factor). A patient is not monitoring his blood pressure. Is this because of a lack of resources to purchase a monitoring device (level 3), or is it because of a lack of dexterity to manipulate the device accompanied by poor vision (level 1 and level 2)? Is it a lack of motivation (level 2)?

The characteristics of the components of self-care agency are addressed in the nursing diagnostic processes, as their relationship to components of the therapeutic self-care demand is evaluated. Assessment and diagnosis of self-care activities may take place at the broad level of self-care operations, the less general level of power components, or the very specific level of foundational capabilities and dispositions.

SUMMARY

Self-care is action. Self-care is accomplished through a series of actions or operations—knowing what to do, making a decision to follow a certain course of action, and acting. Each of these operations requires particular capabilities and dispositions. This complex set of capabilities and dispositions is represented by the term *self-care agency*. Self-care agency is multifaceted. In this chapter, the components of self-care agency are explored. Knowledge related to the structure, development, operability, and adequacy of self-care agency developed in the nursing sciences is essential knowledge for professional nursing practice. In addition, knowledge developed in the social sciences, physical sciences, medical science, and related disciplines is useful in answering nursing questions.

LEARNING ACTIVITY

The preceding discussion has illustrated the complexity of self-care agency and the challenges that nurses face in exploring and understanding the operability in a particular situation. Take time to explore the following articles to help broaden your understanding of the variables and conditioning factors related to the power to engage in self-care.

Anderson, J. A., & Olnhausen, K. S. (1999). Adolescent self-esteem: A foundational disposition. *Nursing Science Quarterly, 12*(1), 62–67.

Argyris, C., & Schön, D. (1978). *Organizational learning: A theory of action perspective.* New York, NY: McGraw-Hill.

Dickson, V., Cameron, J., Johnson, J. C., Bunker, S., Page, K., & Worrall-Carter, L. (2010). Symptom recognition in elders with heart failure. *Journal of Nursing Scholarship, 42*(1), 92–100.

Fleck, L. (2012). The nutrition self-care inventory. *Self-Care and Dependent Care Nursing, 19*(1), 26–34.

Klymko, K. W., Artinian, T., & Price, J. E. Abele, C., & Washington, O. G. (2011). Self-care production experiences in elderly African Americans with hypertension and cognitive difficulty. *Journal of the American Academy of Nurse Practitioners, 23*(4), 200–208. doi:10.1111/j.1745-7599.2011.00605.x

Lauck, S., Johnson, J., & Ratner, P. A. (2009). Self-care behaviour and factors associated with patient outcomes following same-day discharge percutaneous coronary intervention. *European Journal of Cardiovascular Nursing, 8*, 190–199. doi:10.1016/j.ejcnurse.2008.12.002

National Primary Care Research and Development Centre, The University of Manchester in Collaboration with the University of York. (2009). *What influences people to self-care?* Retrieved from http://www.population-health.manchester.ac.uk/primarycare/npcrdc-archive/Publications/WHAT_INFLUENCES_PEOPLE_TO_SELF_CARE_MARCH_2009.pdf

Riley, P. L., & Arslanian-Engoron, C. (2013). Cognitive dysfunction and self-care decision making in chronic heart failure: A review of the literature. *European Journal of Cardiovascular Nursing, 12*(6), 505–511. doi:10.1177/1474515113487463

Swanlund, S. L., Scherck, K. A., Metcalfe, S., & Jesek-Hale, S. R. (2008). Keys to successful self-management of medications. *Nursing Science Quarterly, 21*(3), 238–246. doi:10.1177/0894318408319276

Westlake, C., Sethares, K., & Davidson, P. (2013). How can health literacy influence outcomes in heart failure patients? Mechanisms and interventions. *Current Heart Failure Reports, 10*(3), 232–243. doi:10.1007/s11897-013-0147-7

References

Anderson, J. A., & Olnhausen, K. S. (1999). Adolescent self-esteem: A foundational disposition. *Nursing Science Quarterly, 12*(1), 62–67.

Anstiss, T. (2009). Motivational interviewing in primary care. *Journal of Clinical Psychology in Medical Settings, 16*(1), 87–93. doi:10.1007/s10880-009-9155-x

Argyris, C., & Schön, D. (1978). *Organizational learning: A theory of action perspective.* New York, NY: McGraw-Hill.

Backscheider, J. (1974). Self-care requirements, self-care capabilities and nursing systems. *American Journal of Public Health, 64,* 886–896.

Bandura, A. (1997). Self-efficacy: Toward a unifying theory of behavior change. *Psychological Review, 84,* 191–215.

Britt, E., Hudson, S. M., & Blampied, N. M. (2004). Motivational interviewing in health settings: A review. *Patient Education and Counseling, 53*(2), 147–155. doi:10.1016/S0738-3991(03)00141-1

Davidson, P. M., Daly, J., Leung, D., Ang, E., Paull, G., DiGiacomo, M., & Thompson, D. R. (2011). Health-seeking beliefs of cardiovascular patients: A qualitative study. *International Journal of Nursing Studies, 48*(11), 1367–1375. doi:10.1016/j.ijnurstu.2011.02.021

Furth, H. G. (1977). The operative and figurative aspects of knowledge in Piaget's theory. In B. A. Geber (Ed.), *Piaget and knowing: Studies in genetic epistemology.* London, UK: Routledge & Kegan Paul.

Mason, P. (2008). Motivational interviewing. *Practice Nurse, 35*(3), 43–48.

Medalia, A., & Saperstein, A. (2011). The role of motivation for treatment success. *Schizophrenia Bulletin, 37*(suppl 2), S122–S128.

Meyer, G. A. (2002). The art of watching out: Vigilance in women who have migraine headaches. *Qualitative Health Research, 12,* 1220–1234. doi:10.1177/1049732302238246

Miller, W. R., & Rollnick, S. (2014). *Motivational interviewing: Helping people change* (3rd ed.). New York, NY: Guilford Press. Retrieved from http://www.myilibrary.com.ezproxy1.lib.asu.edu?ID=394471

Miller, W. R., & Rose, G. S. (2009). Toward a theory of motivational interviewing. *American Psychologist, 64*(6), 527–537. doi:http://dx.doi.org/10.1037/a0016830

Moran, A. (2012). Attention theory. In S. Murphy (Ed.), *The Oxford handbook of sport and performance psychology* (pp. 39–43). New York, NY: Oxford University Press.

Morse, J. M., & O'Brien, B. (1995). Preserving self: From victim, to patient, to disabled person. *Journal of Advanced Nursing, 21,* 886–896.

Nursing Development Conference Group. (1979). *Concept formalization: Process and product* (2nd ed.). Boston, MA: Little, Brown.

Orem, D. E. (2001). *Nursing: Concepts of practice* (6th ed.). St. Louis, MO: Mosby.

Prochaska, J., & DiClemente, C. C. (1983). Stages and processes of self-change of smoking: Toward an integrative model of change. *Journal of Consulting Clinical Psychology, 51,* 390–395.

Rollnick, S., & Miller, W. R. (1995). What is motivational interviewing? *Behavioural and Cognitive Psychotherapy, 23,* 325–334.

Ryan, R. M., & Deci, E. L. (2000). Intrinsic and extrinsic motivations: Classic definitions and new directions. *Contemporary Educational Psychology, 25,* 54–67.

Suffet, F., & Lifshitz, M. (1991). Women addicts and threat of AIDS. *Qualitative Health Research, 1*(1), 51–79.

Taylor, S. G., & Renpenning, K. (2011). *Self-care science nursing theory and evidence-based practice.* New York, NY: Springer.

Tomstad, S. T., Söderhamn, U., Espnes, G. A., & Söderhamn, O. (2012). Living alone, receiving help, helplessness, and inactivity are strongly related to risk of under-nutrition among older home-dwelling people. *International Journal of General Medicine, 5,* 231–240.

Wadsworth, B. J. (1984). *Piaget's theory of cognitive and affective development* (3rd ed.). New York, NY: Longman.

White, Peters, & Schim. (2011). Spirituality and self-care: Expanding self-care deficit nursing theory. *Nursing Science Quarterly, 24*(3), 293. doi:1177/0894318411410888

CHAPTER 8

NURSING PRACTICE OPERATIONS

From Diagnosis to Designing the
Patient–Nursing System

Professional nursing practice includes the orderly execution of specific operations. These include diagnosis and prescription, design and planning, production, and control. An approach to nursing diagnosis is presented in this chapter that is most likely quite different than that you are used to. The focus of nursing diagnosis is not on treating a particular health state, but it is on establishing an understanding of relationships among components of the self-care system, self-care practices, conditioning factors, and evidence of an inability to perform the required health-related self-care. Having determined that an actual or potential self-care deficit exists, a prescription or plan for action is developed. Design is a cooperative activity occurring between patient, family, and nurse to determine which components of the prescription will be the target of action, who will participate in the action system, and to allocate roles and responsibilities. Planning is related to activities such as the allocation of resources and obtaining equipment. Production and control are concerned with implementation of the action system and evaluation of effectiveness or recommendation of revisions. Execution of each of these operations, precursors, and components of evidence-based practice is discussed in this chapter.

OBJECTIVES

After reading this chapter, the learner will be able to:

1. Describe nursing practice operations
2. Compare and contrast the traditional nursing process with the focus of nursing practice as viewed from the perspective of self-care deficit nursing theory
3. Demonstrate understanding of the theory of self-care deficit

4. Discuss three types of self-care limitations

5. Distinguish between self-care deficit and self-care limitations

6. Describe the process and outcome of nursing diagnosis from a self-care perspective

7. Explain what is involved in the processes of prescription and design

KEY CONCEPTS   nursing practice operations • self-care deficit • self-care limitations • nursing diagnosis • prescription for action • design

NURSING PRACTICE OPERATIONS

A practice operation is a mental process or a process of a practical nature that is necessary in some form of work or production. Nursing practice includes a series of mental and practical processes by which nursing is produced. These are nursing practice operations. Prior to formalizing nursing theories, the *nursing process* was defined as a problem-solving activity. Problem-based nursing had its origins in this perception of nursing practice, and early conceptions of nursing diagnosis were closely related to those of medicine. The health care professional interviews a person, does a physical assessment, may order some diagnostic studies or tests, and on the basis of this information comes to some conclusion (a diagnosis). Based on this conclusion, a further course of action or no action is prescribed.

You may be familiar with the North American Nursing Diagnosis Association (NANDA) listing or other such listings commonly used in charting and in electronic information systems. These listings are statements of conclusions. These commonly used listings have limitations when working from a self-care perspective, as they do not adequately reflect the action component associated with self-care, nor a consideration of the totality of the components of the nursing system. Many of the items in the listings would be considered conditioning factors and not diagnoses from the perspective of self-care deficit nursing theory. A good test of the utility of the statement for nursing purposes is, "Does it provide direction for nursing action?" The use of such listings limits the opportunity for describing the relationships among the variables that are associated with self-care, which, in turn, provide direction for nursing action.

When viewing nursing practice through the lens of nursing theories, the nursing process is conceptualized as more than the linear problem-solving process that begins with identifying the major concern, collecting data, selecting a diagnostic label that most closely relates to the data collected, and selecting and implementing an appropriate intervention. Rather, from the perspective of the self-care deficit nursing theory, the focus of nursing practice is on the relationships among patient, nurse, and person as well as among the identified variables associated with the power to produce self-care and the knowing and meeting of the therapeutic self-care demand.

The theory of the nursing system, embracing the theories of self-care deficit and self-care, provides direction for each of the operations that are associated with the design and production of the nursing system.

THE THEORY OF SELF-CARE DEFICIT

The theory of self-care deficit, which provides direction for diagnosis and prescriptions, proposes that maturing and mature people may have health-related limitations for actions that are associated with their own or their dependent's health states. As a result, they may be either completely or partially unable to know and/or to meet existent and emerging requirements for care for themselves or for their dependents. In such a situation, that is, when a self-care deficit exists, there may be a role for nursing. The term *self-care deficit* expresses a relationship between two variables—self-care agency and the therapeutic self-care demand. The self-care agency may be greater than, equal to, or less than the self-care demand. When a self-care deficit exists, the power or capabilities to produce the required self-care is less than the demand. It is important to note that *deficit* as used in this theory is neither a derogatory term nor is it meant to categorize a person as deficient. It is not a value judgment. It simply expresses the relationship between the demand, as represented by the right-hand side of the balance scale in Figure 8.1, and the capability, as represented by the left-hand side. In this representation, the demand is greater than the capability; so, a self-care deficit would exist. It should also be noted that the self-care deficit does not negate a health promotion approach. In order to promote health, one must infer some actual or potential limitation and design a program to meet that limitation. For example, a program to combat obesity is predicated on the assumption that the person lacks knowledge about the dangers of overeating, knowledge of basic nutrition to be able to make better choices in selecting food, some limitation in being able to control the source of the food (e.g., "I eat what I am served"), lack of resources, or limitation in accepting themselves as being seriously overweight. An individual who might seek out a health professional for assistance

FIGURE 8.1   Illustration of Self-Care Demand Greater Than Self-Care Agency = Need for Nursing

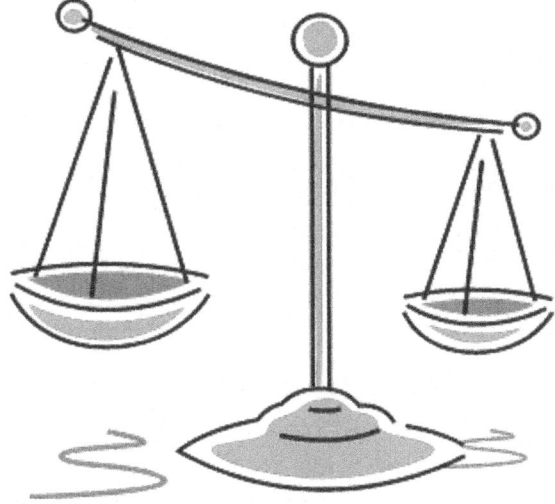

Self-care agency   Self-care demand

in improving health or fitness is doing so on the assumption that more could be done to meet health goals.

SELF-CARE LIMITATIONS

On a day-to-day basis, we take self-care for granted. Only when requirements for self-care change or when a person does not or cannot perform one or more of the self-care operations—acquiring knowledge about required actions, making a decision, and acting—do we ask, *why?* We become aware of specific abilities and conditioning factors that make it possible for a person to perform self-care when we begin to explore the *why not.* We may also become aware of specific factors that are interfering with or limiting the production of self-care—self-care limitations. Some of these self-care limitations have been identified and are presented next. This presentation is not considered complete.

Self-care limitations are factors that affect the ability of the person to perform one or more of the self-care operations of knowing what to do, decision making, or acting. Some of these limiting factors are controllable, whereas others are not.

Limitations of Knowing About How the Body Functions, and the Self-Care Actions Required

There may be a requirement to do things differently than one has been used to. For example:

- Having to change a diet in order to lower cholesterol

- Adjusting to changes in the way a body functions, such as occurs after a stroke

- Integrating into one's regimen a new prescription for helping to manage self-care such as that associated with being newly diagnosed with diabetes

There may be changes in the neurological system, which affect physiological and psychological functioning. These may include sensory deficits, variations in cognitive functioning, levels of consciousness, and rational thinking. Electrolyte imbalances and side effects of drugs and/or use of illegal substances may result in organic disorders affecting thinking or rational behavior. Mental and emotional disorders may affect both development and exercise of components of self-care agency. There may be factors associated with neurochemical pathology that affect rational agency. Cultural beliefs may not be consistent with reality. Limitations such as those mentioned earlier affect knowing when to take action and what action to take, attaching meaning to a situation (sense making), perception, and knowing how to organize an action system, including what is the appropriate or therapeutic sequencing of actions.

Limitations for knowing may also include not having enough information to know what questions to ask or who to ask. People may not have enough accurate antecedent knowledge to reason within a self-care frame of reference. There may be a language barrier or cultural factors that inhibit asking appropriate questions. In addition to interventions directed toward the patient, there may be group or community programs that are designed to assist people in overcoming or managing these limitations.

Limitations for Making Judgments and Decisions

There may be insufficient information on which to base a decision. There may be cognitive components that limit the person's ability to discriminate between options. There may be difficulty deciding what to do or for a number of reasons such as stress, pressure from outside sources, or fear of consequences if a particular course of action is followed. The person may decide on a course of action but then choose not to act. The provision of data is not necessarily the provision of usable information. In order for data to become meaningful, some interpretation is necessary. When an individual understands what he or she has been told, he or she is more able to make an informed decision.

Limitations Associated With Implementing a Course of Action

There are a myriad of reasons that a person might have issues with implementing a course of action. There may be lack of specific skills or resources related to accomplishing the required self-care. A lack of energy has been identified as a limiting factor in exercising self-care agency. There may be other priorities for action, lack of interest, motivation, and persistence to care for self. Culture plays a part in implementing self-care actions as do family values and family system functioning. Outside interferences such as family crises and social disasters are obvious interferences in the exercise of self-care agency. Some foundational capabilities and dispositions may limit the ability to implement a course of action. In a classic work, Backscheider (1974) described limitations for taking action associated with the level of operative knowing of the patients. Health care providers tend to speak in abstract and complex terms. Backscheider described people who are concrete thinkers and designed a clinic for patients with diabetes as a result of her study. Patient education materials have improved since then, but many still use concepts and language that the patient may not understand or know how to use.

OVERVIEW OF DIAGNOSIS AND PRESCRIPTION

Nurses use their investigatory skills and knowledge to find answers to questions that are specific to the focus of nursing, that is, the self-care system of the person under care in a specific environmental situation. In addition to objective information collected through physical assessment and diagnostic studies, the diagnostic process in nursing involves eliciting information about self-care practices from patients and/or significant others. This information is supplemented by information about events, conditions, and circumstances that have occurred and are affecting people in their environmental situations as well as affecting their motivation and ability to engage in appropriate self-care at a particular point in time. Validation of judgments occurs through the interaction and communication between the nurse, the person under care and/or significant others, and other health care providers. This is a complex interpersonal process and, as such, the nature and characteristics of the interpersonal relationships are significant conditioning factors affecting both the questions and the answers. In nursing practice, a description of the relationships may be more helpful than a diagnostic label. The processes of diagnosis and prescription begin with exploring the current self-care system and self-care practices. In theory, diagnosis precedes prescription; in the following discussion, the processes are presented as linear. However, in actual practice, diagnosis and prescription are occurring constantly and almost simultaneously. These processes involve constantly seeking answers to the questions, "What is?" "Why?" "What should be?" and "What can be done?" Both art and science are involved in the information gathering and validation of judgments, and in the interaction and communication that occurs between the nurse, other health care providers, the person under care, and/or significant others. The nature and characteristics of the interpersonal relationships are significant factors affecting both the questions and the answers.

Reflection on the technological, social, and interpersonal dimensions of the situation is a part of this process. Simultaneously, the nurse is collecting data, determining the interrelationships and meaning inherent in the data, and coming to some conclusion based on the facts available. In seeking a solution to any problem, the answer to the question, "What data should be collected?" is determined by the focus of concern, the questions being asked, the knowledge base available to both ask and answer the questions, and theories that provide direction for further exploration.

As described in previous chapters, the focus of concern relates to the proper object of the discipline of nursing—the inability of a person to provide the quantity and quality of required self-care. Questions guiding nursing inquiry include: "What are the purposes of self-care actions at this point in time?" "What actions are required to achieve those purposes (the self-care demand)?" "Is self-care adequate?" "Is self-care agency developed?" "Is it operable?" "Is it adequate?" "What are the requirements for nursing?" More detailed questions, specific to the situation but still reflecting this perspective, guide the investigation related to the specific situation. The information gleaned, in turn, is used in selecting a method of helping and designing a plan of care, which, when implemented, becomes the nursing system.

Prescription involves evaluating related strengths, capabilities, limitations, and working with patients to select the most appropriate actions in relationship to self-care demand. Having determined the presence of a self-care deficit, the next step is prescribing a course of action. What assistance is required? What will the patient be responsible for doing? Are other family members or support people to be involved? What will be the role of nursing? Foundational to prescription is getting an understanding of what the person is willing or unwilling to do. Until the person understands and accepts the need for action, there is little likelihood that he or she will follow through with any plan of action that the nurse may prescribe. The idea of negotiating the self-care demand and prescribing actions that are agreed on by the patient is valuable. As previously noted (Chapter 4), systems thinking requires that one do the right thing even if it is done in a slow way. This is especially important in helping patients manage chronic illness (Table 8.1).

The methods of helping that are appropriate in the situation are a function of the characteristics of the development, operability, and adequacy of the self-care

TABLE 8.1 Components of the Nursing System

Self-Care Deficit	Method of Helping	Patient Actions	Nursing Actions	Nursing Agency
Motivation to quit smoking	Guidance and support	Use telephone support system when tempted to smoke.	Support positive efforts to stop smoking.	Knowledge of strategies to facilitate stopping smoking
Inability to be consistent in regular intake of nutritional requirements	Guidance and support Teaching	Budget for food. Plan meals ahead. Learn about which foods meet requirements. See dentist.	Establish helpful relationship with patient. Facilitate meal planning. Provide information in appropriate format.	Acceptance of patient preferences Accommodation of preferences in meal plan

agency and the capability of involved family members in relation to the nature of the self-care deficit. Selection of the method of helping begins with working with the patient to identify his or her goals. The goal may be as simple as "to stop smoking for a week." What specific action will the person have to take to accomplish that goal? What help is needed from nursing? There may be more than one method of helping employed at any one time. In selecting a method of helping, it is also important to determine whether the required action has an internal orientation such as a need for learning and decision making related to not smoking, or an external orientation such as supporting a person in his or her decision to stop smoking.

Based on the specifics of the self-care deficit(s) and the goals, and having identified the methods of helping that are appropriate, the next step is clarifying the roles of patient, nurse, and others who may be involved. The following process operations are presented as a guide to areas for this exploration. This information is presented in a linear fashion, which is not the way you will be using it in practice. It will not be appropriate to explore every area in every situation. Begin exploration where the person is and through the processes of constant comparison and analysis, proceed from there, dependent on information gleaned and conclusions drawn.

When considering the self-care system, try thinking not about self-care in relation to the specific health state such as "nutrition self-care," "diabetic self-care," or "heart-failure self-care." Think of self-care as a totality influenced by many variables. The person is living in a sociocultural environment with many more factors impacting day-to-day existence and the self-care system than just health state. The person and the nurse within the nursing situation are concerned with management and implementation of the integrated self-care and nursing systems, thus operationalizing the expressions *holistic view, holistic care,* and *holistic nursing.*

THE DIAGNOSTIC PROCESS AND RELATED QUESTIONS

Questions to Be Answered

1. Conditioning factors

- Which basic conditioning factors and/or foundational capabilities and dispositions are currently influencing the actions that the person will have to take to care for self (conditioning the demand)?
- Which requisites are affected?
- How are usual self-care practices affected?
- How are these conditioning factor(s) influencing components of self-care agency?

2. Overview of self-care requisites that are affected in the current situation

- What are current methods of meeting the requisite?
- What is the person's judgment that the requisite is met/unmet?
- What are objective indicators/cues that the requisite is met/unmet?
- What is the nurse's judgment of whether the requisite is met, unmet, or at risk for being unmet?

3. Overview of self-care agency

- What are the self-care limitations?
- Is self-care agency developed? What is the potential for development?
- Is self-care agency operable? What is the potential for operability?
- Is self-care agency adequate to meet affected requisites now or in the future?

4. Calculate the therapeutic self-care demand

- Describe the actions required to achieve the desired self-care goals.
- This involves thinking in three dimensions at the same time: thinking about requisites of concern, conditioning factors affecting those requisites, and interplay among the action systems that are associated with meeting each requisite.

5. Establish preliminary goals for action

- Evaluate/describe the relationship between self-care demand and self-care agency.
- Share description of the relationship with the patient.
- Determine goals of the patient (basis for developing adjusted therapeutic self-care demand).
- Adjust action system based on preceding information.

6. Describe the self-care deficit

- Describe adjusted therapeutic self-care demand.
- Reevaluate the relationship between self-care agency and adjusted self-care demand.
- Describe existing and/or projected self-care deficit.

The data that will inform nursing practice have been presented in a linear fashion—lists of self-care requisites and related actions, lists of power components, and so on. This is not how practice works. Many of the items presented are areas you may already consider in your practice. The model is like a map—it presents a global view of the current and potential concerns in the situation but that is all. In practice, you will begin where the patient is and proceed on a circuitous route by using the "map" to guide exploration while following the clues provided by the patient and your knowledge base as a nurse to get to the end point—determining the nature of the need for nursing.

Selecting a Method of Helping

Helping involves interpersonal communication. It requires establishing a particular type of relationship with another. If a person is unconscious, that communication occurs through touch and voice. If a person is able to participate in the helping relationship through decision making or doing, the responsibilities for the care actions are distributed between the person requiring the care and the helper(s). This helping relationship has moral, ethical, and legal dimensions as well as is affected by cultural beliefs and related rules of appropriateness. The method of helping that is appropriate in the situation is influenced by all of these factors and by the nature of the self-care deficit.

In the situation described next, considering the self-care deficits identified, the appropriate methods of helping would include guiding and supporting, providing a developmental environment, and teaching. Teaching is the appropriate method in relation to meeting the new components of the self-care demand associated with the colostomy. In implementing the teaching process, it would be essential to assess John's current knowledge and understanding of what it means to have a colostomy, how he feels about having a colostomy, his stage of acceptance of this condition, and his readiness to learn. Guidance and support are appropriate in the process of managing his colostomy within the broader context of daily living. Provision of a developmental environment as he adjusts his self-image to the new normal and makes required adjustments is related to interpersonal relationships. In the early stages, there may be a need to act for or do with him in managing the colostomy until the necessary skill level is attained.

DESIGN

"Design is a core process of a professional. . . . [an] intellectual activity that requires both practical experience and theoretical support" (Taylor & Renpenning, 2011, pp. 135–136). "Design occurs in the context of the specific. The elements of design include understanding the operational environment, setting the problem, developing

CASE EXAMPLE

John has just come home from the hospital with a colostomy after a partial colon resection 10 days ago for a malignancy. No follow-up therapy is planned. He is 80 years old, a retired sales person, and lives in an apartment with his wife of 50 years; they have no immediate family in the area. He has all the supplies he needs to look after the colostomy, including a very complete instruction sheet. The discharge information sheet indicates that he has had an opportunity to participate in colostomy care before leaving the hospital, but it does not contain any information about how he is managing his colostomy or how he feels about it. His wife has had no instruction regarding care of the colostomy. That is all I know about him. Where do I start?

Begin where he is—his self-care practices—and as you do so think in three dimensions at the same time (systems thinking) while considering the interrelationships among:

- **The most significant conditioning factors** immediately apparent in the situation—diagnosis of cancer, the colostomy, living with his wife, no family support in the area, and an 80-year-old recovering from major surgery

- **His current self-care practices** and how they are affected immediately and also in the long term by the significant conditioning factors—managing colostomy, disposal of wastes, monitoring skin, regulating elimination, adjusting diet, adjusting to this being the new normal, maintaining social contacts, adjusting to impact of changing health state on lifestyle, age, conditions of living, and previous experiences

- **Using what you know about the** *components of self-care agency* to identify specific strengths and limitations related to making the adjustments to self-care practices that are required in the immediate future. What components of self-care agency will require the attention of nursing?

The result of this constant comparative analysis of relationships leads to a description of the therapeutic self-care demand and an expression of existing or potential self-care deficits.

The nature of the self-care deficit then provides direction for selecting the appropriate method of helping and prescribing a course of action.

Examples of components of the therapeutic self-care demand for John would include the following:

- Adjust content and timing of intake of food in relation to bowel elimination.

- Balance rest and activity, getting enough rest for healing to occur and activity to aid in recovery of regular gastrointestinal (GI) functioning.

- Care for the colostomy per instructions; monitor skin integrity.

- Maintain social contacts.

- Accept self as needing help in managing the changing method of bowel elimination as well as in care of colostomy.
- Know when and how to call for professional help.

Examples of components of self-care agency in relation to self-care demand:

- John has always seen himself as very much in control of himself and his surroundings, able to do what he wants to and when.
- He says he is the decision maker in the family, makes the financial decisions, and so forth.
- He says he has always been basically a private person, keeping his problems to himself, and not reaching out for help.
- John has never been particularly aware of the relationship between bowel habits and eating content or timing, never having had any problems in this area.

Example of expression of self-care deficit:

- He lacks knowledge related to the association between the intake of food and bowel elimination.
- He has had little experience relying on others for assistance and has difficulty reaching out to others and accepting help when required. He has always been the decision maker. This has the potential for a negative impact on the relationship with his wife.

In the case of John, the actions related to meeting the components of the therapeutic self-care demand associated with managing the colostomy and intake of food are pretty straightforward. New knowledge and new skills are required, both of which John is capable of learning. His decision-making pattern is well established and not likely to change. This may be problematic, as he is faced with current and future health-related situations over which he has little or no control. In Chapter 10, the nature of a collaborative care system is described. If John and his wife have a long-established collaborative care system, the nurse must take the roles and functions of both John and his wife into consideration when designing the nursing system.

a design concept, and assessment and reframing" (p. 136). Design is made specific to the individual patient when roles and actions of the nurse and the patient are determined in relation to self-care tasks and adjustments of components of the therapeutic self-care demand. The design may also include direction for regulating, protecting, and developing self-care agency. If working from a self-care perspective in an organizational setting and employing the use of standard care plans, it will probably be necessary to modify the care plan to incorporate the self-care variables into the design of the plan for the individual person. Part of the design process includes incorporation of processes to determine the effectiveness of the nursing system and making adjustments to the system based on information regarding the effectiveness—evidence-based nursing in action that provides the theoretical support.

Planning involves specification of any or all of the following: time, place, environmental conditions, equipment, and supplies required to implement or produce the system. This includes the manpower required for effective production. Adjustment of the plan to accommodate situational changes is part of the process of professional responsibility. Nurses are familiar with the term *nursing care plan*, particularly in institutional settings. Planning follows design and specifies the who, what, where, when, and how the design is to be carried out, as well as the actions to be taken.

Examples of Elements of a Design for a Nursing System

The tasks to be accomplished in designing the nursing system include:

Identifying the self-care tasks to be performed in a coordinated fashion within specified times

Making adjustments in constructing the ongoing therapeutic self-care demand

Regulating the exercise of self-care agency

Protecting powers of self-care agency

Providing for development of self-care agency. (Taylor & Renpenning, 2011, p. 141)

SPECIAL CASE

Once again, we return to the case example of Mrs. Smith, prior to her discharge from the hospital. In designing the discharge plan for Mrs. Smith, the nurse will list the things that need to be done, such as therapeutic exercise of her hip; eating three meals with high protein and calcium; taking pain medication before therapy and before bed; resting in the afternoon for at least 1 hour; drinking water at meals and at least one glass in between each; not drinking water after dinner meal except as needed for taking medications; keeping incision clean and dry by using warm water; cleansing at the sink until wound heals; showering when okayed by MD; observing for signs of infection, such as redness around the incision, or other unusual signs; and keeping track of return appointment times and contact information for care coordinator, nurse practitioner, or physician.

The nurse will help Mrs. Smith decide how she will accomplish these tasks, what other concerns she might have now and in the near future, and ways to adjust her environment to protect herself, such as removing scatter rugs, installing hand holds for the toilet, and adjusting the height of chairs and the bed for ease of sitting and rising.

The professional nurse is responsible for designing the nursing system of care within the context of other systems of care and the context of daily living. A coordinated interprofessional plan is the ideal. When the plan of care is designed, the tasks or work to be done may be delegated to others as appropriate.

LEARNING ACTIVITY

Select a patient situation well known to you. Following the processes described in this chapter, determine the nursing diagnosis and design an appropriate nursing system.

References

Backscheider, J. E. (1974). Self-care requirements, self-care capabilities, and nursing systems in the diabetic nurse management clinic. *American Journal of Public Health*, *64*(12), 1138–1146.

Taylor, S. G., & Renpenning, K. (2011). *Self-care science, nursing theory, and evidence-based practice*. New York, NY: Springer.

CHAPTER 9

PRODUCTION AND CONTROL OPERATIONS AND EVIDENCE-BASED PRACTICE

Production and control are, to a great extent, the managerial functions of nursing. They relate to how care is given to each patient and to a population of patients. You began learning production operations when you first started learning skills in your original program and gained some expertise as you moved forward in your practice. In Chapter 8, we described the operations of designing and planning. The operations discussed here relate to the doing components of nursing. How does the work of nursing get done? How do we make the plan work? The production operations are more familiar; the control operations are usually thought of as evaluation but are more than that. "The nurse manager role is becoming more complex and falling to nurses with less experience. The responsibilities and challenges they face include staffing their units, hiring and coaching employees; meeting quality standards; and ensuring patient and nurse satisfaction" (Trossman, 2015, p. 1).

In this chapter, the link between a conceptual framework for nursing practice and organizational variables related to production and control is addressed. As you progress in assuming more and more professional responsibilities, understanding the relationship between organizational variables and professional practice becomes increasingly important. One of the responsibilities of the professional nurse is providing input into the development of organizational variables that affect both patient care and nursing practice. As an RN, you know that nursing care is provided to individual people within context. To more accurately and efficiently produce and control nursing and as you become more specialized, the description of the clinical population you serve will be viewed with more precision, based on your expanding knowledge and clarified nursing lens. Since knowing the parameters of the population to be served from a nursing perspective is basic to the provision of care to individuals, that process is described and the utility of such descriptions is illustrated. A structure for categorizing data associated with nursing practice that could be incorporated into an electronic patient record is included. The impact of these on evidence-based practice is addressed. The chapter concludes with a perspective on what constitutes the characteristics of professional practice.

OBJECTIVES

After reading this chapter, the learner will be able to:

1. Know the role of the nurse as caregiver and care manager
2. Know the managerial operations for delivery of nursing in patient, unit, or population situations
3. Describe the relationship between organizational variables and professional practice
4. Identify variables of concern to nursing that should be included in electronic health records (EHRs)
5. Describe a population utilizing a conceptual framework for nursing practice

KEY CONCEPTS   production • control • population • appropriate care • profession as manager • data elements and outcomes

PRODUCTION AND CONTROL

Provision of nursing services requires knowing the nursing needs of a person or a population and evaluating nursing action in relation to those needs. The population may be the patients in a hospital unit or nursing home, or the clientele of an agency such as home health or hospice. Description of a population is a precursor to design and production. Although nursing services are provided through the actions of individual nurses, the majority of nursing is provided by nurses employed by health care agencies. Consequently, the health care organizations have had and continue to have a major impact on nursing practice, the organization and development of nursing knowledge, funding for nursing research, and the emergence of evidence-based practice.

The accomplishment of the actions decided on or planned for raises questions for the nurse as to how to proceed with the selected actions: What must I do? What resources are needed and available? Do I need assistance? If so, who is best to help? The nurse then begins to do the work. As the actions are being performed, there is simultaneous evaluation as to the effect of the action on the prescribed outcome and the simultaneous change in the design. The feedback provides the substance for making changes at the time of taking action or in a more purposeful evaluation afterward. Control functions include this evaluation and adjustment not just of particular sets of actions but also of the whole system so that a coordinated system of care is provided. Control operations include monitoring, observation, and appraisal. Is the patient receiving the care required? Are the actions producing the desired effect? What in the system is impeding the care? Would changes in the environment facilitate the caregiving? Is the distribution of actions or work between the patient and the nurse appropriate?

DEFINING A POPULATION

Defining a population from a nursing perspective is an essential component in providing consistent care and in evaluating the effectiveness of nursing intervention or action. Defining a specific population or the characteristics of the members of a group can be the basis for planning care and care delivery systems, developing standards of care, and creating protocols to be used in providing care. From these general descriptions, care can then be particularized for an individual patient. Evaluation of the effectiveness of nursing action is a responsibility of the individual professional nurse as well as of the organizations offering health care services. Measurement of the effectiveness of nursing from a personal as well as an organizational perspective requires answering the following questions:

- What is the condition/variable of concern to us?
- What do we hope to achieve—our expected outcomes?
- How do we expect to achieve these?
- How will we measure our accomplishments?
- How do we determine why we did or did not make a difference?

The term *population* is commonly applied to people who are defined by geography, as in a particular community, city, country, and so on. It may also apply to an aggregate of people who are defined by common characteristics such as homeless people, people in a community with mental illness, surgical patients in a hospital, and residents of a long-term care facility. The process of defining an aggregate or a population begins with selecting an organizing variable such as one or more of the data elements and categories described in Table 9.1.

Nursing has traditionally identified the populations served by medical terms (surgical, obstetrical), location of service (emergency, critical care), age (children, adult health), or medical diagnosis (people with heart failure, people with type 2 diabetes, and postnatal patients). Certainly, people within each of these categories have common requirements for assistance in managing their self-care. However, describing our populations from a nursing perspective focuses on the requirements for nursing that are similar across categories of medical diagnoses and gives us another perspective on the specifics of requirements for nursing services. Standards of nursing care can be developed for the described population, the care delivered can be described, and the outcomes of nursing services can be evaluated. This also emphasizes the need to ensure that the elements in the database reflect the concerns of nursing.

Defining a population can have meaning for the individual practitioner as well as for the health care organization providing nursing services. I would like to share the following personal experience with you.

Community health nurses in an inner-city situation were responsible for the following people with tuberculosis, ensuring that they were cooperating with their treatment. Working with this group of people was challenging, as they had alcohol and substance abuse disorders. The nurses saw their responsibility as more than providing medication at the time the patients came for their welfare checks. They became interested in studying this group further when some university students came for field work. With fresh eyes the students focused on the nutritional

TABLE 9.1 Data to Inform Effectiveness of Self-Care System

- **Conditioning factors**
  - Personal factors
    - Age, sex
    - Residence and environmental conditions
    - Family system factors
    - Sociocultural, education, occupation
    - Socioeconomic factors
  - Patterns of living
  - Health state and health care system
    - Medical diagnosis
    - Nurse-determined conditions
    - Patient's description of health state
    - Family members' description
    - Health care system features
  - Developmental state
    - Patient's goals for the future
    - Objective appraisal future re development
    - Self-management capabilities
    - Factors affecting self-management

- **Data elements associated with self-care requisites**
  - Universal requisites
    - Maintain sufficient intake of air
    - Maintain sufficient intake of water
    - Maintain sufficient intake of food
    - Provide care associated with elimination
    - Maintain balance between rest and activity
    - Maintain balance between solitude and social action
    - Prevent hazards to life, functioning, and well-being
    - Promotion of normalcy
  - Developmental requisites
    - Provide materials for physiological development in accord with stages of physical development
    - Provide environmental, physical, and social conditions to ensure feelings of comfort, safety, sense of closeness to another, and sense of being cared for
    - Prevent sensory overload, sensory deprivation
    - Promote and maintain affective and cognitional development
    - Provide conditions to facilitate development of skills that are essential for living in a society
    - Foster awareness of self as a person within a family and community
    - Regulate physical, biological, and social environment to promote development of skills to manage states of fear or anxiety

(continued)

TABLE 9.1 Data to Inform Effectiveness of Self-Care System *(continued)*

- Health deviation self-care requisites
  - Seeking and securing appropriate medical assistance
  - Being aware of and attending to pathological conditions, including effects on development
  - Effectively carrying out prescribed diagnostic, therapeutic, and rehabilitative measures
  - Being aware of and attending to deleterious or discomforting effects of prescribed therapies, including effects on development

- **Self-care agency**
  - Self-care limitations, capabilities
    - Knowing
    - Decision making
    - Performing self-care
  - Power components of self-care
    - Maintenance of attention and vigilance with respect to self as self-care agent
    - Controlled use of available physical energy for self-care
    - Ability to control the position of the body and body parts for self-care
    - Ability to reason within a self-care frame of reference
    - Motivation for self-care
    - Ability to make decisions about self-care and to operationalize these
    - Ability to acquire knowledge from authoritative sources, to retain it, and to operationalize it
    - Repertoire of cognitive, perceptual, manipulative, communication, and interpersonal skills adapted to the performance of self-care operations
    - Ability to order discreet self-care actions or action systems to achieve self-care goals
    - Ability to consistently perform self-care operations and to integrate them with relevant personal, family, and community living

- **Foundational capabilities and dispositions**
  - Conditioning factors affecting capabilities and dispositions
    - Genetic and constitutional factors
    - Arousal state
    - Social organization
    - Culture
    - Experience
  - Selected basic capabilities
    - Sensation: proprioception and esteroception
    - Learning
    - Exercise or work

(continued)

TABLE 9.1 Data to Inform Effectiveness of Self-Care System *(continued)*

- Regulation of the position and movement of the body and body parts
- Attention
- Perception
- Memory
- Central regulation of motivational, emotional processes
- Knowing and doing capabilities
  - Rational agency
  - Operational knowing
  - Learned skills: for example, reading, writing, counting, reasoning
  - Self-consistency in knowing and doing
- Dispositions affecting goals sought
  - Self-understanding
  - Self-awareness
  - Self-concept
  - Self-value
  - Self-acceptance
  - Self-concern
  - Willingness to meet needs of self
  - Future directedness

- **Community variables/systems with community effect on self-care system**
  - Public policy
  - Environment
  - Legislation
  - Communication
  - Health care policies and available services
  - Power brokers
  - Resources
  - Predominant sociocultural values
  - Transportation

requirements of this patient group. They identified that they were not eating properly and should be taught what foods they should eat and how best to prepare them. The problem was that most of these people did not have access to cooking facilities or storage places for food, and teaching did not seem to be the best approach. The nurses began looking at these patients not as individuals but as a group of people with some common conditioning factors affecting their health. In talking among themselves about these, the nurses came up with three categories:

1. Older men who lived relatively stable lives. They tended to eat at the same food lines, drink in the same bars, and lived in the same rooming house at least for a month at a time.

2. Younger men who abused alcohol and drugs. There were no regular places where they ate and drank, making it harder for the nurses to follow up on them. They did eat at food lines, lived in rooming houses but tended to move frequently.

3. Young women who were often dependent on men for support and companionship. They lived wherever their current man lived. They too ate at food lines. (*Note*: There were no older women.)

The nurses concluded that development of appropriate self-management systems was hindered not just by lack of knowledge but also by the conditions of living, lack of adequate resources, results of drug abuse, and sociocultural orientation. These specifically interfered with:

- Ability to consistently manage self-care

- Ability to reason within a self-care frame of reference

- Motivation for self-care

- Decision making

Based on this information, the nurses constructed a data collection tool that identified what people in each subgroup needed to do to promote specific aspects of their health and the related capabilities. As a result of this project, the information that the nurses recorded changed from physical findings and medication administration to data about self-management abilities, factors interfering with developing or exercising these, and nursing interventions and outcomes.

In analyzing this population, it became evident that action was also required at the community level. Attention was then directed at the quality of food being served at the food lines and was also directed at the housing, as in discussion it became apparent that one of the reasons for moving was poor sanitation. Another by-product of this investigation was recognizing that the group of unstable young men required more nursing time than the remainder of the population.

With the recording system in place that reflected not only nursing time spent on medication administration and physical assessment but also on activities related to improving self-management skills, it would be possible to get a more accurate picture of the relationship between patient requirements and nursing services, including costs and outcomes.

The initial analysis of the data provided an impetus for action at the community level. Incorporation of the data regarding activity aimed at improving self-management for individual patients, and results of intervention strategies provided a database for the planning of nursing services for this population.

The preceding example illustrates that individual nurses can make a difference in the organization. The nurses in this example moved from following their job descriptions as identified in the policies of the organization (monitoring people with tuberculosis in the community) to thinking as professional practitioners, identifying the variables of concern to nursing, and employing systems thinking to analyze the data associated with those variables. This gave them a nursing perspective on the situation rather than a medical or an epidemiological perspective, and the result was a new solution to an old problem. They knew before the project started that self-management skills were an issue across the board in this downtown city center population, but they had no organized way to collect these data or to share this information with those responsible for planning care at the organization level. Use of the conceptual framework in data collection and analysis provided them with this organizing tool.

By developing our own categories, we can facilitate the development of nursing knowledge—people with low self-esteem demonstrating limitations for decision making; or postnatal patients who are eligible for discharge from the hospital but are having difficulty establishing breastfeeding. This information can be incorporated into policies and standards of care. For example, patients ready for discharge who are having difficulty establishing breastfeeding will be referred to a community health nurse or a lactation specialist for follow-up. The development of such standards is important not only in the accreditation process but also to identify variables linked to monitoring quality of practice. Description of the population served from a nursing rather than from a medical perspective also provides nursing with a more precise way of costing nursing services, determining nurse staffing requirements, and ensuring nursing-sensitive outcomes.

Examples of Descriptions of Populations Utilizing Variables of Concern to Nursing

Populations—for example, in a rehabilitation setting—may be identified by the nature of the self-care limitations. For example, the target population for the nursing system comprises people exhibiting one or more of the following limitations:

- Limitation in movement arising from spinal cord injury, brain injury, other neurological impairments, joint replacements, and injury to the musculoskeletal system

- Limitations in cognitive functioning associated with brain injury

- Limitations in adaptation of self and lifestyle associated with physical disability

- Limitations/inability of dependent-care agent to accept/manage the dependent's self-care and/or his or her combined self-/dependent-care system

This description of a population can highlight the need for specific assessment tools and staff development programs.

Or the target population in a community setting may be described as:

Women of child-bearing years who have a baby aged 0 through 28 days. This population includes women who are experiencing or who are likely to experience limitations in their self-care agency as a result of a live birth. In addition, the woman is expected to function as a dependent-care agent for her infant. The self-care requisites may be associated with the following:

- Labor process

- Postpartum healing

- Adaptation to parenting

- Dependent-care agency role
- Integration of infant into the family
- Maintenance of marital bond

Again, identification of the particular requisites that are generally of concern in this population can be linked to the focus of concern in the assessment and service delivery processes.

THE DATA BANK, STANDARDS OF PRACTICE, AND MEASURING OUTCOMES

The following standards of nursing practice illustrate one way that the use of a conceptual framework for practice can facilitate internal consistency between the data elements of an EHR, development of standards of practice, identification of nursing-sensitive indicators, and evaluation of quality of practice.

- Within 24 hours of admission, the nurse has collected data about the patient's perception of his or her problem, evaluated his or her usual patterns of living and self-care practices, and identified the changes in self-care practices that are required as a result of his or her current health state. The sources for this information include the patient, the family, the physician, the health record, and other relevant people.

- Within 24 hours of admission, the nurse will have analyzed the data to determine the current nursing diagnoses (i.e., relationship of self-care agency to the components of the current therapeutic self-care demand in light of current conditioning factors).

- The therapeutic self-care demand will be continuously recalculated, and its relationship to self-care agency will be reevaluated.

- Existing and projected self-care deficits will be recorded appropriately at the change of each shift.

PERFORMANCE REVIEW GUIDELINES

The standards of practice can, in turn, be linked to the performance review guidelines as illustrated in the following items.

An audit of records of patients cared for by this nurse indicates that:

- The data collected include the patient's perception of his or her problem, his or her usual patterns of living and self-care practices, the changes in therapeutic self-care demand brought about by his or her current health state, and his or her capability to meet the demand.

- Current and projected self-care deficits are calculated and recorded for patients within 24 hours of their admission. Revised statements of self-care deficits are recorded as appropriate at each change of the shift.

- The self-care deficit statements include the following components: the limitation for action and the associated basic conditioning factor or foundational capability, as well as the specific action demand.

PROFESSIONAL NURSE AS CAREGIVER

Performing Care as Skilled Expert

Benner's work was published in 1984, and the phrase *novice to expert* came into our lexicon as a way of viewing the development of the self as expert nurse. Her focus was on the process of skill acquisition in nursing. She proposed that skill development proceeded from novice, advanced beginner, competent, and proficient to expert. "It is difficult to appreciate the nonreflective, noncognitive, responsive nature of expert performance and how hugely different this is from the rule-following of beginners and competent-level performers" (Day, 2009, n.p). Dreyfus (2007) describes expert performance as "arational"—not only irrational but also not analytic or calculative; experts live in a world of affordances and solicitations that "[call] forth a flexible response to the significance of the current situation" (p. 1144) and afford the possibility of a certain response. In contrast to expert practice, the practice of a novice, an advanced beginner, and a competent nurse consists of the "analytic behavior of a detached subject, consciously decomposing his environment into recognizable elements, and following abstract rules" (Dreyfus & Dreyfus, 1986, p. 35). The expert engages in "involved skilled behavior based on an accumulation of concrete experiences and the unconscious recognition of new situations as similar to whole remembered ones" (p. 35). Day expresses concern regarding rules-based nursing as depriving nursing of experts. He suggests that as evidence-based practice and standardization of nursing interventions become more the mode, there is less necessity; as a result, fewer opportunities exist for nurses to rely on their clinical judgment. Rather than helping nurses learn from experience, more rules are created when the judgment of nursing appears to have resulted in deterioration in a patient's situation. This continuing creation of rules for nurses to follow limits development of clinical expertise. Thus far, we have presented you with a rational, analytic, and reasoned process with the occasional caveat that it does not work this way in the real world or that there are ways to facilitate the use in practice. This occurs through the development of expertise by sustained practice within a defined area of expertise, reflection on occurrences and outcome by one's self, with others, and through formal and continuing education. The use of a conceptual framework facilitates the development of expertise; as one continues to add pieces of data through education, reflection helps to see the relationships and patterns between and among these discrete items. The development of tacit knowledge as discussed in Chapter 3 is part and parcel with developing expertise. Continued repetition of actions and rule following does not facilitate development of expertise. There are instances when rule following and standardized practice are necessary for patient safety, but even in these instances, the development of expertise is needed for the relational aspects and for the evaluation of the outcomes of following the rules. "Expert nurses are infinitely adaptable in their responses to the situations at hand because they are able to engage in situated, context-driven reasoning" (Day, 2009, n.p.).

Schön (1983) proposed two ways of reflecting. The first is *reflection-on-action*, which involves thinking through a situation after it has happened. Second, the nurse incorporates *reflection-in-action* as a regular part of practice as expertise develops.

As the nurse accumulates greater volume and range of experiences, he or she goes beyond routine application of rules, facts, and policies and procedures. Through reflection-on-action and reflection-in-action, expertise is developed and the nurse is able to view experiences from a variety of perspectives. (Bobay, Gentile, & Hagle, 2009, n.p)

Another dimension of performing as a skilled expert is that of the moral and legal responsibility one has to the patient. We owe our patients the highest level of care possible. We should aim at providing that and not making it a habit to be satisfied with any other level of care; however, the standard of reasonable and prudent care needs to be considered. Chapter 13 develops this topic in more detail.

Appropriate Caring

From a nursing perspective, appropriate care is that care that reaches the objectives of nursing, helping a person maintain or regain his or her self-care system in response to changing demands. There are many aspects to the concept of *appropriate care*, defined as "suitable for a particular person, condition, occasion, or place; fitting" ("Appropriate," n.d.). The literature identifies categories such as age or developmentally appropriate, culturally appropriate, and medically appropriate. There are two types of appropriateness: appropriateness of a service and appropriateness of the setting in which care is provided (i.e., inpatient vs. outpatient or home care; Lavis & Anderson, 1996).

Age and Developmentally Appropriate Care

According to The Nurse Agency, it is required by the Joint Commission on the Accreditation of Healthcare Organizations (JCAHO) "that any healthcare providers who have patient contact be competent in age appropriate characteristics and needs. JCAHO requires that all individuals with patient contact receive education and training related to the characteristics and needs of the age groups with which they come into contact" (Nurse Agency, 2005). Seminal work done by Erikson (1959) on stages of developmental needs across the life span and by Piaget (1972) on cognitive development are excellent resources for age-related characteristics. Other age/developmental cohorts with age-related issues are premature infants, newborns, developmentally disabled, adolescents, and the elderly. Erikson and Erikson (1997) added a stage to address the developmental needs of the elderly or aging.

Culturally Appropriate Care

By learning the core cultural values of the major ethnic groups represented in their practice, nurses and social workers can provide better care. Each family caregiving case provides a professional with an opportunity to correct, validate, or expand his or her knowledge base and comfort level with people of different cultures (Webb, 2008).

Everyday, difficulties can arise when caring for people from different ethnic and cultural backgrounds, especially when they speak little or no English. A client trusts a nurse but if the nurse does not demonstrate that he or she trusts the client, then the clinical intervention undertaken will in some way create an unnecessary barrier. Respect is the basis for trust; without it, "trust will be expressed superficially and the nurse will only receive from the client lip-service, a cultural communication technique where the client tells the nurse what they think the nurse wants to know, or hear. A client from another culture has to trust otherwise there will be little or no respect for the work the nurse initiates" (Lane-Krebs, 2012, p. 26).

Nurses are similar to others in society, and they have personal values, beliefs, and attitudes that could negatively affect the ways they provide care. Nurses need to be encouraged to sincerely examine personal values and to reflect on personal bias that might conflict with professional responsibilities. Appropriate health care is that in which the expected clinical benefits (e.g., improved symptoms) of care outweigh the expected negative effects (e.g., adverse drug effects) to such an extent that the treatment is justified ("Appropriate Care," n.d.).

In the United States, there is a legal definition for *appropriate care* related to the Medicare program. For the purposes of determining quality of care, appropriate care means that the patient received all the care he or she was eligible to receive. Appropriate Care Measure (ACM) is a score devised by the Center for Medicare and Medicaid Services (CMS). Using established criteria, a score is determined to evaluate hospital performance. "Overall appropriate care measure is the total percentage of heart attack, heart failure, pneumonia, surgical care, stroke, venous thromboembolism, and at-risk patients who received all recommended treatments and preventive measures based on their clinical condition" (Pennsylvania Health Care Quality Alliance, 2008–2013). There are appropriate measures identified for each of the seven targeted groups listed earlier. These reflect accepted standards of care, based on current scientific evidence. Given the structure of health care reimbursement systems in the United States, where payment for services by the physician is based to a great extent on procedures or services performed (fee-for-service model), there is a need for vigilance on the part of the consumer and other providers regarding unnecessary procedures. In October 2015, the *New York Times* reported on a situation of medically unnecessary procedures (Creswell, 2015). Elaborate bureaucratic systems are being proposed and implemented in an attempt to ensure patients receive necessary and appropriate care, which is especially focused on Medicare and Medicaid clientele.

Appropriate Level of Care

The patient should receive the appropriate level of care as well. Having a patient in a unit and providing a higher level of care than is required is not only costly but also may deprive patients of the expert nursing care that the staff in the more appropriate unit could provide. There are also costs associated with caring for a patient who requires a higher level of care than is provided in a particular unit. There are issues regarding transfer from nursing home to hospital or from hospital to nursing home. What is the appropriate level of care for a patient on life support with a poor prognosis of recovery?

Another issue related to level of care is the economic cost to the individual as well as to society. In the United States, what happens if a person is not able to afford a higher level of care when medically needed? Or when the patient would benefit from home care after discharge from the acute-care setting but it is neither available nor affordable?

The interesting thing about level of care is that it is a matter of the level of nursing care that is required for the patient that determines the appropriate level as much as or more than the medical condition. Decades ago, nurses were proposing progressive patient care (PPC) models. There would be various units for different care requirements, and the patient would be moved from one unit to another as he or she progressed or was less able to care for himself or herself. PPC was pioneered and advocated by RADM Faye Glenn Abdellah (Ret.), USPHS, EdD, ScD, RN, FAAN, the first nurse and woman to serve as Deputy Surgeon General of the United States. Her ideas were presented in her works, *Patient Centered Approaches to Nursing* (Abdellah, 1960) and *Better Patient Care Through Nursing Research* (Abdellah & Levine, 1965). The American Academy of Nursing honored her in 2012 as a living legend, crediting her with having "forever changed the focus of nursing theory from disease-centered to patient-centered" (ANA, 2016). In the contemporary landscape of health care, her influence is seen everywhere but at the time of her works there were no such things as post-anesthesia recovery units, intensive- or critical-care units, or step-down units. She used nursing problems to differentiate levels of care. Patient-centered care now tries to focus on the needs of the patient as the differentiating factor. In an analysis of Adbellah's work, there is criticism that the holistic care of a patient is not taken into consideration. The differentiation of levels of care is primarily related to nursing requirements that are correlated with other health and illness states.

Working With Non-Nursing Personnel in Performance of Care

In the majority of health care settings, much of the direct care is performed by others than the professional nurse (e.g., LPNs, CNAs). As part of both production and control operations, the nurse is responsible for the kind and quality of care given. This is true whether or not the nurse is in a managerial role. These responsibilities are probably well known to you at this time in your career. Other courses in your curriculum will aim at increasing your clinical leadership knowledge and understanding of your responsibilities.

Care of Self

We care, because we're nurses, but we're people, too. In order to be an effective caregiver, the nurse needs to be in the best health possible, working through stressful situations and within institutional constraints. This aspect of caregiving is important enough that a chapter on care of self is included in this book. Chapter 14 identifies care of self as a nursing imperative and proposes strategies for managing stress.

PROFESSIONAL NURSE AS MANAGER

One of the common courses in RN–BSN or accelerated degree programs is that of leadership and management in nursing and health care. Given that this is emphasized later in your program, we will just give an overview at this time. The work unit, be it hospital, clinic, nursing home, or other, is best viewed as a system with many sub-systems. The roles and functions of the manager are elements of the relationships between and among these elements. Factors influencing the system include the environment, philosophy of institution, and a myriad other factors. As you move from direct caregiver to broader managerial roles, you will increase your under-standing of the significant factors such as governmental regulations. There are many new roles emerging for nurses to be involved in managing the patient's care or the health needs of populations described in Chapter 11.

Some of these more contemporary roles are those of care coordination, case management, or care management. As an example, one of the U.S. corporations, Group Health Cooperative in Seattle, Washington, includes care management nurses and details their responsibilities. They work together with hospitalists and clinical teams (Box 9.1).

BOX 9.1 Roles and Responsibilities of Care Management Nurses at Group Health

Our care management nurses and hospitalists monitor a member's inpatient care. Care management nurses are available by phone to assist patients and clinical teams in outpatient settings.

Their responsibilities include:

- Ensuring that the member's physician is aware of or involved in the case
- Facilitating the flow of information between the hospital and Group Health
- Assisting hospital discharge planners
- Confirming coverage through review services or customer service
- Facilitating the use of Group Health or contracted providers
- Answering member questions about coordination of care
- Facilitating high-quality, cost-effective use of medically appropriate resources
- Initiating and participating in patient-care conferences and utilization review committees
- Educating internal and external staff about case management and care coordination
- Orienting new contracted providers to Group Health

Coordination of Care

Care management nurses review admission reports and coordinate with hospital social workers and discharge-planning staff to ensure early identification of high-risk patients and timely discharge planning. After discharge from acute-care

---

(*continued*)

BOX 9.1   Roles and Responsibilities of Care Management Nurses at Group Health *(continued)*

facilities, our nurses continue to coordinate care. Our nurses also call the patients approximately 48 hours after discharge to ensure that their transition to home is going well and that follow-up appointments have been made. If a patient is having difficulty, the care management nurse will facilitate a same-day appointment to avoid readmission to the hospital.

Case Management

Our nurses serve as case managers for members whose needs are complex or when resource allocation decisions are required. Case management may cross many settings throughout an episode of illness or treatment. Case management nurses can follow a medically fragile patient after discharge to ensure smooth transition to the next level of care. They are also able to work with patients in advanced stages of chronic illness to understand how to cope with their disease and provide symptom management.

Interhospital Transfers

Care management nurses coordinate planned weekday transfers between contracted inpatient hospital units. They also ensure that hospital staff have the necessary information to facilitate after-hour transfers.

Admission and Continued-Stay Review

We review hospital, skilled nursing facility, nursing home, and home health admissions for clinical need and appropriateness and to identify coordination of care needs. Continued-stay reviews focus on high-risk diagnoses, variance from length-of-stay guidelines, and coordination of care needs. Many of our plans require pre-authorization for planned admissions.

Our care management nurses work closely with a facility's utilization review staff to conduct reviews and coordinate care. If the admission or continued stay appears to be inappropriate, our nurses, in conjunction with the patient and the multidisciplinary team, develop an alternative plan. Our nurses may request a second-level physician review to determine the reason for decertification.

Source: National Quality Forum (2016).

Interdisciplinary Collaboration

Interdisciplinary care is one of the newer trends in health care. Because most participants in multi- and interdisciplinary ventures were trained in traditional disciplines, they need to learn to appreciate the differing of perspectives and methods. Jessup (2007) clarifies the distinction between multidisciplinary and interdisciplinary care teams. Most nurses are used to participating in multidisciplinary teams that "utilize the skills and experience of individuals from different disciplines, with each discipline approaching the patient from their own perspective" (p. 330).

"Interdisciplinary team approaches, as the word itself suggests, integrate separate discipline approaches into a single consultation. Individuals from different disciplines ... are encouraged to. ... [step] out of disciplinary silos to work for the best outcome for the patient" (p. 330). In order to practice within either a multi- or an interdisciplinary team, the nurse must be knowledgeable and confident in the discipline. When reading the literature or discussing the types of team care, it is helpful to know the differences.

Care Coordination

The U.S. Agency for Healthcare Research and Quality (AHRQ) defines and describes *care coordination* as "deliberately organizing patient care activities and sharing information among all of the participants concerned with a patient's care to achieve safer and more effective care. This means that the patient's needs and preferences are known ahead of time and communicated at the right time to the right people, and that this information is used to provide safe, appropriate, and effective care to the patient" (Improving Primary Care Practice, 2015). Programs for care coordination are typically a part of primary care and an aspect of the CMS "medical home" initiative. The National Quality Forum of Institute of Medicine (IOM, 2004) notes, "The U.S. healthcare system is fragmented, with patients, families, and caregivers forced to navigate an increasingly complex system filled with inefficiencies. Lack of care coordination leads to serious complications, including medication errors, preventable hospital readmissions, and unnecessary pain and suffering for patients." There are a number of goals and initiatives underway to resolve these issues, one of which is looking to transforming the work environment of nurses.

Participation in Decision Making

Although nursing is practiced in a one-to-one relationship between patient and nurse, much of what the nurse does and thinks about on a daily basis in the workplace is influenced, shaped, and even controlled by organizational variables. There is an organizational structure with job descriptions. These prescribe scope of practice, extending to day-to-day activities. They influence distribution of power and decision making. The professional nurse has a responsibility to share in the decision making within the organization. It is the responsibility of the individual professional to share the views of his or her profession with the management, to ensure that the policies, procedures, job descriptions, and educational opportunities instituted by the management facilitate meeting the goals of professional discipline and facilitate practice of the individual practitioner. When nurses do not make their views known collectively, they become invisible in the organization decision-making process.

For example, patients are admitted to the hospital because they require highly skilled technical interventions by a variety of professionals, including nurses. Many patients are discharged while still in need of care by those same professionals, particularly nurses. Nurses have lost the power to make decisions in that area. However, follow-up care may be needed. It is here that nurses can have a major impact. Establishment of an efficient communication system regarding follow-up is the responsibility of the organization. Professional nurses are responsible for making the needs for nursing and nursing interventions visible by ensuring that information specific to nursing assessments and prescription for nursing intervention is incorporated into the communication system. Although nurses may not have direct decision making in regard to the timing or criteria for patient discharge, they can influence decision making through collaboration and interprofessional practice. As these modes of practice become more accepted, and nurses have the opportunity through participation in policy development to practice nursing to the full extent of their professional education, better decisions can be made.

Decision Making and the Recording System

In analyzing patient records in relation to elements of concern to nursing that can be used to inform outcomes of nursing actions, requirements for nursing services, and costing of nursing services, it quickly becomes apparent that these data are missing. This has been reflected in the failure of patient classification systems to have meaning for practitioners at the bedside and to be useful tools for allocating staff.

EHRs are becoming increasingly significant in health care systems. The systems are limited in attention to variables that are indicative of sociocultural and interpersonal dimensions of the nursing system, as well as systems of self-care and self-management capabilities. The validity and reliability of these systems has been a discussion point of many articles in the nursing literature. The American Academy of Nursing on Policy recommended that "EHRs capture and permit sharing of contextual patient information, promote shared decision-making, enhance appropriate interprofessional planning/providing of health care services and facilitate monitoring of patterns of health and outcomes of care for entire populations" (Sullivan, 2015, p. 614).

Recording systems serve several purposes in an organization. They are essential for the communication of care produced and outcomes achieved. As the number of professions represented in the health care system has increased, the health information needs associated with it have become increasingly complex. The EHR has improved communication of patient-related data between various health professionals and service organizations. It has the potential for providing a base for evaluating quality as well as for establishing costs of many aspects of patient services. However, in its present form, it has some limitations for nursing and patient management of self-care.

When the groundwork was being laid for development of the EHR, the patient record at the time was a primary source for the kind of information to be included. Also, nursing activity was analyzed to get an understanding about the data that should be included in reference to the nurse's daily activities. Nursing theory and conceptual frameworks for nursing practice were just beginning to be discussed. Apart from attending to "nursing implications" related to the medical diagnosis or physician orders, direction for understanding nursing practice was limited. Physician order entry systems, recording of laboratory data, were structured and easily converted into electronic form and costing of these services could easily be identified. The data representing the concerns of nursing were primarily in a narrative form, lacking structure. At that time, systems for integrating narrative data into the electronic record were in the early stages of development. These data became the basis for the classification systems associated with staffing. The success of linking diagnostic-related groupings to patient stay in hospitals to determine costs led to an increased interest in developing similar classifications for nursing. The theoretical bases for developing nursing diagnostic categories did not exist so these classification systems were developed from a task base or from data related to the practice of medicine.

Heslop and Lu (2014) found that current recording systems do not adequately reflect the totality of the concerns of nursing can only be remedied by nurses. The current record does not make provision for incorporating data associated with the caring component, the social and interpersonal dimensions, and the components associated with patient self-management. The lack of this information is highlighted in the difficulty associated with connecting quality of nursing care and nurse-sensitive outcomes. They found there is a lack of agreement on definitions of indicators, data collection, and analysis, all of which call into question the validity and reliability of conclusions. They identified two main categories of outcomes: (a) structural outcomes associated with service delivery (e.g., hours of nursing care per patient day, nurse staffing) and (b) outcomes related to patient variables (e.g., prevalence of pressure ulcer, falls, nosocomial selective infection, patient/family satisfactions). From a professional perspective, are these the best descriptors of nursing excellence and of the contribution of nursing to health care that we can put forth to the public and the funders of nursing services? What does that say of us as a discipline with a discreet body of knowledge and as independent professional practitioners?

An issue of concern for the profession is that as a result of lack of meaningful data in feedback reported to nurses, they are not particularly engaged with quality monitoring.

Heslop and Lu (2014) have some suggestions about the electronic record that could be helpful:

- Development of effective and sustainable information systems...that include nursing-sensitive indicators will benefit national approaches to enhance health care performance.

- The concept of nurse-sensitive outcomes not linked to a nursing conceptual framework—"has bearing upon the meaningfulness and boundaries of the concept and relevance to clinical practice" (p. 2470).

- Nurse-sensitive outcomes remain invisible within information systems. Undesirable clinical behaviors persist without recourse to some sort of interventions.

DATA ELEMENTS AND OUTCOME MEASUREMENTS

Identification of data elements that are significant to nursing practice is a beginning step in designing a patient electronic record to facilitate measuring outcomes. Two categories of data elements derived from work associated with self-care deficit nursing theory are illustrated in Figure 9.1, and their utility for nursing practice is shown.

FIGURE 9.1 Structure of Elements of Concern to Nursing.

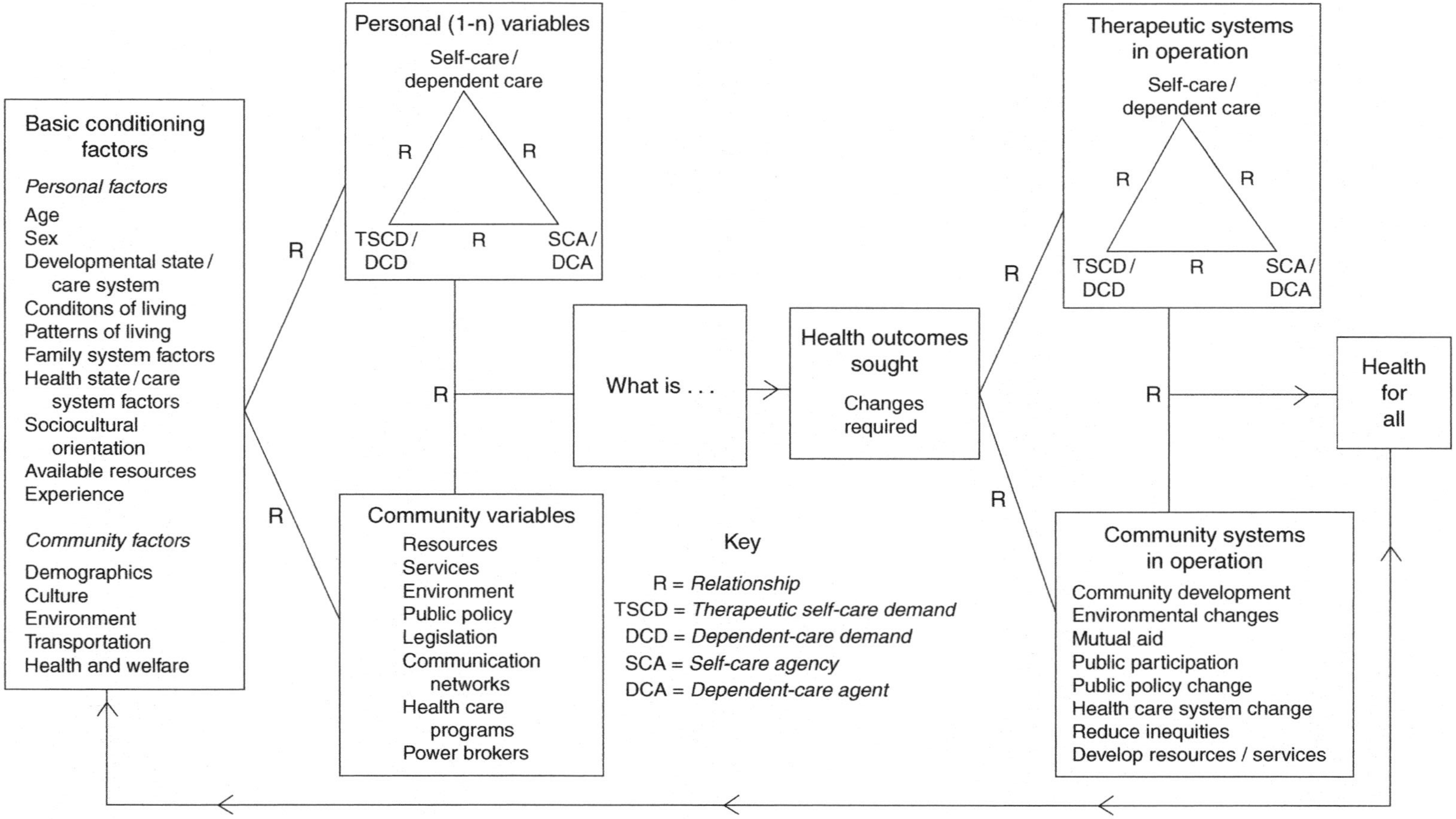

163

In Table 9.1, the data elements associated with self-care deficit nursing theory that provide information about the effectiveness of the self-care system were presented in a structured format. In Table 9.2, outcome categories relative to patient action and to nurse action are proposed. Data elements consistent with Figure 9.1 would be collected, and meaning could be attached to those elements by utilizing the structure in Table 9.2.

A care plan such as that in Table 9.3 for a person with respiratory dysfunction could be constructed from patient data elements included in the information system. Outcomes of nursing actions and patient actions could also be in the design of the information system by addressing elements in the structure in Table 9.1.

Inclusion of data elements identified and designing the system to allow practitioners to explore possible relationships and outcomes have the potential for generating nursing diagnoses (Bliss-Holtz, 1996). This type of internal consistency is dependent on the integration of a nursing theory, a conceptual framework, and system design.

TABLE 9.2   Self-Care Deficit Nursing Theory Outcome Categories

Patient
- Self-management system
  - Adequate or taking action to modify
  - Integrated into a broader system of living

- Therapeutic self-care demand (actions to meet requisites)
  - Calculates
    - What needs to be done
    - How—best methods to use
    - Time sequence
    - Equipment
  - Adjusts as necessary
  - Actions performed
    - Quantitatively—complete
    - Qualitatively—how well, consistency

- Self-care agency
  - General self-care agency
    - Developed
    - Exercised
    - Adequate
  - Self-care operations performed
    - Knowing
    - Decision making
    - Acting

(continued)

TABLE 9.2   Self-Care Deficit Nursing Theory Outcome Categories *(continued)*

- Power components
- Dependent-care system
  - Adequate or taking action to modify
  - Dependent-care operations performed
    - Knowing
    - Decision making
    - Acting
  - Development of dependent-care agency
  - Dependent-care system integrated into self-care system of dependent
  - Dependent-care system and self-care system of dependent integrated into daily living
  - Dependent-care system and self-care system of caregiver integrated into daily living
  - Cooperation and coordination between caregivers if more than one

- Basic conditioning factors
  - Environment—conditions of living—managing/modifying
  - Health state/system factors—managing
  - Family system factors—managing/modifying
  - Personal sociocultural factors—managing/modifying

Nursing
- Nursing system
  - Identified self-care limitations
  - Self-care deficits overcome, compensated for
  - Self-care agency maintained, protected
  - Self-care agency increased
  - Dependent-care system established, operable, adequate

- Regulating/monitoring basic conditioning factors
  - Condition, prevention of complications
  - Therapy, effects, results
  - Bodily functions, elimination, etc.
  - Safe, protective use of equipment
  - Safe, protective, supportive physical, social, and psychological environment
  - Coordination of communication with other health care services
  - Availability, adequacy of follow-up services

Adapted from Allison and McLaughlin-Renpenning (1999). Used with permission.

TABLE 9.3   Components of Care Plan for Persons With Respiratory Dysfunction

Maintains an Adequate Intake of Air	Capabilities to Be Assessed
Practices bronchial hygiene techniques • Performs deep breathing and coughing exercises regularly • Protects others from exposure to infections • Consults with nurse/physio re effectiveness of technique as required	Motivation to take preventive action as opposed to reacting to a crisis Capability of performing skills related to breathing and coughing, preventing spread of infection Knowledge required to monitor effectiveness of breathing and coughing exercises Knowledge regarding how, when, and who to contact for assistance
Incorporates breath-control strategies into daily routine • Uses breath-control techniques effectively	Knowledge and skill regarding performance of pursed lip and diaphragmatic breathing, inspiration/expiration ratio control, stacking, and positioning strategies Motivation to take required action

LEARNING ACTIVITIES

1. Using SCDNT, describe the characteristics of the patients that are currently your responsibility.
2. Identify expected outcomes of nursing services for this population.
3. Review patient records to determine if data related to these is available. If not, what steps would you as manager take to remedy the situation?

References

Abdellah, F. G. (1960). *Patient–centered approaches to nursing.* New York, NY: Macmillan.

Abdellah, F. G., & Levine, E. (1965). *Better patient care through nursing research.* New York, NY: Macmillan.

Allison, S. E., & McLaughlin-Renpenning, K. (1999). *Nursing administration in the 21st century.* Thousand Oaks, CA: Sage Publications, Inc.

American Nurses Association. (2016). RADM Faye Glenn Abdellah, (Ret.), USPHS, EdD, ScD, RN FAAN, 2012 Inductee. Retrieved from http://www.nursingworld .org/fayeglennabdellah

Appropriate. (n.d.). Retrieved from http://medical-dictionary.thefreedictionary.com/ appropriate

Appropriate Care. (n.d.). Retrieved from http://www.thefreedictionary.com/appropriate

Benner, P. (1984). *From novice to expert: Excellence and power in clinical nursing practice.* Menlo Park, CA: Addison-Wesley.

Bliss-Holtz, J. (1996). Using Orem's theory to generate nursing diagnoses for electronic documentation. *Nursing Science Quarterly, 9*(3), 121–125. doi:10.1177/089431849 600900311

Bobay, K., Gentile, D. L., & Hagle, M. E. (2009). The relationship of nurses' professional characteristics to levels of clinical nursing expertise. *Applied Nursing Research*, *22*(1), 48–53. doi:10.1016/j.apnr.2007.03.0015

Creswell, J. (2015, October). A small Indiana town scarred by a trusted doctor. *The New York Times*, p. BU1.

Day, L. (2009). Evidence-based practice, rule-following, and nursing expertise. *American Journal of Critical Care*, *18*(5), 479–482. doi:10.4037/ajcc2009147

Dreyfus, H. L. (2007). Why Heideggarian AI failed and how fixing it would require making it more Heideggarian. *Artificial Intelligence*, *171*, 1137–1160.

Dreyfus, H. L., & Dreyfus, S. E. (1986). *Mind over machine: The power of human intuition and expertise in the era of the computer*. New York, NY: The Free Press.

Erikson, E. H. (1959). *Identity and the life cycle*. New York, NY: International Universities Press.

Erikson, E. H., & Erikson, J. M. (1997). *The life cycle completed* (Extend version ed.). New York, NY: W. W. Norton.

Heslop, L., & Lu, S. (2014). Nursing-sensitive indicators: A concept analysis. *Journal of Advanced Nursing*, *70*(11), 2469–2482. doi:10.1111/jan.12503

Improving Primary Care Practice. (2015). Rockville, MD: Agency for Healthcare Research and Quality. Retrieved from http://www.ahrq.gov/professionals/prevention-chronic-care/improve/index.html

Institute of Medicine. (2004). *Keeping patients safe: Transforming the work environment of nurses*. Washington, DC: National Academies Press.

Jessup, R. (2007). Commentaries: Interdisciplinary versus multidisciplinary care teams: Do we understand the difference? *Australian Health Review*, *31*(3), 330–331.

Lane-Krebs, K. (2012). Recognising difference: The need to develop culturally appropriate care. *Australian Nursing Journal*, *19*(9), 26.

Lavis, J. N., & Anderson, G. M. (1996). Appropriateness in health care delivery: Definitions, measurement and policy implications. *Canadian Medical Association Journal*, *154*(3), 321–328.

National Quality Forum. (2016). Effective Communication and Care Coordination. Retrieved from http://www.qualityforum.org/Topics/Effective_Communication_and_Care_Coordination.aspx

Nurse Agency. (2005). Age appropriate care. Retrieved from http://www.thenurseagency.com/new%20docs/AgeAppropriateCare2005.pdf

Pennsylvania Health Care Quality Alliance. (2008–2013). *Our measures, appropriate care.* Retrieved from http://www.phcqa.org/measures/category.php?category_id=5

Piaget, J. (1972). *The psychology of intelligence*. Totowa, NJ: Littlefield.

Schön, D. A. (1983). *The reflective practitioner*. New York, NY: Basic Books.

Sullivan, C. G. (2015). Putting health in the electronic health record: A call for collective action. *Nursing Outlook*, *63*(5), 614–616. Retrieved from http://dx.doi.org/10.1016/j.outlook.2015.08.003

Trossman, S. (2015, September/October). Preparing for the boomer effect. *American Nurse*, *47*(5), 1, 7.

Webb, R. (2008). Culturally appropriate care. *American Journal of Nursing*, *108*(9 Suppl), 30.

PART III

BEYOND THE SELF

By definition, *caregiving* involves two or more people: one in need of assistance and the other providing care. There are many and diverse arrangements for providing assistance to others. When there are two or more people who are the focus of the nurse or who are intimately involved in the personal situation of the patient, the dynamics of the nursing system change, as does the unit of analysis. The nursing system is more complex. A unit of more than two, referred to as multi-person, has additional aspects and is described in the chapters on family and community.

CHAPTER 10

DEPENDENT-CARE AND COLLABORATIVE-CARE SITUATIONS

This chapter presents the basics of nonprofessional caregiving and the development of appropriate nursing systems when there are two nonprofessional people involved in the care system. The focus of this chapter is on the basic unit of care, the dyad—that is, two people who are the focal point of the care situation.

OBJECTIVES

After reading this chapter, the learner will be able to:

1. Define and give examples of a multi-person unit
2. Distinguish between dependent- and collaborative-care situations
3. Identify legal situations that may define the relationships between people
4. Explain the significance of communication, decision making, and reciprocity within collaborative and dependent care
5. Discuss the issue of caregiver stress and how this also may impact the recipient of dependent care
6. Explain what is meant by cycle of dependency
7. Demonstrate an understanding of factors to be considered in assessment of a dependent-care situation
8. Describe the ways in which nurses can intervene in a dependent-care system
9. Apply the essential elements or diagnostic processes related to dependent care

KEY CONCEPTS   multi-person unit • dyads • dependent care • collaborative care • cycle of dependency • diagnostic processes related to dependent-care operations

DYADS ARE COMPLEX SYSTEMS

Multi-person units, such as couples, parents, and families, are understood through the use of systems theory and complexity concepts. Dyads are viewed as systems. Energy is exchanged, and the change in one part leads to a change in the other parts. Complexity encompasses factors of self-organization; emergence; system characteristics, including information flow; and sense making (Chapter 1). Nursing can often provide invaluable assistance when two people (a dyad) are faced with a health challenge as they work to organize and make sense of what is needed and how best to do this within their broader systems of living.

Sometimes, people choose to help one another, whereas at other times it is a role assigned to them by the culture or society. When dealing with a unit, the nurse must decide who gets services and who needs to be helped first. A mother brings a child into the emergency department (ED) because of a fall; he probably has a broken arm. The mother is on the verge of a panic attack. Who does the nurse tend to first? How is that decision made? In your education and practice experience, you can likely relate many stories or cases where there are two people involved. The critical element in working with dyads is that both people have a claim to your actions. And your nursing actions will be designed to meet the requirements of both people.

Legal and Personal Relationships

In order to establish a nursing system, both the legal and personal relationships between the individuals need to be understood. When two people present themselves as an integral unit—such as mother and child, husband and wife, spouses, family members, guardian, and so on—the nature and legitimacy of that relationship is to be established. Who is ill or injured or in need of care? What is the relationship of the people, one to another? Socially? Legally? In different settings, this may be noted by an admissions clerk or a receptionist. Or the individuals themselves may so clarify, perhaps by a simple introduction: "This is John, my spouse." In a minority of situations, a more legal clarification may be needed. For example, who is the legal custodial parent of a child? Does an adult child have the authority to make decisions for an elderly parent? Does a person with severe mental illness have a guardian who needs to make decisions regarding the person's care? How do you incorporate wishes of an underage child into the care system? Issues of legality are discussed further in Chapter 13. For now, suffice it to say that we in general, unless presented with information to the contrary, assume that a legitimate relationship exists as presented by the patients. As part of the nursing process, details about the relationship may become necessary. Things such as the extensity, intensity, duration, and continuity of interactions will influence the development of the nursing system.

Dependent and Collaborative Care

There are two primary dyadic relationships: dependent and collaborative. It is often the case that nurses deal with more than one person; most patients are members of a family or some other close relationship. In earlier chapters, the family is described as a conditioning factor or the context within which dyadic care is given with the identified patient as the central focus of the nursing system. Later, the family will be described as a unit of service. From the perspective of family systems theory, the *family* is defined as a small group of closely interrelated and interdependent individuals who are organized into a single unit so as to attain specific purposes, namely, family functions or goals (Freidman, Bowden, & Jones, 2003). The foundation of nursing when caring for two or more people is in the relationships between and among those people. A major difference in the two situations, dependent or collaborative, lies in the established relationship. In a dependent-care situation, one person relies on another for some or all of his or her care. In a collaborative situation, both people share the responsibilities of caring for self and other in a mutually agreed-upon or accepted manner. Models and theories that are foundational to understanding collaborative and dependent care in nursing practice include models or theories of personalism, deliberate action and action system, helping, interpersonal interaction, adult learning, technology, and parenting (Young, Taylor, & Renpenning, 2001). Although there are similarities between parenting and dependent care, parenting is more than dependent care and not all dependent care is done as a component of parenting. The application of these foundational ideas occurs in experiences with infant, child care, adolescent, adult, and older adult health situations.

Communication, decision making, and reciprocity are described as factors conditioning the shared care within a dyad. Shared care as a concept is synonymous with collaborative care and dependent care. Sebren (2005) suggests these factors as areas for developing interventions to assist the dyad in overcoming limitations. These are not only described in terms of the dyad but would also be useful in working with the family of which the dyad is a part (see Chapter 12). Some resources to assist in addressing these factors include focusing on family strengths and resilience (Olson, Larsen, & McCubbin, 1982; Walsh, 2006), and learning to help facilitate difficult conversations between and among family members (Harris, 2009; Keating, Russell, Cornacchione, & Smith, 2013; Wallace, 2015).

Importance of Caring for Self While Caring for Others

The importance of caring for self while caring for another is emphasized by many authors. Stress associated with caring for someone with dementia has been well documented (Furlong & Wuest, 2008; Son et al., 2007). Furlong and Wuest (2008) focused on the issue of caring for a person with declining self-care abilities, specifically Alzheimer's disease. The caregiver often foregoes attending to many aspects of self-care because of involvement with "the other." Effects of caregiver stress have been found to be especially detrimental for women who provide care for family members (Butts et al., 2014; Penning & Wu, 2015). Lack of caregiver self-care not only has a negative effect on the caregiver but also negatively impacts the care recipient as well. This is to be expected when viewed from a systems perspective, as the change in one part will lead to a change in another part of the system. For the nurse dealing with the dyad as a unit of service, interventions with one element may produce the desired outcome of reducing stress for the other person. If the nurse changes the environment within which the care is being given, it is possible that the stress on the caregiver may be reduced or the opposite might occur. Any change has the potential to increase stress, though the intention was its reduction.

Caregiver burden, caregiver stress, and *caregiver strain* are terms used to describe the physical, emotional, and financial toll of providing care. Four areas where there is research on caregiver burden are: "care-giver health outcomes, differential impacts of social support, care giving for family members with dementia, and balancing work and care-giving responsibilities" (Gwyther & Strulowitz, 1998, p. 432).

Caregiver strain and burden have been described by the Oncology Nursing Society (ONS, 2014) as encompassing the difficulties of assuming and functioning in the caregiver role as well as associated alterations in the caregiver's emotional and physical health that can occur when care demands exceed resources. The society has also developed an evidence-based discussion of the topic and identified only two recommended interventions: (a) cognitive behavioral interventions and approaches, and (b) psychoeducational interventions. Multicomponent interventions are likely to be the most effective at reducing caregiver strain and burden, because they use a variety of techniques to address the caregivers' needs (Honea et al., 2008). The ONS also has an evidence-based practice guideline for managing caregiver strain and burden (Becze, 2008).

A guide for practitioners to assess and intervene in instances of caregiver burden includes asking questions such as, "Do you feel that you are under a lot of stress? What aspects of your day are the most stressful? Have you been feeling more anxious and irritable lately? Are you getting help from family and friends"? (Parks & Novielli, 2000, n.p) There are a number of instruments that are available online that aid in measuring caregiver burden.

COLLABORATIVE SELF-CARE

The idea of a collaborative care system is relatively simple. Examples are evident in everyday life and practice. Inherent in collaborative self-care is a concept of shared work, resulting in negotiated roles for integrating and performing actions to meet the individuals' requirements for self-care. Collaborative-care systems usually occur between adults. Simple examples of sharing in responsibilities include a couple wherein one member may choose to be a primary decision maker about self-care and the other may provide the material resources (Geden & Taylor, 1999). The wife of a diabetic man may take responsibility for managing the man's diabetic care, developing menus, monitoring his health status, and maintaining records. The husband may either cede this responsibility to his wife completely or actively monitor what is happening and participate in making choices. Although the pattern or distribution of actions may vary, the action system requires that both members make a contribution to the system of care. A nurse may be involved in helping a couple develop their care system, perhaps as a diabetes educator. Teaching only Mr. X, the person with diabetes, how to manage his care is usually less effective than working with the collaborative-care partners. If Mrs. X traditionally does the cooking and shopping, she needs to make changes in how she does this to accommodate his needs as well as her own. Therefore, it is essential to assess the roles that each person plays in a collaborative-care situation.

A traditional collaborative-care system is a unique whole that is formed through the informal or formal negotiation for care by two adults. When one partner is hospitalized or becomes incapacitated, this has a negative impact on the self-care system of the other person. When in a collaborative-care system one person becomes ill and is no longer able to collaborate in the production of care, the other is confronted with the need to take on those self-care actions to meet the demands that are no longer met through the prior system. The nurse may be instrumental in helping them adapt to the changing situation or in transforming the existing system into a dependent-care system. This is often the major focus in discharge planning and home health care. Initially, it may be necessary to adapt the existing care system to meet the new demands. With time, the focus might be on transforming the care system, perhaps through changing the living arrangements or environment.

One couple's description of their collaborative-care systems summarizes the tension that often exists. Two people, Jim and Deb, have a collaborative care system. Together, they have learned that the "relationship . . . is a complicated one indeed. Deb is not Jim's slave. Jim is not Deb's child. Deb has a life independent of Jim. Jim has a life independent of Deb. The intersection of their lives . . . is a relationship and, like all human relationships, it is sustained by their mutual effort" (Stephenson, 2007b, pp. 36–37). Another couple noted, "It's amazing the challenges you don't think of until they confront you." And another couple, Roy and Alice, know "that the days ahead are uncertain—they both are old. But that's okay. Whatever lies ahead, they will ace it together, taking care of each other as best they can" (Stephenson, 2007a, pp. 81–82).

The essential elements of the collaborative-care system are the same as those identified in an individual's self-care system. The difference lies in the ways in which the requisites are met, as illustrated in Figures 10.1 and 10.2 (Geden & Taylor, 1999, p. 330).

The nursing actions, based on knowledge of the requisites and agency of each person, may be directed toward one or the other or both people. In a collaborative-care system that is highly integrated, it is sometimes difficult to separate out the components of the self-care systems of the individuals. This may become necessary when the health state or environment of one or the other undergoes change. Mr. and Mrs. Adams have a functioning collaborative-care system established during their 50 years of married life. The ways in which they have worked together are well established and evolved through the years as they aged. After a catastrophic event, such as cerebrovascular accident, the functional roles changed. If the inability to care for self is significant, the care situation may change to one of dependency rather than to one of collaboration. Or there may need to be renegotiation of the roles and tasks assumed by each member. The nurse may play an important role in assisting with these negotiations or in identifying the need for further modification while always keeping in mind the two people in the unit. In this instance, the care system was transformed into a dependent-care system. When Mr. Adams was discharged home, he was dependent on Mrs. Adams for almost all of his care, which she was able to do with the assistance of home health workers. Over time, he regained his functional abilities so that they were again in a collaborative-care system.

FIGURE 10.1   Collaborative-Care System: Theoretical Model

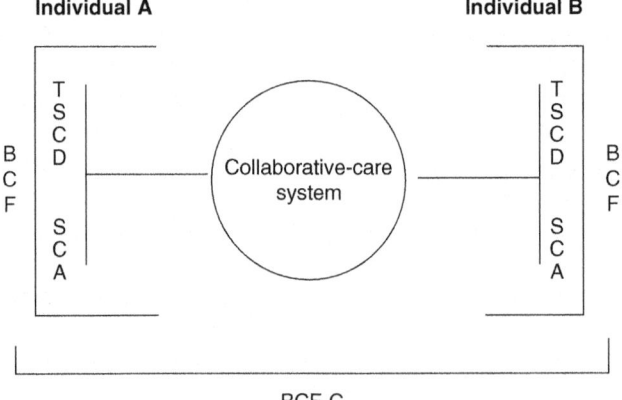

BCF, basic conditioning factors; BCF-C, couple's basic conditioning factors; SCA, self-care agency; TSCD, therapeutic self-care demand

FIGURE 10.2   Collaborative-Care System: Shared Work

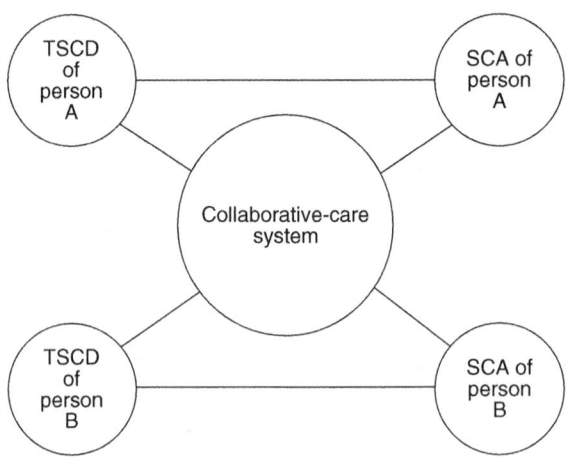

SCA, self-care agency; TSCD, therapeutic self-care demand

DEPENDENT-CARE SYSTEMS

What makes a dependent-care situation different from the care systems previously discussed? It is similar to situations of self-care insofar as the basic components of requirements and agency are the core elements. Unlike individual and collaborative-care systems, dependent-care systems exist when one person acts on behalf of another and there is no requirement that the dependent person actively negotiate or participate in his or her own care or care of the other. The dependent person may contribute to his or her own self-care as he or she is able to (Taylor, Renpenning, Geden, Neuman, & Hart, 2001). When more than one dependent caregiver is involved in a situation, although the relationship at any one point is time is dyadic, the system is more complex with the addition of each caregiver. There are extra demands placed on the dependent person, as he or she must accommodate to the differences in interpersonal relationships with each different caregiver as well as to the difference in caregiving skills and actions.

Before the nurse can proceed, the nature of the dependency needs to be clarified. Dependency is a relationship between two people in which one person requires something from another. The basis of the dependency may be social and/or legal. It occurs within the context of a particular social unit, commonly the family. The provision of assistance and the nature of the assistance to be provided are a function of the general culture and the culture of the specific groups. No person can exist apart from a human community (Ashley & O'Rourke, 1989, p. 7). Humans cannot develop either physically or psychologically without constant interactions with other humans and interpersonal relationships. Human contact is needed for continuing development or maintenance of the social self. When people are unable to care for themselves, a state of dependency exists.

Cycle of Dependency

Dependency is not an all-or-none state. Everyone begins life dependent on others for life-sustaining care. As each person grows and develops, the amount and kind of assistance varies until the individual is independent and able to care for self. The healthiest state is considered to be interdependent, meaning that we can not only act independently as we are able to do so but also ask for help when needed, that is, when we are ill or going through some other problem. By choice or circumstance, that person may develop some kind of shared system—collaborative or dependent. As they age, there is an increasing likelihood that there will be movement toward more dependence on others for care.

People Who May Be Involved in Dependent Care

Though the dependent-care unit is described as a dyad, that is, the dependent person and the responsible person, most dependent-care situations include other people as well. It may be a family that includes both parents and maturing children/siblings in care activities. It might be an extended family with nonrelated people providing care—neighbors, friends, or people employed to provide some care services.

Legal dependency may refer to a child and parents. If the parents are not married, one person is designated as the custodial parent and is the dependent caregiver. In adults with diminished capacity because of infirmity, another person will be identified as the guardian or caretaker. There are obvious complexities in many of these situations that require legal counsel. For example, Mr. Jones has three children: two daughters and one son. If Mr. Jones is unable to care for himself at home, which child, if any, has the right or responsibility for becoming the dependent caregiver? In many families, the tasks of dependent care are amicably negotiated between family members. When there is disagreement within the family, a legal determination may be required. How the nurse interacts with the various family members is a function of these relationships and agreed-upon roles.

Whoever is the responsible person, there are certain roles and tasks that are appropriate. Tables 10.1 and 10.2 identify the roles and tasks expected of the people in the dependent-care situation.

When assessing a situation or designing a nursing system in such situations, the roles the individuals are assuming or might assume are to be considered. For example, the dependent person is always seen as a person with likes and dislikes, abilities and limitations. As recipients of care, they need to be willing to accept the ministrations of others and work along with them to accomplish goals. The dependent-care agent (DCA) is a person in a relationship not only with the care recipient but also with other members of the family. When assuming the role of caregiver, for example, they need to be cognizant of the prior relationship with the other. Children who are caring for dependent parents frequently experience difficulty with changing roles.

Some things that condition the roles and actions in dependent-care situations include "the differences in the aspiration of interacting persons; and the organization or lack of organization of the positions and roles of interacting parties" (Donahue-White, 1997, p. 455). One woman cites the nature of her caring relationship with a dependent elderly family member as "trying to take care... in a manner that not only preserves... her independence, but also, without compromising her care, preserves [her] sense of independence" (Stephenson, 2007a, p. 39).

The specific tasks to be performed are a function of the self-care requisites, self-care agency, and the dependent-care agency of the responsible person or caregiver. In assessing what might be attributes of the dependent-care system, there are many factors to be considered. These factors may form the basis for discharge planning for a patient who is about to leave an institutional care setting.

From a nursing perspective, the need for provision of dependent care is first a function of the self-care demand of the dependent person and second a function of the caregiver or responsible person's ability to provide needed care, referred to

---

TABLE 10.1   Dependent-Care Units: People and Roles

People	Roles
The person who is dependent	• Individual • Person in relationship • Recipient of care • Participant in care
The dependent-care agent	• Individual • Person in relationship • Provider of care (directly or as manager or coordinator)
Other caregivers	• Individual • Person/people in relationship • Provider of care

Adapted from Geden and Taylor (1999).

TABLE 10.2 Factors to Be Considered in Assessing the Dependent-Care Situation

Object of Assessment	Variables to Be Considered
Patient	• Level of performance of activities of daily living (ADL) • Ability to work with body • Cognitive ability • Compliance/adherence level • General health state • Emotional stability • Level of anxiety • Level of energy • Presence of symptoms • Motivation • Perspective on interpersonal relations—acceptance of care • Perception regarding competence of caregiver • Perceived relationship to caregiver
Primary dependent-care agent	• Intact mental processes • Desire to help • Cognitive ability • Physical limitations • General health state • Ability to work with another's body • Emotional stability • Motivation • Level of anxiety • Level of energy • Perceived relationship with patient
Home environment	• Presence of necessary facilities • Access to support by other people or agencies • Facilities for privacy • Availability of resources
Technical/equipment	• Need for manipulation of special demand • Complexity of tasks • Critical observations needed • Expected duration of tasks • Number of activities necessary • Amount of coordination of activities • Amount of equipment needed

Adapted from Geden and Taylor (1999).

as *dependent-care agency*. Development of a care system for the unit requires that the nurse evaluate the development, operability, and adequacy of dependent-care agency. What are the capabilities and limitations of the one person to provide good care to another? In the instance of a new mother–infant dyad, the mother will provide all the care needed by the infant as well as take care of her own self-care requirements. This is a skill with which many new mothers need assistance. So although the infant is unable to care for self, the mother often has limitations in her ability to provide dependent care as well as in tending to her own self-care. It is critical, then, for the nurse to assess both the mother's dependent care and self-care agency and to provide nursing assistance as needed.

Other examples of dependent-care systems include the care systems between an adult and a child with a disability, an elderly person with an adult child caretaker, or two elderly adults, one of whom is incapacitated. As the dependent person's self-care system changes, the characteristics of the dependent-care system will also change. With the infant growing and developing, the mother teaches the child age-appropriate actions for care of self while continuing to take actions needed to maintain the health and well-being of the child. With the adult child/parent unit, the reverse may be occurring; instead of giving the dependent more opportunities to care for self, the care system may be requiring more intervention on the part of the adult child to maintain the health and safety of the older parent. The role of the nurse in these situations may begin as one of support and education to both the dependent and the responsible person in the form of developmental, behavioral, or informational assistance, eventually transitioning to one of providing direct care to the dependent. An interesting phenomenon in dependent-care systems that exist over time is the incorporation by the person who is dependent on the care being given by others into their own perception of their self-care capabilities. Anecdotally, one nurse reported the response of a woman when asked by the MD how she was doing. She responded, "I'm doing just fine. I'm eating well, I get out when I need to, and I'm taking my medications...." The reality of the situation was quite different. None of those activities would be getting done if it were not for the skill of the caregiver, though the dependent person's perspective was that of caring for self.

The elements of a dependent-care system are shown in Figure 10.3.

As in all multi-person systems, the complexity increases as a function of the number of people involved and the nature of the relationships. Similarly, a nursing system in dependent-care situations is also more complex (Figure 10.4).

See Box 10.1 for the essentials of developing a dependent-care system or the diagnostic processes related to dependent-care operations (estimative, transitional, and productive).

Mrs. Smith was living alone and being independent. She was in neither a dependent- or collaborative-care system. We can speculate that in her early adult life she might have been in a collaborative-care system with her husband and was the dependent caregiver for her son. After she injured herself, had surgery, and was discharged from rehabilitation, what kind of care system was appropriate for her? Because of her limited mobility, she is socially dependent. Her son agreed to take the responsibility of caring for her, though not legally responsible, as she is still able to make decisions. Should her mental status deteriorate, that could change.

What are the characteristics of the dependent-care system established for Mrs. Smith? In the previous chapters, her self-care abilities and limitations are described. Her son has a fully

FIGURE 10.3   Basic Dependent-Care System

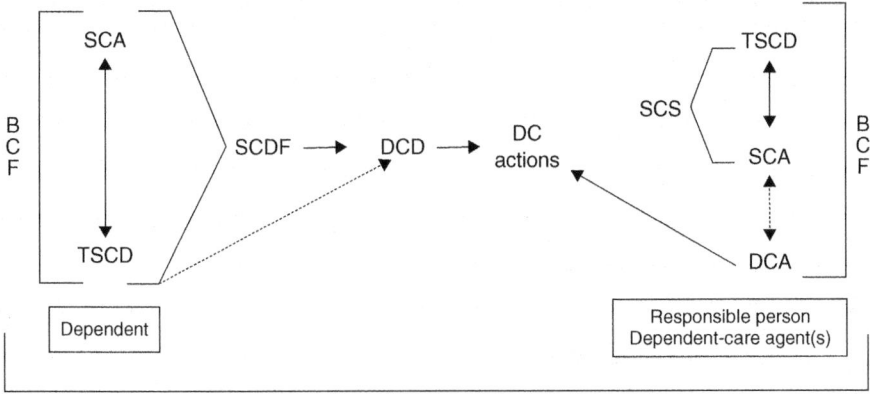

BCF, basic conditioning factors; DC, dependent care; DCA, dependent-care agent; DCD, dependent-care demand; SCA, self-care agency; SCDF, self-care deficit; SCS, self-care system; TSCD, therapeutic self-care demand

FIGURE 10.4   Elements of a Nursing System in Dependent-Care Situations

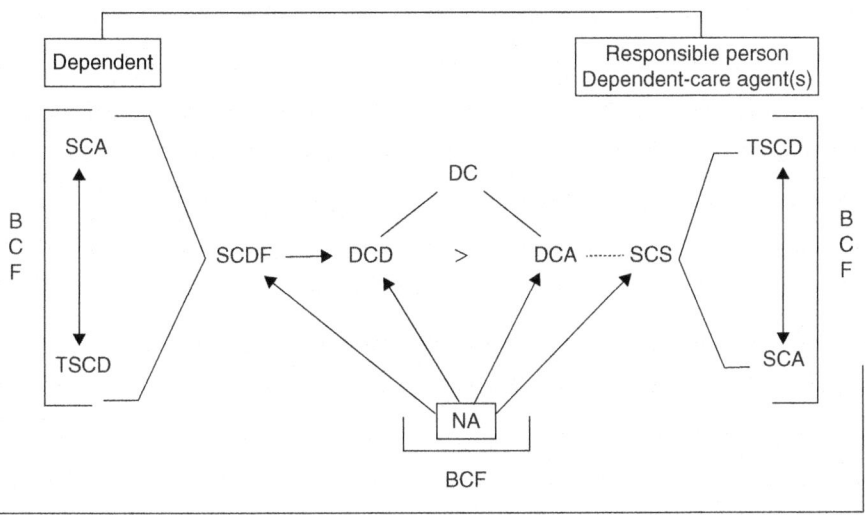

BCF, basic conditioning factors; DC, dependent care; DCA, dependent-care agent; DCD, dependent-care demand; NA, nursing agency; SCA, self-care agency; SCD, self-care demand; SCDF, self-care deficit; SCS, self-care system; TSCD, therapeutic self-care demand

functioning self-care system. He is able to provide the necessary care for Mrs. Smith with the help of others. His dependent-care agency is both developed and adequate.

Parenting and Dependent Care for Ill Child

When the dependent is a child with an illness or developmental disability, the dependent-care system established by the family is more complex. There are the

BOX 10.1   Essentials of Developing a Dependent-Care System

- Specifying the TSCD of the dependent person
- Evaluation of adequacy of SCA of the dependent person
- Evaluation of the adequacy of the DCA
- Meeting components of TSCD of the dependent person
- Regulating the exercise of SCA of the dependent person
- Regulating the exercise of the DCA

DCA, dependent-care agent; SCA, self-care agency; TSCD, therapeutic self-care demand

usual aspects of parenting and, for an ill child, need for another care system. In a study of parents with children with cancer, parents were found to provide for the universal and developmental self-care requisites but were not comfortable dealing with the illness-based requisites (Burley-Moore & Beckwitt, 2004). Parents often express a need for assistance with supportive/educative/developmental requisites of ill children, especially when the care is being given at home. Education from health care providers, including accurate information about the child's disease and treatment, helped them provide care to their child; it helped them feel more in control. Counseling by the nurse on the use of parental care methods to alleviate symptoms (both traditional comfort measures and use of prescribed medications, including medications to stop nausea and vomiting, pain, etc.) and hydration (monitoring fluid intake) are helpful. For example, traditional comfort measures used by parents in the United States and across cultures (as related to diet/nutrition) include methods such as adding flavoring to food items, changing the variety of foods, providing small frequent meals, and offering soft or liquid diets. Other comfort measures that parents/caregivers provide (as related to mind/body control) include talking, reassurance, drawing, playing, singing, watching a favorite show with family, allowing/assisting child with his/her computer games and other electronic tools, use of body massage, bathing, cold compresses on the forehead, and so forth. Reinforcement of these parental caregiving methods by providers is basic (Williams, Williams, & Williams, 2014). They described the family as being divided into two groups—the sick child and the healthy siblings; the needs of each can be vastly different, which can create difficulties for parents. Parents also described needing grandparents or family friends to do many things for the healthy siblings that they would usually do themselves (Williams et al., 2014).

The responsibilities of the parent–DCA of the child with asthma are described as requiring four sets of action (Cox & Taylor, 2005, p. 252). The sets of actions shown in Table 10.3 illustrate the complexity of caring for a child with asthma. In addition, these actions are performed in the context of a family and an overall system of living. As the child matures, there is the added responsibility of assisting the child to successfully learn about and manage his or her own care.

Caring for one's self is difficult. Caring for another is even more complex.

TABLE 10.3   DCA's Actions Related to Asthma

Process: DCA takes appropriate, sequenced, and timely actions

Four sets of action that must be taken at the right time and in the right amount by a competent DCA to achieve the outcome of adequate control of asthma symptoms

Competent Action Set 1: Detects, interprets, and monitors meaningful symptoms	Competent Action Set 2: Regulates and administers medications	Competent Action Set 3: Identifies and avoids environmental triggers	Competent Action Set 4: Appropriately seeks medical advice in a timely manner
DCA believes the diagnosis of asthma is relevant.	DCA has appropriate medications prescribed.	DCA is aware of relevant triggers.	DCA has access to medical treatment.
DCA has the ability to appraise.	DCA has medications and supplies available at all times.	DCA pays attention to symptoms associated with confounding illnesses that trigger asthma exacerbations.	DCA has a relationship with a health care provider who makes self available for medical concerns.
DCA is aware of and able to discriminate meaningful asthma symptoms.	DCA is skilled in medication administration.	DCA understands and uses strategies to identify and avoid triggers.	
DCA keeps time available to assess and to take action.	DCA is knowledgeable in asthma medications, purpose, duration of action, dosing, and when it is appropriate to repeat doses.	DCA understands and uses protective strategies that minimize trigger exposure.	

DCA, dependent-care agent.

LEARNING ACTIVITIES

1. When faced with a dependent-care situation, how would you begin the diagnostic process? Use a systems perspective.
2. In a dependent-care situation, what is the basis for determining the actions to be taken?
3. What is the difference in how you would approach a dependent-care situation as compared with a collaborative-care situation?

References

Ashley, B., & O'Rourke, K. (1989). *Healthcare ethics: A theological analysis* (3rd ed.). St. Louis, MO: Catholic Health Association of the United States.

Becze, E. (2008). *Putting evidence into practice to manage caregiver strain and burden.* Pittsburgh, PA: Oncology Nursing Society.

Burley-Moore, J., & Beckwitt, A. E. (2004). Children with cancer and their parents: Self-care and dependent-care practices. *Issues in Comprehensive Pediatric Nursing, 27*(1), 1–17. doi:10.1080/01460860490279518

Butts, B., Gary, R., Dunbar, S. B., Higgins, M. K., Miller, A., & Corwin, E. (2014). Caregiver stress and cardiovascular disease risk among female family caregivers of persons with heart failure. *The Journal of Cardiovascular Nursing, 29*(5), 390.

Cox, K. R., & Taylor, S. G. (2005). Orem's self-care deficit nursing theory: Pediatric asthma as exemplar. *Nursing Science Quarterly, 18*(3), 249–257. doi:10.1177/08943 18405277528

Donahue-White, P. (1997). Understanding equality and difference: A personalist proposal. *International Philosophical Quarterly, 37*(4), 441–456.

Friedman, M. M., Bowden, V. R., & Jones, E. G. (2003). *Family nursing: Research, theory, and practice* (5th ed.). Upper Saddle River, NJ: Prentice Hall.

Furlong, K. E., & Wuest, J. (2008). Self-care behaviors of spouses caring for significant others with Alzheimer's disease: The emergence of self-care worthiness as a salient condition. *Qualitative Health Research, 18*(12), 1662–1672. doi:10.1177/ 1049732308327158

Geden, E. A., & Taylor, S. G. (1999). Theoretical and empirical description of adult couples' collaborative self-care systems. *Nursing Science Quarterly, 12*(4), 329–334.

Gwyther, L. P., & Strulowitz, S. Y. (1998). Care-giver stress. *Current Opinion in Psychiatry, 11*(4), 431–434. doi:10.1097/00001504-199807000-00012

Harris, J. J. (2009). Family communication during the cancer experience. *Journal of Health Communication, 14*(suppl 1), 76–84. doi:10.1080.10810730902806844

Honea, N., Brintnall, R. A., Given, B., Sherwood, P., Colao, D. B., Somers, S., & Northouse, L. (2008). Putting evidence into practice: Nursing assessment and interventions to reduce family caregiver strain and burden. *Clinical Journal of Oncology Nursing, 12*(3), 507–516. Retrieved from https://cjon.ons.org/cjon/12/3/putting-evidence-practice%c2%ae-nursing-assessment-and-interventions-reduce-family-caregiver#sthash.QMF6tjIO.dpuf

Keating, D. M., Russell, J. C., Cornacchione, J., & Smith, S. W. (2013). Family communication patterns and difficult family conversations. *Journal of Applied Communication Research, 41*(2), 160–180. doi:10.1080/00909882.2013.781659

Olson, D. H., Larsen, A. S., & McCubbin, H. I. (1982). Family strengths. In D. H. Olson, K. I. McCubbin, H. Barnes, A. Larson, Muxen, M., & M. Wilson (Eds.), *Family inventories: Inventories used in a national survey of families across the family life cycle* (pp. 121–136). St. Paul, MN: University of Minnesota, Family Social Science.

Oncology Nursing Society. (2014). Caregiver strain and burden. Retrieved from www .ons.org/practice-resources/pep/caregiver-strain-and-burden.

Parks, M., & Novielli, K. (2000). A practical guide to caring for caregivers. *American Family Physician, 62*(12), 2613–2620.

Penning, M. J., & Wu, Z. (2015). Caregiver stress and mental health: Impact of caregiving relationship and gender [Abstract]. *The Gerontologist.* doi:10.1093/geront/gnv038

Sebren, M. (2005). Shared care, elder and family member skills used to manage burden. *Journal of Advanced Nursing, 52*(2), 170–179.

Son, J., Emo, A., Shea, D. G., Femia, E. E., Zarit, S. H., & Parris Stephens, M. A. (2007). The caregiver stress process and health outcomes [Abstract]. *Journal of Aging and Health, 19*(6), 871–877. doi:10.1177/0898264307308568

Stephenson, C. (2007a). In sickness and in health. In Jamakaya (Ed.), *A celebration of caregiving: Portraits and stories.* Milwaukee, WI: IndependenceFirst.

Stephenson, C. (2007b). Sustained by mutual effort. In Jamakaya (Ed.), *A celebration of caregiving: Portraits and stories.* Milwaukee, WI: IndependenceFirst.

Taylor, S. G., Renpenning, K. E., Geden, E. A., Neuman, B. M., & Hart, M. A. (2001). A theory of dependent-care: A corollary theory to Orem's theory of self-care. *Nursing Science Quarterly, 14*(1), 39–47.

Wallace, C. L. (2015). Family communication and decision making at the end of life: A literature review. *Palliative & Supportive Care, 13*(3), 815–825. doi:10.1017/S1478951514000388

Walsh, F. (2006). *Strengthening family resilience* (2nd ed.). New York, NY: Guilford Press.

Williams, P. D., Williams, K. A., & Williams, A. R. (2014). Parental caregiving of children with cancer and family impact, economic burden, nursing perspectives. *Issues in Comprehensive Pediatric Nursing, 37*(1), 39–60. doi:10.3109/01460862.2013.855843

Young, A., Taylor, S. G., & Renpenning, K. (2001). *Connections nursing research, theory, and practice.* St. Louis, MO: Mosby.

CHAPTER 11

MEANING OF FAMILY IN NURSING

In every conceivable manner, the family is link to our past, bridge to our future

—Alex Haley

Family nursing begins as an extension of the content on dependent care in Chapter 10. Dependent care and parenting were described in the context of the primary dyad with responsibility for caring. In this chapter, that idea is extended to focus on the family and its role in maintaining health and well-being. The family will first be described as a conditioning factor to the individuals that comprise the family unit. Family-centered nursing is the appropriate nursing system in these instances. Second, the family will be considered as a unit of care or of service, as a whole system, that is, Family Systems Nursing. The family may be a factor that conditions the therapeutic self-care demand and self-care agency of the family member who is the identified patient; it may be the setting within which dependent care is provided; or it may be the unit of service for which nursing is provided. The systems concepts that are presented in earlier chapters form the basis for the analysis and discussion. Much of the knowledge the nurse has regarding family is from the foundational sciences or antecedent bodies of knowledge such as sociology or psychology. In this chapter, we look at the family as it relates to the proper object of nursing. As you know by now, nursing is complex in so far as the aspects or dimensions of individuals are concerned. As we move from a consideration of the individual as self to the family and community, the complexity changes.

OBJECTIVES

After reading this chapter, the learner will be able to:

1. Define *family*
2. Describe important elements of Family Systems Theory

187

3. Identify various types of family structure
4. Differentiate between family function and family functioning/processes
5. Identify types of family function
6. Describe nursing in family situations in terms of self-care
7. Demonstrate an understanding of family as a basic conditioning factor
8. Differentiate between family-centered nursing and Family Systems Nursing

KEY CONCEPTS   family • Family Systems Theory • family structure • family function • family functioning/processes

GENERAL CONSTRUCTS RELATED TO FAMILY

The family is conceptualized as a self-defined group of two or more individuals who consider themselves to be a family. Someone once said of the family: They are the people you cannot get away from, or from another perspective, maybe those who you choose to be with. Although the members may be physically and geographically separate by choice or circumstance, there are genetic and/or emotional bonds that influence health and well-being. Family is a relational concept. The family's structure consists of recurrent patterns of interaction that its members develop over time, as they accommodate to each other (Minuchin Center, 2012).

Family Systems Theory, derived from General Systems Theory, which has been discussed throughout this book, provides a view of the family as "a dynamic, interactive unit that undergoes continual evolvement in structure and function" (Miller-Keane, 2003). There are subsystems within the larger family unit, such as the dyads described in Chapter 10; for example, mother and child, mother and father, and brother and sister. There are also suprasystems, such as the community and various community structures, including school, church, and others. Historically important family systems theorists include Murray Bowen and Salvador Minuchin. A major concept in Bowen's (1976, 1978) work is differentiation, which is defined as the ability to operate as an autonomous person without feeling unduly influenced or overly responsible for family/significant others. Differentiated individuals can separate themselves from significant others while remaining emotionally connected (Johnson & Waldo, 1998). Bowen suggested that patterns of differentiation are passed down through generations. People who are not sufficiently differentiated may either remain fused with a family member/members or cut themselves off emotionally. An "emotional middle ground" (p. 406) whereby individuals develop and maintain their own separate identities while still remaining engaged with family/significant others is considered ideal. The core concepts addressed by Minuchin are disengagement (excessively rigid relationship boundaries) and enmeshment (diffuse or vague, ambiguous boundaries), whereas clear boundaries would define the norm (Johnson & Waldo, 1998). However, it is important to consider that these constructs represent family relationships primarily within Western societies. For example, in a review of Family Systems Theory and cross-cultural research, within the structure of Japanese families, it is common that mother–child relationships are extremely close and dependent, which might appear as enmeshment from a Western perspective. Also, the fact that marital partners in Japanese society often do not seek to spend time alone as a couple does not indicate that there is a problem in the relationship. And nonverbal forms of communication are to be relied on rather than verbal expression (Rothbaum, Rosen, Ujiie, & Uchida, 2002).

A family may be viewed according to its structure or how it is organized. How the family is configured, who is included in its membership, and how relationships are patterned or formed within the family are potentially important factors to consider when health care is being planned for a family member or for the entire family (Mosby, 2009). The most commonly identified family structure has been that of the nuclear family, consisting of two parents who are usually married and their children. Other types of family structures, in addition to the nuclear family, include single-parent family, extended family, childless family, step family or blended family, and grandparent family (Blessing, n.d.). Additional family structures have been identified in recent years, including, among others, adopted family, biracial or multiracial family, conditionally separated families due to factors such as military service or hospitalization, gay or lesbian family, and immigrant or migrant family (Edwards, n.d.). When working with families, our own family structure may influence the way that we view others. It is important to be aware of this and to maintain an open and nonjudgmental attitude toward family structures different from our own.

A family may also be considered from the perspective of family function, and family functioning and processes. Family function addresses the assigned sociocultural roles of the family, that is, how the family views and manages reproductive issues (abortion, infertility, artificial insemination, surrogate parenting), socialization, affective matters (e.g., nurturance, sense of belonging), economics, and health care (Kaakinen & Hanson, 2015). Family functioning and processes, on the other hand, are those ongoing interactions through which the tasks and goals of the family are accomplished. This includes roles such as provider, housekeeper, and child care. Disruptions or shifts in these roles secondary to illness or injury can lead to role strain, conflict, and overload, which are discussed in Chapter 10. Other family processes include communication, decision making, coping, and family rituals and routines that provide "organization and give meaning to family life" (p. 30). Compared with family structure and function, family functioning and process seem to have the greatest impact on the overall health and well-being of the family. So, when illness or other stressors arise, these factors need to be addressed (Kaakinen et al., 2015).

Family and Nursing

Before nursing became an established profession, the locus of caring was the family within a specific culture and community. As the sciences of caring, illness, and relationships evolved, so too did the role of family and community in regard to caring. Even now, the definition of *family* with its concomitant roles and responsibilities is changing. Different cultural groups understand *family* in different ways. Nursing also has developed its knowledge base as related to the family. Acceptance of the family as an essential component of nursing care has always existed. In the 20th century, a body of knowledge about families began to take on greater importance with the recognition that a family as a unit or system could be the focus of interventions. Over time, family nursing became a specialty field within the profession of nursing. The term *family* is used to symbolize a conceptual system lens that accounts for the interaction, reciprocity, and relationships between multiple systems levels. These include the illness, the ill individual, the family, the nurse, and the larger systems within which they are nested. When "families, groups, organizations, and communities as interactional units with a plurality of persons as components are conceptually appropriate extensions of the concepts of client and person in nursing, then all other domain concepts, including all steps of the nursing process, need to be specified to reflect these extended definitions" (Schultz, 1987, p. 79).

The classical works on the family by Minuchin and Bowen, introduced earlier, provide much of the theoretical basis for the knowledge and interest of nursing in families. Minuchin developed structural family therapy by using a systems approach. The family's structure consists of recurrent patterns of interaction that its members develop over time, as they accommodate to each other (Minuchin Center, 2012). Bowen's (1978) Family Systems Theory views the family as an emotional unit, and it uses systems thinking to describe the complex interactions in the unit; the focus is on the emotional independence of the family. The work of these scholars provides a framework to view the individual as a part of the family (Haefner, 2014).

As we focused on the individual, the family was viewed as a context or basic conditioning factor (Chapter 5). When we considered Mrs. Smith, she and her son were described as a family of two, living in different places while remaining in a close relationship. A dyad is the simplest form of family. There are many more constellations of people and relationships that constitute family. When we conceptualize the family as a system (the whole is greater than the sum of the parts), the nursing process takes on a different nature. Though the proper object is unchanged, that is, self-care requirements and limitations, the manifestations of the elements are expressed differently.

Systems theory and later application of systems theory to families (Whitchurch & Constantine, 1993) offer ideas about how to conceptualize families as relational systems and subsystems in a new way. The family has primary responsibility for the development of character and capabilities of each and all of its members. The interdependence of human beings leads us to understand that the well-being or functionality of the unit can be an end in itself. Family well-being goes beyond that of the separate individuals to include the quality of their interactions and the outcomes of those interactions for the unit as a whole. All the methods of helping described in Chapter 4 are relevant when working with individuals or dyads within a family. Although the needs of the care recipient may be the primary reason for nursing, the relational aspects of the family will give direction to the selection of helping methods.

Family as System

Family Systems Nursing can be conceptualized as focusing on the whole family as the unit of care. The focus is always on the interaction and the reciprocity. It is not "either/or" but rather "both/and." Family Systems Nursing is the integration of nursing, systems, cybernetics, and family therapy theories (Wright & Leahey,

1990, p. 149). "Involving families in a systemic, relational way in health care is called many different things within the literature, depending on the context of the practice and the healthcare provider: family-focused practice, family centered practice, family health and healing, family nursing, Family Systems Nursing, systemic health care, family medicine, medical family therapy, medical social work, and so on" (Bell, 2009, p. 124). Family Systems Nursing requires nurses to make "a conceptual shift, even a paradigm shift, to account for interaction and reciprocity between health/illness suffering and family functioning, the interaction between themselves and the families in their care, and also consider the larger systems within which families and health care provider interact" (p. 126). The nurse using Family Systems Nursing is adept at assessing multiple systems levels and at choosing interventions that target the systems level that offers the greatest possibility for health and healing; that is, the intervention might target the individual, the relationship between two or more family members, the relationship between the family and the nurse or other health care providers, the health care system, society and culture, or some combination of these. Family Systems Nursing is a specialty level of practice. However, at any level of practice, the nurse should be aware of the systemic approach to care.

Following the use of systems concepts, the family is considered a complex, adaptive system. Family nursing can be conceptualized as focusing on the whole family as the unit of care. Concentration is on both the individual and the family simultaneously. The focus is always on the interaction and the reciprocity. In working with families, we acknowledge each family member's view as equally valid and recognize that a single event, situation, or activity can be perceived in different ways by each.

When the family as a unit is the system, there are subsystems and suprasystems discussed earlier that need to be a part of the analysis. Each individual member is a subsystem; dyadic relationships between siblings or between husband and wife may also be subsystems. Large entities within which families operate such as an extended family or a social or cultural group may be considered supra- or mega systems. Information and energy flow between these elements. As a unit, the family functions (i.e., the purposes for the family system) that are relevant to nursing include:

- The socialization of family members as self-care and dependent-care agents
- The recognition of therapeutic self-care demands of individual family members and the development of strategies to meet these demands, including:
  - Awareness of changes occurring in the person and the environment
  - Knowledge of conditioning effects of these changes on the health state
  - Knowledge of ways of meeting therapeutic self-care demands and skills and motivation to meet these
  - Awareness of the conditioning effect of the interrelationship of family members on the therapeutic self-care demands and abilities of each individual family member
- Access to, control, and management of resources needed to meet therapeutic self-care demands and health care needs of family members
- The integration of the aspects of self-care and dependent care into an overall satisfactory plan of living and development for the family (Taylor, 1989, p. 135).

These functions form the basis for assessment of the family. There are four assessment dimensions: individual subsystems, family interaction patterns, unique characteristics of the whole, and environmental considerations (Whall, 1981). A professional nurse has the knowledge base to establish a nursing system with family considerations.

Family as Basic Conditioning Factor

When an individual is the unit of care, or identified patient, the family has meaning to the nurse as a factor that conditions the self-care demands and abilities of the individual. Self-care is learned within the family. The family conditions the specific values of self-care requisites. The family may be a resource available to be used by the individual or for managing self-care requirements.

In looking at the family as a factor that conditions the individual's self-care system, it is also helpful to consider the family as the context in which dependent care occurs. Though the focus from the perspective of nursing may be on the dyad, many dyadic relationships are within families. An example of the family as a basic conditioning factor can be found in a study by Dalton and Matteis (2014). They found that nonsupportive family behaviors, such as nagging, increased the likelihood of older adults not engaging in self-care management related to exercise. This is consistent with the findings of other studies. Deimling, Smerglia, and Schaefer (2001) examined the effects of family environment and decision making on caregiver depression. The care recipient's physical and mental impairment are direct sources of stress for the caregiver. Often, the caregivers' spouses themselves have frailties that limit their ability to provide care and to withstand the rigors of caregiving and the experience of the decline of the spouse or partner. Family caregivers engaged in home-based end-of-life care describe their "experiences dialectically as: prioritizing needs–ignoring needs, feeling connected–feeling isolated, and juggling to manage–struggling to survive" (Ward-Griffin, McWilliam, & Oudshoorn, 2012, p. 491). The literature frequently refers to this as family-centered nursing.

Family Unit as Focus of Nursing Care

As part of providing nursing care for the family unit, the elements of the system and the subsystems need to be assessed or described. The family has a unity, constituted from its members, that is substantially different in structure and function from the individual members. Assessment will include the determination of the primary reason for considering the family as a system. This is illustrated in the example used by Taylor (1989). The Burke family comprises a mother, a father, and two siblings, one of whom is chronically ill. During a home visit, the nurse assessed that the mother was meeting the therapeutic self-care demand of the ill child and the well sibling, but she was not attending to her own care. Mr. Burke, the father, was meeting his own demands but he was unable to assist in the care of other family members. Mrs. Burke was experiencing deficits in maintaining normal relationships with her husband. As a result, she was not meeting affectional needs with her husband. He, in turn, was not participating in meeting the dependent care needs of the children or in assisting his wife to meet her self-care and other personal needs. Affectional functions of the family are disrupted because of the dependent-care and self-care situations. This family situation, then, constitutes a legitimate nursing situation in which interventions are directed toward the mother's self-care deficits and the ill child's self-care demands. Appropriate interventions might range from increasing the father's dependent-care agency directed toward the wife and children to the extreme of removing the ill child from the home setting to decrease demands on the family. If, after these self- and dependent-care demands are resolved, the affectional functions of the family remain disrupted, the situation would likely require the assistance of a family counselor rather than a nurse. The approach used in Family Systems Nursing views a situation in a similar manner but begins with a more integrated relational methodology developed in the specialty.

In developing a Family Health System, Anderson (2000) proposes that the nursing perspective of family health should link family structure, function, and health variables (including both wellness and illness) and incorporate the biopsychosocial and contextual system aspects of nursing while viewing the family as a unit and considering individual health issues of the family. (p. 105)

She notes that "family health incorporates the collective and the interaction of individual health with the collective" (p. 106). Figure 11.1 illustrates the complexity of nursing when the family is the unit of service. The assessment and intervention at this level as proposed by Anderson is specialty-level practice, but a baccalaureate-prepared nurse can incorporate these ideas into any areas of practice (Figure 4, Taylor, 1989).

FIGURE 11.1   Family as Unit of Service

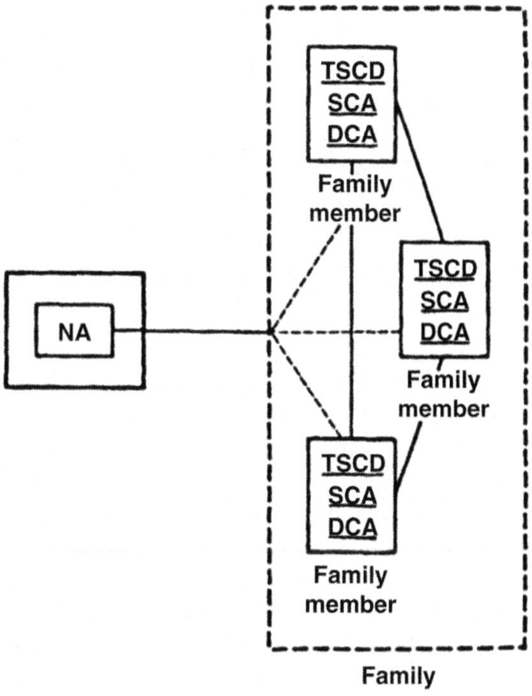

DCA, dependent care agency; NA, nursing agency; SCA, self-care agency; TSCD, therapeutic self-care demand.

Family and Self-Care

Schumacher (1996) studied family caregiving during chemotherapy for cancer in adults with a focus on family caregiving role acquisition. She emphasized the dyadic nature of family-based illness care and the shifting patterns of self-care and caregiving as characteristic of illness care during this event.

HeretoHelp is a website of the British Columbia Partners for Mental Health and Addictions Information (HeretoHelp, 2014). They have a workbook that talks about "ways families can look after their own well-being while caring for a family member. It is important that caregivers remember their own health is equally important." The workbook suggests that family members learn to take care of themselves so that they remain well for their own sake and to better provide care to the other. See more at: www.heretohelp.bc.ca/workbook/family-self-care-and-recovery-from-mental-illness

An interesting article by Deependra and Niehof (2013) illustrates the need to look at the demands and agency of all people in the family as individuals and as a system before invoking strategies for helping. Their study assessed the relationship between women's autonomy and husbands' involvement in maternal health care. They suggest that a strategy to increase or improve "inter-spousal communication could also improve maternal health practices and outcomes by reducing disagreement between the spouses on matters pertaining to maternal health" (p. 10).

Scollan-Koliopoulos (2004) saw individuals perform self-care in the family and noted that multiple family members tend to share similar habits related to diet and physical activity. Obesity has been shown to run in families. This is reflective of the system dynamics within the family. The emotional symptoms of an individual are an expression of the emotional symptoms of the family, which are often embedded in patterns of behaviors from past generations (Haefner, 2014).

Looking at the family and self-care from a cross-cultural perspective is described in the work by Gallant, Spitze, and Grove (2010). Patterns of chronic illness self-care behaviors for older African Americans, Latinos, Asian Americans, and American Indians in the United States were examined. This led to identifying the need for nurses to know the cultural differences, notably culturally patterned.

A review of the literature on family and self-care shows it to be of worldwide interest. There are articles related to the topic from countries of Canada, China, Japan, Nepal, the Netherlands, Singapore, Taiwan, Thailand, Turkey, and the United States.

In summary:

> When the family is viewed as a basic conditioning factor, the nurse is concerned with the identification of the effect of the family on the patient's need for self-care and the extent to which the family can assist the family member who is the patient in meeting his self-care demands and needs for assistance. When the family is viewed as the setting within which dependent care is given, the nurse is concerned with the conditioning effects of the family on both the dependent and the dependent care givers. When the family is the unit of service, the nurse is concerned with the interactive existent or projected effects of the meeting of the therapeutic self-care demands of the individual family members on the overall family functioning. (Taylor, 1989)

Initially, Mrs. Smith and her son were a nuclear family. However, given that both are adults and do not live in the same residence, the nature of the family has changed. They are a relational dyadic family. There appears to be a close relationship between Mrs. Smith and John. It would help to know whether John was assisting his mother out of a sense of duty or out of affection, as this will condition his participation in her care, both now and in the future.

One of the conclusions regarding the family is that a major influence on the development and facilitation of self-care and family systems is the community. Chapter 12 examines the community and population-based nursing.

LEARNING ACTIVITIES

1. Diagram your family as a system. What are the structural elements? What are the relational elements, that is, family function and family functioning/processes?

2. Using the diagram, show what happens when one family member becomes ill.

3. Choose three different cultural groups. Compare and contrast how each of these groups views the definition and role of the family.

References

Anderson, K. H. (2000). The family health system approach to family systems nursing. *Journal of Family Nursing, 6*(2), 103–119. doi:10.1177/107484070000600202

Bell, J. M. (2009). Family systems nursing: Re-examined. *Journal of Family Nursing, 15,* 123–129. doi:10.1177/1074840709335533

Blessing, M. (n.d.). *Types of family structures.* Retrieved from http://family.lovetoknow.com/about-family-values/types-family-structures

Bowen, M. (1976). Theory in the practice of psychotherapy. In P. Guerin (Ed.), *Family therapy: Theory and practice* (pp. 42–90). New York, NY: Gardner Press.

Bowen, M. (1978). *Family therapy in clinical practice.* New York, NY: Jason Aronson.

Dalton, J. M., & Matteis, M. (Fall, 2014). The effect of family relationships and family support on diabetes self-care activities of older adults: A pilot study. *Self-Care, Dependent-Care and Nursing, 21*(1), 12.

Deependra, K. T., & Niehof, A. (2013). Women's autonomy and husbands' involvement in maternal care in Nepal. *Social Science and Medicine, 93,* 1–10. doi:10.1016/j.socscimed.2013.06.003

Deimling, G. T., Smerglia, V. L., & Schaefer, M. L. (2001). The impact of family environment and decision-making satisfaction on caregiver depression: A path analytic model. *Journal of Aging and Health, 13*(1), 47–71. doi:10.1177/089826430101300103

Edwards, J. O. (n.d.). *The many kinds of family structures in our communities.* Retrieved from https://www.scoe.org/files/ccpc-family-structures.pdf

Gallant, M. P., Spitze, G., & Grove, J. G. (2010). Chronic illness self-care and the family lives of older adults: A synthetic review across four ethnic groups. *Journal of Cross-Cultural Gerontology, 25*(1), 21–43. doi:10.1007/s10823-010-9112-z

Haefner, J. (2014). An application of Bowen family systems theory. *Issues in Mental Health Nursing, 35*(11), 835–841. doi:10.3109/01612840.2014.92125741

HeretoHelp. (2014). Family self-care and recovery from mental illness. Retrieved from http://www.heretohelp.bc.ca/workbook/family-self-care-and-recovery-from-mental-illness

Johnson, P., & Waldo, M. (1998). Integrating Minuchin's boundary continuum and Bowen's differentiation scale: A curvilinear representation. *Contemporary Family Therapy, 20*(3), 403–413. doi:10.1023/A:1022429332033

Kaakinen, J. R., & Hanson, S. M. H. (2015). Family health care nursing: An introduction. In J. R. Kaakinen, D. P. Coehlo, R. Steele, A. Tabacco, & S. M. H. Hanson (Eds.). *Family health care nursing: Theory, practice, and research* (5th ed., pp. 3–32). Philadelphia, PA: F. A. Davis.

Miller-Keane. (2003). *Miller-Keane encyclopedia and dictionary of medicine, nursing, and allied health* (7th ed.). Cambridge, MA: Harvard University Press.

Minuchin Center. (2012). About structural family therapy. Retrieved from http://www.minuchincenter.org/structural_family_therapy

Mosby. (2009). *Mosby's medical dictionary* (8th ed.). St. Louis, MO: Elsevier.

Rothbaum, F., Rosen, K., Ujiie, T., & Uchida, N. (2002). Family systems theory, attachment theory, and culture. *Family Process, 41*(3), 328–350. doi:10.1111/j.1545-5300.2002.41305.x

Schultz, P. R. (1987). When client means more than one: Extending the foundational concept of person. *Advances in Nursing Science, 10*(1), 71–88.

Schumacher, K. L. (1996). Reconceptualizing family caregiving: Family-based illness care during chemotherapy. *Research and Health, 19*(4), 261–271.

Scollan-Koliopoulos, M. (2004). Consideration for legacies about diabetes and self-care for the family with a multigenerational occurrence of type 2 diabetes. *Nursing and Health Sciences, 6*(3), 223–227. doi:10.1111/j.1442-2018.2004.00196.x

Taylor, S. G. (1989). An interpretation of family within Orem's general theory of nursing. *Nursing Science Quarterly, 2*(3), 131–137. doi:10.1177/089431848900200308

Ward-Griffin, C., McWilliam, C. L., & Oudshoorn, A. (2012). Relational experiences of family caregivers providing home-based end-of-life care. *Journal of Family Nursing, 18*(4), 491–516. doi:10.1177/1074840712462134

Whall, A. (1981). Nursing theory and the assessment of families. *Journal of Psychiatric Nursing, 19*, 30–38.

Whitchurch, G., & Constantine, L. (1993). "Systems Theory." In P. Boss, W. Doherty, R. LaRossa, W. Schumm, & S. Steinmetz (Eds.), *Sourcebook of family theories and methods: A contextual approach.* New York, NY: Plenum Press.

Wright, L. M., & Leahey, M. (1990). Trends in nursing of families. *Journal of Advanced Nursing, 15*, 148–154. doi:10.1111/j.1365-2648.1990.tb01795.x

CHAPTER 12

COMMUNITY AND NURSING

This chapter is concerned with the interrelationship between nursing and the community. *Community* is commonly defined as a unified body of individuals with common interests and who are living in the same geographical area. A community can be considered a conditioning factor, as introduced in Chapter 5. A community can also be viewed as the place of work and the focus of nursing action. The self-care system and systems concepts introduced in the previous chapters continue to be the basis for analysis and discussion as the interrelationship between nursing and the community is explored. Much of nursing in the community takes place within an interdisciplinary environment, thus adding another dimension to the analysis of situations and relationships.

OBJECTIVES

After reading this chapter, the learner will be able to:

1. Describe various ways of conceptualizing a community
2. Describe responsibilities of the community with regard to health-related self-care
3. Differentiate between public health nursing, home care nursing, and nursing when the community is the unit of service
4. Define population health
5. Describe his or her perception of the unique contribution of nursing in the community

KEY CONCEPTS   community systems and self-care systems • unit of analysis • community as conditioning factor • community as relationship • community as aggregate • community-based nursing service • population health

THE COMMUNITY AS SYSTEM

Changes are occurring in the way we view a community. Nursing has traditionally accepted that the community is the locale of services. For the sake of clarity, the community is seen as a collection of individuals who may be bound by a shared locale, interest, or other factor. A community is also an expression of relationships, a feeling of wanting to be with other people or one of caring about the other people in a group. The development of this feeling is sometimes a strategy used by nurses to accomplish certain outcomes within the group, recognizing that one person's caring can lead to a change in another or in the whole group. Considering *the community* or *a community* as a group or a system of some various size and composition is not the same as *a developing community*, though they are related terms. As noted in Chapter 1, globalization is leading us to see a community in broader parameters both in how we see the community and in the need to develop a more cohesive feeling of a community. Global health care addresses health issues within the largest and most complex community system, not just the locale. The purposes of global health care are health for all. This is a newly developing multidisciplinary area. A related area of health care is international health, which focuses on a more definable locale.

The *community* may be defined as a complex system, with elements, relationships and interactions, and feedback and energy exchange. Setting the level of the system allows us to see the community at several levels. When the system is defined as a person living within an identified group, the concept of the community as a basic conditioning factor can be developed. The place where the person resides and the environmental conditions surrounding the person have a direct impact on the health of the members of the community. Knowledge of these factors and the conditioning effect that they may have on health care enables providers to design either strategies that may impact each person as an individual or strategies that affect all. If the community is located near a source of water contamination, the intervention could be at the individual level—having everyone boil the water before use. On the contrary, the source of contamination can be removed, thereby enabling all in the geographical area to be healthy.

Community and Self-Care

The proper object of nursing as a discipline does not change when considering the role of nursing in relation to population health. Although the variables associated with the inability of people to provide the amount and quality of required self-care are still of concern, the focus is on improving the health of people and populations through changes that are associated with the community systems in operation that impact the self-care system. This includes collecting and analyzing data about social determinants of health, poverty, education, and so on (see Chapter 2), and their impact on the self-care system. What impact do policies related to the health care system, funding for the system, availability of services, and so on, have on population health, health of individuals, and self-care systems? Eastlake community in Atlanta, Georgia, and communities that were rebuilt after Hurricane Katrina in New Orleans, Louisiana, are strong evidence of the relationships among the architecture of a community, its recreational facilities, and the impact that these have on the safety and health of its members. The question to be answered in developing programs to enhance population health is, "What changes in community systems are required to achieve health for all?"

Levels of Systems and Community-Based Nursing

The community system may be at the level of the individual, family, or community, and intervention strategies may target any one of these. Relationships within communities may range from close and personal to more impersonal. Attention to all of the levels that may be simultaneously present makes the nursing situations in the community very complex. Nurses in a community work with:

- Individuals within the context of family and community and within a particular environment

- Individuals and their caregivers in a dependent-care system that is also within the context of family and community and within a particular environment

- Groups within the context of a particular community and within a particular environment

- Community conceptualized as a system and as people in relationships

DATA COLLECTION AND ANALYSIS

The nurse collects data at the level of, and about, one or more of the following systems: the individual, the family, the group, and the community. She examines those data for meaning and then may decide whether the intervention is appropriate at the level of one or more of the following: the individual, the family, the group, or the community. In deciding what data are relevant, what meaning to attach to those data, and how to design appropriate interventions, nursing brings together both nursing theory and theory from related disciplines. In determining what data are relevant and how to analyze them, the particular interest of the discipline of nursing remains centered around "the inability of persons to provide continuously for themselves the amount of required self-care." Data are only data until they are interpreted and given meaning. Nurses use nursing theory as a pair of glasses through which to view the situation and to make sense of it. They also use the knowledge base developed by other disciplines but use it to answer nursing questions—questions about the relationship between the community and the self-care system. In addition to the methods of helping that were previously discussed, they also employ methodologies such as community development and political processes to achieve the goals of nursing.

VARIABLES OF CONCERN

The broad spectrum of variables to be considered when integrating a community-based focus into nursing practice is illustrated in Figure 9.1 (see Chapter 9). The data collection and analysis processes are interdisciplinary ventures, with the contribution of nursing being to ensure that items affecting self-care are included in both data collection and analysis activities.

WHAT IS

Data are collected about the variables on the left-hand side of the figure, facilitating an understanding of the community as a meta system or a suprasystem, with many systems and subsystems, all of which impact the components of self-care systems. These data are used to determine *what is*.

- What are the characteristics of the self-care systems of individuals making up the community?
- How are basic conditioning factors and the conditioning effects of community variables affecting self-care systems and self-care practices of members of the community?
- What are the goals, values, and beliefs regarding health and self-care?
- What conditions are limiting the abilities of people to meet their health and self-care goals within their beliefs and values?

HEALTH OUTCOMES SOUGHT AND IDENTIFYING CHANGES REQUIRED

The next step is to determine *what should be* so that desirable health outcomes can be identified and changes required could be specified to achieve the goal of "Health for All." On the right-hand side of the figure, the elements of concern that are involved to achieve the goals are identified. The target for intervention may be at the level of the self-care systems of individuals, the dependent-care system, the family, or the community systems in operation. Interventions within this model are very much an interdisciplinary activity. Specific nursing services may include teaching, guiding, supporting, community development, and programs to accomplish the empowerment of individuals and groups.

Nurses could participate in developing strategies to facilitate the development and exercise of self-care agency. These could include identifying groups that are at risk for being unable to meet self-care requisites and develop strategies, providing screening programs, supporting development of appropriate public policies in reference to factors that limit development or exercise of self-care agency, working to ensure funding for programs, and so on, to facilitate meeting requisites. They can also assist people in gaining access to available programs and services and in participating in those services.

Nurses usually do not use the "doing for" helping methods in a community situation. When their focus is on small groups, their role is to help their patients manage their health issues. This relates to finding answers about the knowledge, decision making, and acting capabilities of patients and the factors affecting each of these. Do they know what to do? If not, do they have the resources to acquire that knowledge? Are the decisions they are making and the actions they are taking appropriate? If not, why not? Is helping the nurse's role in the particular situation? Or, should some other health care provider be included? Answering the last two questions, in particular, requires a clear understanding of nurses' contribution within the complex interdisciplinary environment. As is noted throughout the book, nurses need to be able to talk about what they contribute, making that contribution both visible and explicit. This is particularly important in the consideration of nursing and the community, because medicine and epidemiology have been the predominant paradigms guiding data analysis and program planning.

Community as Place of Nursing Services

In North America, nursing in the community was traditionally referred to as *public health nursing (PHN)*, which was concerned with prevention, guided by principles of epidemiology, and practiced within the medical paradigm. PHN involves working with communities and populations as equal partners, and focusing on primary prevention and health promotion (American Nurses Association [ANA], 2007). Most often, the public health nurse works for an official or governmental entity.

The distinction between PHN and community nursing as addressed in the literature is not clear. *Community nursing* refers to the broader field that incorporates the public health and has both health promotion and health care foci. (Kulbok, Thatcher, Park, and Meszaros [2012] describe the history of PHN and evolving roles.) Community dimensions of practice skills focus on communication, collaboration, and linkages between public health nurses and the many stakeholders in a community (Quad Council of Public Health Nursing Organizations, 2011).

In many situations, the role of the nurse in the community includes responsibilities related to both communities and to individuals. Included in these are school nurses, parish nurses, and occupational health nurses. Community health nurses "should have a broad understanding of health issues and be comfortable with autonomy, change, and uncertainty. Nurses entering this specialty must highlight not only their clinical skills, but also their critical thinking, advocacy, and analytical abilities" (Meadows, 2009, p. 19).

Home health or home care nursing is concerned with treatment provided in the home, an extension of or in place of an inpatient setting. In many cases, nursing provided in the home reflects a predominantly medical paradigm. This is to such an extent that access to nursing services very often requires a referral by a physician or supervision of the practice of nursing by a physician. In the United States, this physician control is frequently required to get reimbursement for the care or for the nurse to even be able to provide the nursing care needed by the patient or the patient's family. Also, home care nurses could be educated in diploma or associate degree programs. This may not be so in other jurisdictions where a different reimbursement system is in place.

The term *PHN* is gradually being replaced in many countries by *community nursing*, as the latter is a more inclusive term reflecting the increasing scope and volume of nursing services being provided in the community. This is occurring in large part because of the emphasis on self-care and the responsibility of nursing in facilitating self-care in the management of chronic health issues. This requires a rethinking of the educational requirements for nursing. The educational requirements for people providing public health and for those providing community nursing services have been different. For a long time, public health nurses were required to have a minimum baccalaureate degree. The current standard is that of the BSN for entry to practice, with specialty practice requiring additional education for both public health and community nursing. The current impetus for increasing the educational base of nurses has resulted from:

- Changes in health care delivery systems
- The recommendation that nurses practice to the full degree of their potential
- The broader understanding of the determinants of health
- The moves to operationalize a changing definition of health
- Recognition of the requirement for interdisciplinary consultation and cooperation

All of these have an impact on the knowledge and skills that are required to practice nursing in the changing health care environment. In the community, the nurse is very often the only health-related practitioner present in a given situation.

Community as Unit of Service: Population Health

The current focus of the community as a unit of service is on population health. What is population health? It has been defined in many ways in the literature. Sharfstein (2014, pp. 640–643) presents a whimsical overview of some of the variations:

- 2003 "health outcomes of a group of people," the purpose of which was to broaden considerations related to public policy in the United States to include underlying causes of illness that have been also described as social determinants of health
- 2012 "population health strategy," an insurance product whose goal was to enroll as many people as possible
- "Population health solutions," which range, for example, from health coaching to accreditation to surgical device management
- American Hospital Association perspective, which includes evidence-based health services related to prevention, quality of care, patient safety, and coordination of services across the health care continuum
- 2012 psychiatric researchers use the term in relation to prevention of mental illness
- Information technology (IT) companies use the term in reference to analysis of data
- *Population* is defined as a person's possession of a particular insurance benefit card
- Currently, health care providers use the term in reference to their client base

Sharfstein concludes that, as a result of the shifting definition of *population health*, people are losing the purpose of introducing the term, which was to address the result of socioeconomic inequities both locally and worldwide. The term *population health* has meaning when public health principles are retained, when attention to those left behind because of inequities is included, and when there are coordinated efforts to address underlying determinants of illness.

In the following discussion, population health is considered as being concerned with health outcomes for a group of individuals and with the distribution of such outcomes within the group. The achievement of goals that are associated with population health is an interdisciplinary activity, with each discipline bringing to the table a particular focus associated with the proper object of that discipline.

Conceptual Models Associated With Population Health

Governing bodies and people who are responsible for health-related policy development, program design, and funding decisions find conceptual models to be useful organizers in the processes that are related to the decision making and analysis of data. These models identify factors that affect health behaviors and propose relationships among those factors. There are many such models in the literature. Some have been developed by health professionals, others by professional associations, and still others by government agencies. In the following discussion, two models are presented as examples. The first is a model proposed by two nurses, Fawcett and Ellenbecker (2015). It is still in the theoretical stage. The second model was developed by an interdisciplinary body; the discussion includes examples of its use by the Canadian governments and other health care authorities to inform policy and program development. Both of these models had their origin in the same documents that contain answers to the following three questions:

1.   On *what* should we take action? Strategies for population health that indicated action should be taken on the full range of health determinants.

2.   *How* should we take action? The Ottawa Charter on Health Promotion (1986) sets out a range of comprehensive action strategies.

3.   With *whom* should we act? Both the documents just mentioned indicate that action must be taken at various levels within society to accomplish change.

You are invited to explore the nursing literature for other models that focus on nursing practice.

A CONCEPTUAL MODEL OF NURSING AND POPULATION HEALTH

Fawcett and Ellenbecker (2015) propose a conceptual model of nursing and population health that is concerned with the intersection of nursing, represented by nursing activities and population health. The components of this model are:

- Upstream factors—socioeconomic factors and physical environment

- Population health factors (viewed at the population level)—genetic, behavioral, and physiological factors, resilience, and health state

- Health care system factors—providers, organizations, institutions, payers, and policies

- Nursing activities—population-based nursing practice processes, culturally appropriate wellness promotion, restoration, maintenance, and disease prevention

- Population health outcomes—population-level wellness, disease burden, functional status, life expectancy, mortality, and quality of life.

Fawcett then proposes that upstream factors, population factors, and health care system factors are interrelated. These factors are all related to nursing activities.

Nursing activities are not described or related to a proper object of the discipline of nursing. Rather, nursing activities are described as activities that are carried out through nursing practice processes and "directed to promote or restore and maintain wellness across the life course and to prevent disease" (Fawcett & Ellenbecker, 2015, p. 288). The nursing practice processes of assessment, planning, intervention, and evaluation are the vehicles for nursing practice. Methodologies for these processes are similar to those that are formalized in nursing conceptual models and theories.

Self-care deficit nursing theory and related research that has been conducted worldwide could be useful in developing research proposals to test the relational propositions associated with this conceptual model. Fawcett suggests that population-based nursing research begins with "descriptions of theory concepts representing upstream factors, population factors, health care systems factors, and current population health outcomes" (p. 291). Scholarly activities related to self-care deficit nursing theory could be helpful in advancing these activities past the beginning stage. Much work related to the concepts identified in the propositions, their inter-relationships, and their meaning for nursing practice has been done by scholars in their studies that are associated with self-care deficit nursing theory. In particular, the specification of the theory of the nursing system that embraces the theories of self-care and self-care deficit can provide direction for research related to the proposition "nursing activities mediate the relations of upstream factors, population factors, and health care system factors to population health outcomes" (p. 291).

AN INTEGRATED MODEL OF POPULATION HEALTH AND HEALTH PROMOTION

The public health agency of Canada is one of the government agencies that has published a model related to population health. This model integrates population health and health promotion. It is not specific to any one discipline but reflects the interdisciplinary origin of the model. It is consistent with the overall perspective of the goals of nursing practice from the perspective of self-care deficit nursing theory as depicted in Figure 3.1. This three-dimensional model was developed further, including accessing communication theory for an explanation of societal levels at which action can be taken. These include:

- Individual, family, and friends
- Community—people with common interests or geographic setting, workplace, school, and so forth
- Sector/system—education, income support, housing, and so forth
- Society as a whole

These variables have then been further specified within the three-dimensional model as shown in Figure 12.1. The website includes details about the model and the strategies for using it. (It can be retrieved from www.publichealth.gc.ca). Note

FIGURE 12.1 The Population Health Promotion (PHP) Model.

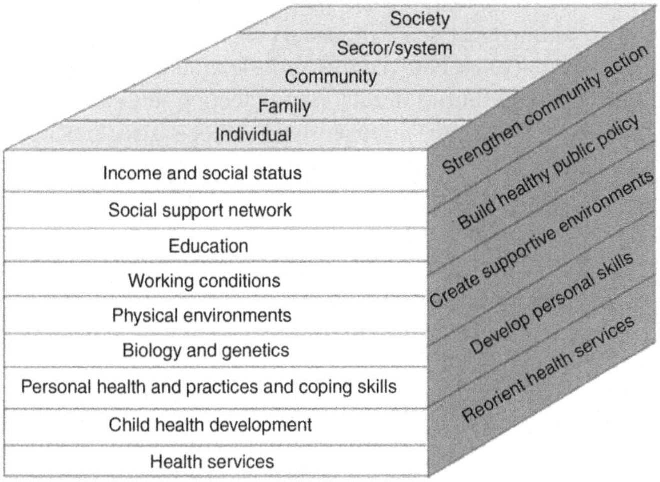

Adapted from the Public Health Agency of Canada (2001). Adapted and reproduced with permission from the Minister of Health.

that it would be very easy to articulate a conceptual framework for nursing practice and the strategies for using the model as presented on the website.

USING THE MODEL IN MAKING SENSE OF POPULATION HEALTH ISSUES

Identifying the variables of concern and constructing a conceptual framework that represents these variables is a beginning step in making sense of the data to be collected and of the complexity associated with understanding the significance of the interrelationships among the many variables. The next step is analyzing those data and drawing some conclusions about the significance of possible interrelationships. Theories such as general systems theory, complexity, and intersectionality that were introduced in Chapter 4 are employed. There are examples of these theories in the nursing literature. McPherson and McGibbon (2010) propose the principles of intersectionality as a lens to examine child mental health inequities; the root causes, including social determinants of health and other inequities related to racism and sexism; and public policy. Green (2013) suggested that intersectionality can be useful in understanding relationships between conditioning factors, self-care agency, and dependent-care agency in vulnerable individuals and multiperson units.

COMMUNITY CONTEXT AND SELF-CARE NURSING THEORY

The utility of nursing theory and systems theory in the design and implementation of a nursing system for a vulnerable population—school children with disability—is described by Green (2013). She emphasizes the interdisciplinary aspects of nursing practice in the community and describes the direction for design of a nursing system in the community, which involves the individual, the family, and dependent-care, aggregate, and community variables. The utility of the systems theory for analyzing the data and constructing the nursing system is highlighted. The article makes reference to universal self-care requisites of populations. However, since only individuals can have self-care requisites, these should be more properly named "responsibilities of communities in relation to meeting self-care requisites."

The model also forms a basis for exploring evidence-based practice. It supports the view that addressing the health of populations is an interdisciplinary responsibility, with each discipline bringing to the table a slightly different perspective depending on the proper object of that discipline but concerned with all of the elements of the model. It also illustrates the complexity of the interrelationships among the variables and provides some indication about the nature of the data required for policy development and evidence to support program development and professional practice.

THE MODEL IN PRACTICE

As a result of the Lalonde Report (1974), the Ottawa Charter (1986), and other previously discussed changes in the understanding of health and the social determinants of health, Canada has undergone major reform in the organization of its health services and related policy initiatives. One of these innovations has been the merging of health services under regional authorities in a public/private partnership delivery model. The Vancouver Coastal Health Regional Authority is one such body (Vancouver Coastal Health, 2014). This organization utilized the model developed by Public Health Canada to provide direction in developing goals, organization design, and programming with a population health focus.

RESEARCH POTENTIAL ASSOCIATED WITH THE MODEL

The documentation accompanying the model highlights that research studies should address health issues, underlying factors, the interventions, and the intended or unintended impact of the interventions. The Vancouver Coastal Health website (www.vch.ca) includes reports of research being conducted at the community level in relation to population health goals. Experiential knowledge gained through practice is an important component of evidence-based practice as well as of formative and summative evaluation studies related to the policies and projects directing practice. Nurses are busy people. They are busy doing. They do not spend much time sharing experiences, successes, and failures related to their practice with one another. This is a major impediment in the development of the knowledge base of nursing.

NURSING AGENCY AND POPULATION HEALTH

The Institute of Medicine (IOM, 2013) recognized that with all the changes in society, an inclusion of our expanding understanding of the determinants of health and the interdisciplinary nature of program development nurses would require an expanded skill set. Two examples of programs related to population health and that illustrate the nature of this skill set are presented. Think of your own knowledge and capabilities. What additional knowledge and skills would you require to be a forceful and effective representative of the nursing discipline in the development and implementation of the programs?

The following are examples of integrated programs of health in a population:

- Promotion of health of school-aged children is given in a program to help young people develop a positive self-image; involving families in the education process; ensuring schools and communities are healthy places; developing an educational system that supports realization of students' full potential; providing funding to achieve the foregoing (Public Health Agency of Canada, 2001)

- "Insite" (http://supervisedinjection.vch.ca/) is an example of a setting and a program that is directed at a targeted population that has political overtones. The arguments pro and con about the existence of the program are reflections of basic values about personal versus societal responsibility, cultural mores, political views, and so forth. Health officials in the city of Vancouver, Canada, recognizing that dealing with drug addiction was a multipronged issue requiring more than treatment facilities, reduced the incidence of deaths related to drug overdoses and dirty needles from 200 in 1995 to 35 per year from 2003 to 2008 by introducing a safe injection site (Milloy, Kerr, Tyndall, Montaner, & Wood, 2008). People using the site have free access to counseling, nurses, social workers, legal aid, and job information. This site has been a source of disagreement between the federal government and local health officials, as implementation of the site was not consistent with federal laws governing management of issues related to illicit drugs. This has resulted in extensive evaluation and the conclusion in 2015 is that the science is in and the Insite is successful. Prior to this science being so definite, the issue ended up at the supreme court of Canada with the court ruling that the law should be set aside in this instance; the court ruled in favor of safe injection sites.

Collecting Data to Inform Population Health Policies and Strategies

Health-related data collected and analyzed through the lens of epidemiology have long been the basis for developing health-related policies. The bulk of data available largely reflects a disease orientation and the concerns of medicine. With the recognition of the social determinants of health and a broader definition of health, this narrow database and associated quantitative research methods are being recognized as having limitations for informing social determinants of health and policy development, and for understanding health-related behavior (IOM, 2013). Data collection in population health should reflect the requirements of each of the participating disciplines.

To date, nursing concerns have been largely considered the same as medical concerns. The data required by nursing to address the proper object of the discipline have been largely inferred from medical or social data. The variables of concern in day-to-day patient–nurse interactions are identified in Table 9.1 and have been explored in detail in previous chapters. Places for considering these data are included in the health promotion model presented in Figure 12.1. It is imperative that these data be made a part of the electronic health care record so that there is a basis for including the perspective of the discipline of nursing in addressing the social determinants of health, establishing policies, developing programs, and implementing action plans to move closer to the goal of "health for all." However, this will not happen without nurses acting as advocates for broadening the elements included in the databases. Examples of research that could be conducted with a broader database and an integrated electronic medical record include:

- The number of homeless people within a particular geographic area; their access to food, water, sleeping conditions; and the incidence of severe respiratory infections
- The range of problems encountered by first-time mothers in relation to feeding their newborns, the length of time during which problems persist, and the incidence and characteristics of issues related to growth and development in the first 3 years of life

---

LEARNING ACTIVITIES

1. Read "Application of the Self-Care Deficit Nursing Theory: The Community Context" (Green, 2013).

    As you read this article, pay particular attention to the application of systems thinking in relation to:

    - The various levels of system within the community
    - The systems approach to analyzing the data
    - The systems approach in constructing the nursing systems for the two children

2. Select a population of people in your community with religious or cultural beliefs that are considered different from the norm. What are the predominant beliefs in this group in regard to women's autonomy and husbands' involvement in maternal health care? What would you do in designing prenatal services, including an education program to accommodate/influence these beliefs?

3. In your nursing practice or in your personal life, you have undoubtedly come across individuals who refuse certain treatment options because of religious and/or cultural beliefs. Analyze one of those situations by using the framework for practice presented in this book. If you had known of such a framework, what would you have done differently at the time?

4. Access www.publichealth.gc.ca again. This time, think about the model in relation to your own practice. Review the values and assumptions underlying the model and the examples of how to work with the document. Identify the significance that such a model could have in your own practice (Public Health Agency of Canada, 2001).

References

American Nurses Association. (2007). *Public health nursing: Scope and standards of practice.* Washington, DC: American Nurses Publishing.

Fawcett, J., & Ellenbecker, C. H. (2015). A proposed conceptual model of nursing and population health. *Nursing Outlook, 63*(3), 288–298. Retrieved from http://dx.doi .org/10.1016/j.outlook.2015.01.009

Green, R. (2013). Application of the self-care deficit nursing theory: The community context. *Self-Care, Dependent-Care & Nursing, 20* (1), 5–15.

Institute of Medicine (IOM). (2013). *Capturing social and behavioral domains in electronic health records: Phase 1.* Washington, DC: National Academies Press.

Kulbok, P. A., Thatcher, E., Park, E., & Meszaros, P. S. (2012). Evolving public health nursing roles: Focus on community participatory health promotion and prevention. *The Online Journal of Issues in Nursing, 17*(2), 1. doi:10.3912/OJIN.Vol17No02Man01

McPherson, C., & McGibbon, E. (2010). The determinants of child mental health: Intersectionality as a guide to primary health care renewal. *Canadian Journal of Nursing Research, 42*(3), 50–64.

Meadows, P. (2009). Community health nursing. *American Journal of Nursing, 109,* 19 doi:10.1097/01.NAJ.0000343102.62178.80

Milloy, M. J., Kerr, T., Tyndall, M., Montaner, J., & Wood, E. (2008). Estimated drug overdose deaths averted by North America's first medically-supervised safer injection facility. *PLoS One, 3*(10), e33519.

Public Health Agency of Canada. (2001). An integrated model of population health and health promotion. Retrieved from http://www.phac-aspc.gc.ca/ph-sp/php-psp/ php3-eng.php

Quad Council of Public Health Nursing Organizations. (2011). *Core competencies for public health nurses.* Washington, DC: Author.

Sharfstein, J. M. (2014). The strange journey of population health, *The Milbank Quarterly, 92*(4), 640–643.

Taylor, S. G., & McLaughlin, K. (1991). Orem's general theory of nursing and community nursing. *Nursing Science Quarterly, 4,* 153. doi:10.1177/089431849100400407

Taylor, S. G., & Renpenning, K. M. (2001). The practice of nursing in multiperson situations. In D. Orem (Ed.), *Nursing concepts of practice* (6th ed., pp. 348–380). St. Louis, MO: Mosby.

Vancouver Coastal Health. (2014). Retrieved from http://www.vch.ca

CHAPTER 13

ETHICAL AND LEGAL ASPECTS OF NURSING

Those who are members of a profession take on responsibilities for their actions in line with the dictates of society and the purpose of the profession. There are many sources that provide guidance for the nurse to act rightly. This chapter looks at the basic precepts of law and ethics and the current status of the nurse in these areas. Nursing practice comprised the actions of the nurse in interaction with many others. As an RN, you know the scope of practice and essential laws within the jurisdiction within which you reside. As you continue your formal education, there are some differences you should be aware of, notably a change in the reasonable person standard. If you pursue a master's or doctoral degree after your BSN, there are a number of additional requirements.

OBJECTIVES

After reading this chapter, the learner will be able to:

1. Describe the major elements of decision making in nursing
2. Identify the primary purpose for legislation and regulatory policies in nursing
3. Identify four sources of law
4. Distinguish between criminal and civil law
5. Distinguish between intentional and unintentional tort and provide examples of each
6. Explain the relationship between personal injury, negligence, malpractice, and the reasonable person standard
7. Explain what is meant by self-regulation of the profession and how this is accomplished

8. Identify two core standards that are necessary for legal nursing practice
9. Distinguish between ethics and morals

KEY CONCEPTS   credentialing • tort • intentional tort • unintentional tort • negligence • malpractice • ethics • morals • moral distress • moral courage

THE CONDUCT OF NURSES

Practice = actions; Actions = choices; Choices = consequences

As a structured, identified entity within a social system, a profession demands certain standards of behavior. There are rules that must be followed and choices that need to be made. These decisions are made for the good of the patient first and foremost. The necessary requirements for a profession include possession of a distinct knowledge base and some standards to which its practitioners can be held accountable. Nursing theory addresses the first requirement for a distinct body of knowledge, whereas professional organizations and regulatory bodies address the second requirement. Another often-cited characteristic of a profession is that it serves a social need and is self-regulated. Self-regulation occurs through governing boards or councils that comprise primarily nurses, members of the public, and various professional organizations. Professional organizations self-regulate through application of agreed-upon standards for accreditation and certification for education and practice. The privilege to do nursing and to call one's self a nurse is governed by society through laws, regulations, and expectations of ethical professional behavior. Various laws and regulations establish the parameters within which a person may legitimately establish a relationship that is referred to as a nurse–patient relationship. Not all political jurisdictions are at the same level of control and differentiation among practitioners of nursing or people working in the helping services. The International Council of Nurses (ICN) was established in 1899 to work on these issues. The ICN is a federation of more than 170 national nurses' associations (NNAs), representing nurses in 130 countries. It is the world's first and widest-reaching international organization for health professionals, working to "ensure quality nursing care for all, sound health policies globally, the advancement of nursing knowledge, and the presence worldwide of a respected nursing profession and a competent and satisfied nursing workforce" (ICN, 2015). The status of regulations regarding health workers for each country can be found on the ICN website. Many professional organizations developed their own Codes of Ethics to be used within their jurisdiction, such as in the United States and Canada. The American Nurses Association (ANA) Code of Ethics and other information is located at www.nursingworld.org, and the Canadian Nurses Association (CNA) can be found in both English and French at www.cna-aiic.ca. Though different in statement or semantics, the essential values are congruent.

DECISION MAKING IN NURSING

There are three critical dimensions to decisions within the profession of nursing—*clinical, legal,* and *ethical.* The primary focus of this book is that of clinical decision making from a nursing perspective. Recognizing that a good decision will integrate all of these dimensions, this chapter explores the legal and ethical dimensions. As health care is changing, the requirements for providers are also changing. This is particularly true as one moves into advanced practice positions. The perspectives of law and ethics in this chapter are those of a Western society. Other cultures and societies may have differing viewpoints.

NURSING AND LAW

As an RN looking to elevate your level of practice, you are already familiar with much of this material. It is presented to aid in focusing the discussion. As in other areas, there is constant change and evolution. The legal status of the nurse took a major step in the early 20th century with the organization of nurses and the formalization of nurse practice acts. In 1903, North Carolina became the first state in the United States to permit licensing of nurses, and New York became the first state to mandate licensing (Miller & Pollitt, 2010). With the work of the ICN and other organizations, progress has been made to legitimize nursing worldwide. As health care systems change and relationships between provider and patient as well as between provider and provider change, there comes a renewed need to become acquainted with the legal aspects of nursing practice and the ramifications of these. An example in the United States is the Health Insurance Portability and Accountability Act (HIPAA) regulations regarding privacy.

As the scope of nursing practice evolved into areas of specialty practice, certification and credentialing through the American Nurses Credentialing Center (ANCC) in conjunction with specialty organizations were formalized.

> The mission of the American Nurses Credentialing Center (ANCC), a subsidiary of the American Nurses Association (ANA), is to promote excellence in nursing and health care globally through credentialing programs. ANCC's internationally renowned credentialing programs certify and recognize individual nurses in specialty practice areas. (ANCC, 2015)

In 2015, the ANCC was certifying nurses in 12 areas of nurse practitioner specialties, 10 clinical nurse specialist areas, and an additional 27 other specialty certifications (ANCC, 2015). All of these require advance education and experience in the specific clinical area. For the ICN, *credentialing* refers to the designation that a person, program, or institution has met established standards and is so recognized. Other terms related to *credentialing* include *licensure, registration, accreditation, approval, certification, recognition*, or *endorsement*. Credentials are typically not permanent, are frequently reviewed, and may be revoked according to Styles and Affara (1997) as cited in ICN (2009).

The essential documents of any profession serve as the foundation for legislation and regulatory policy making that help assure the public's safety. In the United States, nursing practice is typically defined by the state nurse practice act and governed by a board of nursing, but other laws and regulations may also impact practice, and other boards may play a role. Included in these are the ANA Scope and Standards of Practice, Federal and State Laws and Regulations, and Institutional Policies and Procedures. For nurses practicing in the United States, each state has its own requirements for licensure, credentialing or certification, and practice. The ANA developed scope of practice and model nurse practice acts. The National Council of State Boards of Nursing (NCSBN, 2015) provides "education, service and research through collaborative leadership to promote evidence-based regulatory excellence for patient safety and public protection." This organization's website is a basic source for information on the law and regulatory practices along with the official page of your state's board of nursing. The Nursing Licensure Compact allows nurses in participating states to recognize the nursing licenses issued by other participating states, and this is sometimes referred to as reciprocity. Both states in question must be participants in the Nursing Licensure Compact. There are 24 states in the Nursing Licensure Compact, with one more set to join and a few states exploring the possibility. (In the United States, if your state is not involved in the reciprocity exchange, for each new state you go to, you must go online to their board of nursing (BON) and download the appropriate forms for endorsement.) The title advanced practice nurse (APN) is a restricted title, that is, legal certification is required. Certification gives the nurse additional rights and responsibilities. The standard for judging care is different than that used in judging an RN's actions. In Canada, issues of registration and regulation belong to the provinces. The 10 provincial/territorial RN regulators have chosen the NCSBN as the provider of the Canadian RN entry-to-practice exam, starting in 2015.

Basic Legal Concepts

There are basically four sources of law: constitutional, common (case), statutory, and administrative. Aspects of each of these are relevant to the practicing nurse. With the implementation of the Affordable Care Act (ACA) in the United States, there is an ever-increasing number of administrative rules and regulations that impact the practice of nursing. Common law or case law is derived from "decisions previously made by courts and not imposed by legislatures or other government officials" (Common Law, n.d.). It uses principle-based reasoning that "uses the circumstances of a case to evaluate the laws that are applicable" (Common Law, n.d.). The similarities of previous cases or precedents are heavily relied on. When a particular conduct is considered dangerous to society or its citizens, it is identified as a crime through laws. Crimes are punishable by fines, imprisonment, or other methods (Criminal Law, 2015).

There are two types of law: criminal and civil. Criminal law deals with people who have been accused of acts that harm society. Civil law involves disputes that arise when people think they have been harmed by someone else's actions. In a criminal trial, the government prosecutes a person accused of a crime. In a civil law, the court case stems from a lawsuit. Most lawsuits fall into one of the four branches of civil law. Those branches are contract law, property, family law, and personal injury law. Each deals with particular kinds of legal disputes.

A contract is an agreement between two or more parties to exchange something of value. If one party to a contract fails to keep his or her promise, the other party can sue him or her. In that suit, the second party claims to have been injured in some way by the failure of the other to follow the contract. Many everyday actions result in contracts without signing any papers. Employment is usually contractual. As an employee, the agency is held responsible for acts of the nurse following the doctrine of *respondeat superior*, a Latin term meaning "let the superior reply"

("Reasonable Person," 2016). It describes the legal relationship between an employer and employee. When the necessary legal relationship exists, the employer may be liable for the acts of the employee that are committed within the scope of employment. Nurses working in hospitals and for organizations are usually covered by the institution's liability policy. However, as nurses become more independent and entrepreneurial, personal liability issues are more important to the nurse.

Personal injury law involves wrongful actions that cause injury to another person or damage to his or her property. These cases are called *torts*. There are two types of torts. An intentional tort is a deliberate act that results in harm. Though uncommon, there are instances where nursing personnel were accused and convicted of crimes. The second tort is that of negligence, careless or reckless behavior; it occurs when someone does something that a reasonable person would not have done. Negligence also exists when a person fails to do something that a reasonable person would have done. Disagreement over whether or not an action is reasonable can lead to a lawsuit (Grant & Ballard, 2013). Negligence by a professional is called *malpractice*. In order to prove nursing malpractice, it is usually necessary to prove that the nurse was negligent. Proving negligence involves showing that the standard of care was not met. Standards of care developed by the profession, particular institution, or other recognized entity such as within the ACA form the basis for the reasonable person judgment. In addition, there are other factors such as level of education and experience that may alter the level of care expected. *Reasonable person*, a standard used in negligence cases, recognizes that the prudent or reasonable person behaves in a way that is legally appropriate. If one does not behave at least as a reasonable person would, he or she is considered negligent. One judged negligent may be held liable for damages caused by his or her actions ("Reasonable Person," 2001–2015). In professional malpractice, the reasonable person is established through existing standards and expert testimony by a person with similar education and experience. An AD-RN or a BSN-prepared nurse may be judged by a different standard than an APN.

Malpractice is a form of negligence that occurs when a licensed professional, such as a nurse, fails to provide services as per the standards set by the governing body ("standard of care"), subsequently causing harm (Malpractice vs. Negligence, n.d.), a form of non-intentional tort. A review of cases provides additional information and interpretation of the issues or disputes. There are many cases to be found on the web. Three examples are: www.nursingcasestudy.com; www.nursinglaw.com; and www.legalmatch.com/law-library/article/nursing-malpractice.html

Self-Regulation: The NCSBN

The jurisdiction of the state board of nursing, or similar governing organization, besides licensing the individual nurse, extends to promoting safe practice by licensed nurses. This is done through monitoring, investigating, and disciplining. This is part of the self-regulation of the profession:

Accountability is the foundation of professional development and a critical attribute in the nursing profession. Licensed nurses are accountable to the agency that grants them the authority to practice. Through disciplinary processes, boards of nursing serve as forums for patients, families, employers, and others to resolve concerns about nursing practice. (Sheets, 2005, pp. 83–84)

Requirements for maintaining licensure typically include good moral character, continuing clinical competence or continuing education, the absence of a criminal record, language proficiency, and compliance with specific provisions of the jurisdiction's nursing laws. Nurses are held responsible by boards of nursing for being familiar with the rules and regulations that govern their practice, and all nurses are advised to periodically review the laws and regulations, as well as any professional guidelines, advisory opinions, newsletters, practice alerts, or other nursing board publications for all states or territories in which they are licensed. Common misconceptions regarding licensure are identified and refuted by Brous (2012a). These misconceptions include:

- Nursing boards are nursing advocates.
- Private conduct is not relevant to one's performance in a professional capacity.
- Disciplinary action taken by a state pertains only to that state.
- Licensure is a right.

The converse of each of these is true. Nursing boards are responsible for the health of the citizens. They do not act as advocates for the nurse. Disciplinary action in one state is an impediment to practice in another state. Private conduct such as use of recreational drugs may have an impact on your professional status. And a license to practice is a privilege; it is not a right but it does carry with it duties and responsibilities, spelled out in the relevant nurse practice act. This includes defining the scope of practice within which the RN can function.

CORE STANDARDS

There are two core standards for legal practice: competency and good moral character. *Competence* is defined by the NCSBN as including the ability of the nurse to "integrate knowledge, skills, judgment and personal attributes to practice safely and ethically" (NCSBN, 2015, Article 2). Standards of care are tools against which competency can be measured. Good moral character is included in some state nurse practice acts, even though it is not a trait that can be concretely specified (Kim, Kjervik, & Foster, 2014). Indirect measures such as honesty, fairness, respect for the rights of others, and respect for the laws of the state and nation may be indicators of an individual's good moral character. Similarly, good moral character can be manifest in the absence of things such as criminal convictions, professional misconduct, fraud, deception, and misrepresentation. Further elucidation of these standards is found in documents of the NCSBN and ANA.

Some contemporary areas where issues may occur for nurses are in the beginning and end of life, sexual misconduct, discrimination, and child and elder abuse. Misuse of drugs and medication errors are also areas of concern. Appropriate actions taken by the nurse as a part of usual practice behaviors can mitigate the likelihood of incidents occurring. Included in the list presented by Brous (2012b) are good communication skills and practices, continuing education, resolving conflicts between job descriptions and legal scope of practice, maintaining professional boundaries, and maintaining professional liability insurance. There are many situations that have both legal and ethical components. Abortion is legal but may not be considered ethical; right-to-die laws are being enacted to the moral distress of many. Issues of confidentiality, relationships with patients, and matters related to consent, especially in the treatment of minors, are also difficult areas for health care professionals.

ETHICS AND NURSES

Etiquette, Ethics, and Morality

Good moral character is a matter for both legal and ethical consideration. Although used to make judgments about the nurses' legal status, it is also a part of nursing ethics. The development of nursing ethics evolved along with the evolution of nursing as a profession. In early times when nursing was viewed as a charitable undertaking, the belief was that "good" people performed "good" acts. A good nurse was committed to the ideal of doing what was right. Being of the highest character, the good nurse was disciplined by moral training and could be relied upon to do her duty in service to others. The Nightingale pledge taken by many nurses in the first 70 years of the 20th century had the nurse solemnly pledging:

> I solemnly pledge myself before God and in the presence of this assembly, to pass my life in purity and to practice my profession faithfully. I will abstain from whatever is deleterious and mischievous, and will not take or knowingly administer any harmful drug. I will do all in my power to maintain and elevate the standard of my profession, and will hold in confidence all personal matters committed to my keeping and all family affairs coming to my knowledge in the practice of my calling. With loyalty will I endeavor to aid the physician in his work, and devote myself to the welfare of those committed to my care. (Yates, n.d.)

The pledge was named in honor of Nightingale, was composed in 1893 by Mrs. Lystra E. Gretter and a Committee for the Farrand Training School for Nurses, Detroit, Michigan, and was considered a form of the Hippocratic Oath taken by physicians (Yates, n.d.).

The Nightingale Pledge was a statement of the ethics and principles of the nursing profession. The pledge was recited at capping, pinning, or graduation ceremonies. In recent decades, the pledge has either been dropped or substantially altered because of its reference to loyalty to physicians. "Nursing is an autonomous profession and any loyalty should be to protect the patient, even in the face of physician opposition" (Yates, n.d.).

Early on, nursing ethics was virtually indistinguishable from nursing etiquette and the performance of duty. Attributes of the "good" nurse are discussed in Chapter 1 and included forms of polite behavior, such as neatness, punctuality, courtesy, and quiet attendance to the physician. A shift in the understanding of nursing ethics accompanied the shift in roles from loyalty to the authority of the physician now to independent clinical decisions in patient care, including ethical decisions. It is recognized that nurses face ethical challenges in everyday practice and therefore need to strengthen the ethical foundation of nursing to address the ethical pressures resulting from disparities in human, social, and financial resources in health care, and the pervasive nature of moral distress in nurses' work. Questions about ethics have been asked for millennia and are still being examined today. There is much in the literature on the topic of ethics, bioethics, medical ethics, and nursing ethics and how they relate to one another. There are ethical theories based on rights and justice, whereas others are focused on responsibilities, caring, and virtue.

Ethics refer to how a nurse is to act in a given situation; morals overlap with ethics and refer to personal beliefs and cultural values. Both ethics and morals relate to right and wrong conduct. Although they are sometimes used interchangeably, they are different. Morals refer to an individual's own principles regarding right and wrong conduct. Morality is a personal compass of right and wrong. Ethics refer to rules provided by an external source. These can be found in codes of conduct in workplaces or religious principles that provide a social system or a framework for acceptable behavior. Ethics are external standards that are provided by institutions, groups, or the culture to which an individual belongs. Nurses, lawyers, policemen, doctors, and others follow an ethical code laid down by their profession, without regard to their own feelings or preferences (Ethics vs. Morals, n.d.). This is a source of difficulty for some professionals as they work to reconcile personal beliefs with professional expectations.

Advocacy, accountability, collaboration, and caring are foundational moral concepts for nurses' principled, ethical decision making (Fry & Johnstone, 2002). They are important, because they enjoy a firm place in nursing standards and ethical statements throughout the history of the nursing profession and help define the ethical dimensions of the nurse–patient relationship (Fry, 2004).

The nursing literature tends to view ethics from two opposing perspectives: one of justice/rights/responsibilities and one of caring/relationships/situational. The principles identified by Beauchamp and Childress (2009) are viewed as coming from a rights perspective. Some nurse–ethicists have interpreted advocacy as the ethical principle that justifies what nurses do to protect the human dignity, privacy, choice (when applicable), and well-being of the patient (Fry & Johnstone, 2002). Two general ethical principles—respect for human dignity and fidelity—are described as being rooted in the advocacy concept.

Other principles or concepts that are cited in bioethics as relevant to nursing ethics include:

- Autonomy—self-determination, freedom
- Justice—fairness to all people, equal treatment
- Fidelity—faithfulness to commitments made to self and others
- Beneficence—doing good
- Nonmaleficence—do not harm
- Veracity—truthfulness

Virtue ethics has been identified as the current theory that is favored in nursing (Tschudin, 2010). It is described as person based in that it looks at the moral character of the person carrying out an action, rather than at ethical duties and rules, or at the consequences of particular actions (BBC, 2014). The idea of character of the person has been important to nurses for a long time. Early writers of nursing textbooks, such as that by Harmer (1922), focused on good character as a fundamental criterion for being a nurse.

Newham argues that although one can learn the principles of action, applying them requires experience of the world. He further argues that a consequentialist approach is appropriate for nursing. It is the outcome of actions that is important. One can be a good person and still not do the right thing (Newham, 2015). Would a principle such as truth-telling mean that every patient needs to know the true extent of his or her illness or may some information be withheld at times? If a patient makes a choice that you find morally indefensible, what are your duties to the patient? To yourself? In making decisions or selecting actions, people reflect on whether a way of acting is good or desirable, and whether it is more desirable or less desirable than other ways of acting to achieve a goal.

In evaluating ethical practice, Gastmans (2014) poses the question to be answered as "does the nursing behavior—attitude or act—contribute to the human dignity of all people involved in a particular care practice?" (p. 505).

There are five principles identified by Hunter (2010) as important, namely, confidentiality, collaboration, compassion, competence, and care. Of these, care is the most frequently cited as the essential ethical frame for nursing.

Ethics of Caring

The development of an ethic of caring is credited to Carol Gilligan and Nel Noddings. Noddings' first sole-authored book, *Caring: A Feminine Approach to Ethics and Moral Education* (1984), followed close on the 1982 publication of Carol Gilligan's groundbreaking work on the ethics of care, *In a Different Voice* (Gilligan, 1982). The ethics of care is focused on how to respond to the needs of others in complicated real-life scenarios. Think of this approach as mainly involving concepts such as responsibilities, compassion, and relationships. Noddings (1984) argues that the caregiver (one-caring) must exhibit *engrossment and motivational displacement*, and the person who is cared for (one-cared-for) must respond in some way to the caring (p. 69). Engrossment refers to thinking about someone in order to gain a greater understanding of him or her. She considers it as similar to empathy but more personal. The one-caring cannot determine appropriate actions until he or she understands the personal and environmental situation. This level of understanding is a precursor to caring.

The ethics of care recognizes context rather than universal rules. The context of a situation is very important in determining how we should respond. For example, think of a situation where you have to decide how to address too many family obligations in your life. You have to consider the context of the specific situation, your needs, and the needs of others. Rather than focusing on the consequences of actions or our duties, caring ethics considers our response to other people in various circumstances. Although the character of the person is an important aspect and influences the actions, being a person of good character is probably not enough when making ethical decisions.

Codes of Ethics

The professional codes of ethics give direction to the standards expected of nurses. The ICN, ANA, and CNA have developed codes of nursing. Though expressed slightly differently, the essentials are similar. The ICN code states that "Nurses have four fundamental responsibilities: to promote health, to prevent illness, to restore health and to alleviate suffering. Inherent in nursing is a respect for human rights, including cultural rights, the right to life and choice, to dignity and to be treated with respect" (ICN, 2012).

In 2015, the ANA presented the newly revised Code of Ethics for Nurses with interpretive statements. The professional nurse has a moral obligation to know the principles that constitute these standards.

Nurses seeking to create exemplary practice environments refer to the ANA's Foundation of Nursing series to guide them in their daily practice, thinking, and decision making. These three authoritative texts on nursing provide essential information on the foundation of the profession. The series helps you to better understand the scope of the practice and professional standards of nursing, become better prepared to meet the challenges of everyday practice, and grasp the implications and importance of nursing within society. This series includes *Nursing: Scope and Standards of Practice* (3rd Ed.), *Guide to the Code of Ethics for Nurses: Interpretation and Application* (2nd Ed.), and *Guide to Nursing's Social Policy Statement: Understanding the Profession From Social Contract to Social Covenant.* These can be obtained through the ANA (www.nursebooks.org/Homepage/Featured-Items/Essentials-of-Nursing-Practice-Package.aspx).

Ethical Decision Making

A model for ethical decision making is presented here. Basically a standard decision-making model or process, this or similar rubrics for ethical decision making are valid for whatever ethical theory you are operating from. The difference is found in how the problem is framed in ethical terms, and the application of ethical principles to gain meaning. Although you may personally subscribe to a particular theory, in most clinical situations a combination of approaches will be used, particularly as interprofessional practice increases.

In an ethical decision-making model:

1. Identify the problem.

2. Identify the stakeholders or people involved in the situation.

3. Collect information.

4. State the options.

5. Apply ethical principles to the options.

6. Make the decision.

7. Implement the decision.

8. Evaluate the outcome.

Institutional ethics committees or consultants are important in proposing solutions to ethical dilemmas or concerns. In most cases, the deliberations are conducted by a multidisciplinary team to make recommendations. The committee is presented with a situation in which there is a lack of certainty or disagreement about the situation. A formal decision-making model such as the one presented earlier is used in most instances to clarify the facts and principles of concern. The selection of action is up to the person who has the right to make the decisions in that particular situation.

MORAL DISTRESS AND MORAL COURAGE

In the clinical setting, the decisions are generally made by the physician with patient (if possible) and family input. In many instances, there is little or no input from the nursing staff. The nurse may not be in agreement with the decisions made for the patient. "Moral distress is a critical, frequently ignored, problem in healthcare work environments. Moral distress occurs when you know the ethically appropriate action to take, but are unable to act upon it or you act in a manner contrary to your personal and professional values, which undermines your integrity and authenticity" (American Association of Critical-Care Nurses Public Policy, 2008, p. 1). Nurses feel a loss of integrity and dissatisfaction with their work environment. Organizational cultures may stifle ethical behavior. The individual may be either apathetic or unwilling to face the difficult decisions or may fear the social isolation or rejection by his or her peers (Kidder, 2005, p. 211). It takes courage to stand up to these forces, but such action is necessary if one is to maintain his or her own integrity. Moral distress is discussed in more detail in Chapter 14.

Murray (2010) noted that nurses "face ethical dilemmas on a regular basis. Shortages in the numbers of clinicians to deliver patient care, inadequate staffing levels, cost containment measures, consolidation of healthcare organizations, and ineffective leadership have resulted in the escalation of ethical dilemmas nurses face today in healthcare environments" (n.p.). Overcoming or managing moral distress requires moral courage. Moral courage is seen in individuals who, when they uncover an ethical dilemma, explore a course of action based on their ethical values, and follow through with a decision as to the right course of action regardless of the possible consequences this course of action might present.

APPLICATION OF MODEL

The ethical decision-making model described earlier is similar to the steps of any problem-solving rubric. The differences lie in (a) framing the problem in the terms of the choices to be made from an ethical perspective, and (b) using ethical principles to direct choices and to evaluate the outcome of the choice. For example, while working in a critical care unit, in the rush of activities you notice that a mistake was made by another nurse. You do not think that it will cause harm to the patient, but what are you to do? Is honesty necessary when something goes wrong? If you report it, your colleague will be reprimanded for the error and failure to self-report.

LEARNING ACTIVITIES

1. Should a nurse befriend a former patient when that patient sends a friend request on Facebook? Is this a legal or an ethical issue?
2. Discuss the ethical pressures resulting from disparities in human, social, and financial resources in health care.
3. Give examples of moral distress in nurses' work.

References

American Association of Critical-Care Nurses Public Policy. (2008). *Moral distress.* Retrieved from http://www.aacn.org/WD/Practice/Docs/Moral_Distress.pdf

American Nurses Association. (2015). *Code of Ethics for Nurses with interpretive statements.* Retrieved from http://nursingworld.org/MainMenuCategories/EthicsStandards/CodeofEthicsforNurses/Code-of-Ethics-For-Nurses.html

American Nurses Credentialing Center. (2015). Retrieved from http://www.nursecredentialing.org/FunctionalCategory/AboutANCC

BBC. (2014). *Virtue ethics.* Retrieved from http://www.bbc.co.uk/ethics/introduction/virtue.shtml

Beauchamp, T., & Childress, J. (2009). *Principles of biomedical ethics* (6th ed.). New York, NY: Oxford University Press.

Brous, E. (2012a). Common misconceptions about professional licensure. *American Journal of Nursing, 112*(10), 55–59.

Brous, E. (2012b). Professional licensure protection strategies. *American Journal of Nursing, 112*(12), 43–47. doi:10.1097/01.NAJ.0000423512.68887.8d

Common Law. (n.d.). Retrieved from http://www.wisegeek.com/what-is-common-law.htm

Criminal Law. (2015). Retrieved from http://criminal.findlaw.com/criminal-law-basics/criminal-law-basics.html#sthash.o2QRkXFu.dpuf

Ethics vs. Morals. (n.d.). Retrieved from http://www.diffen.com/difference/Ethics_vs_Morals

Fry, S. T. (2004). Nursing ethics. In S. G. Post (Ed.), *Encyclopedia of bioethics* (3rd ed., vol. 4). New York, NY: Macmillan. Retrieved from http://go.galegroup.com.proxy.mul.missouri.edu/ps/i.do?id=GALE%7CCX3402500384&v=2.1&u=morenetuomcolum&it=r&p=GVRL&sw=w&asid=ec3faf629b3098af2da1010bf917ba79

Fry, S., & Johnstone, M. J. (2002). *Ethics in nursing practice: A guide to ethical decision making* (2nd ed.). Oxford, UK: Blackwell Science.

Grant, P. D., & Ballard, D. C. (2013). *Fast facts about nursing and the law: Law for nurses in a nutshell.* New York, NY: Springer.

Gastmans, C. (2014). Sexual expression in nursing homes: A neglected nursing ethics issue. *Nursing Ethics, 21*(5), 505–506. doi:10.1177/0969733014531530

Gilligan, C. (1982). *In a different voice: Psychological theory and women's development.* Cambridge, MA: Harvard University Press.

Harmer, B. (1922). *Textbook of the principles and practice of nursing.* New York, NY: Macmillan.

Hunter, K. (2010). *Nursing-ethics—5 of the most important principles.* Retrieved from http://ezinearticles.com/?Nursing-Ethics—5-of-the-Most-Important-Principles&id=3783446 or http://EzineArticles.com/3783446

ICN. (2009). *Nursing matters fact sheet, credentialing.* Retrieved from http://www.icn.ch/images/stories/documents/publications/fact_sheets/1a_FS-Credentialing.pdf

ICN. (2012). *Preamble to the code.* Retrieved from http://www.icn.ch/images/stories/documents/about/icncode_english.pdf

ICN. (2015). Global database. Last updated April 10, 2015. Retrieved from http://www.icn.ch/what-we-do/global-database

Kidder, R. M. (2005). *Moral courage.* New York, NY: HarperCollins Publishers.

Kim, K. K., Kjervik, D. K., & Foster, B. (2014). Quality indicators for initial licensure and discipline in nursing laws in South Korea and North Carolina. *International Nursing Review, 61*(1), 35–43. doi:10.1111/inr.12069

Malpractice vs. Negligence (n.d.). Retrieved from http://www.diffen.com/difference/Malpractice_vs_Negligence

Miller, W., & Pollitt, P. (2010). North Carolina, pioneer in American nursing: Passage of the first nurse registration law in the United States. *American Journal of Nursing, 110*(2), 70–71. doi:10.1097/01.NAJ.0000368066.92921.be

Murray, J. S. (2010, September). Moral courage in healthcare: Acting ethically even in the presence of risk. *Online Journal of Issues in Nursing, 15*(3), Manuscript 2. doi:0.3912/OJIN.Vol15No03Man02

National Council of State Boards of Nursing. (2015). Retrieved from https://www.ncsbn.org/about.htm

Newham, R. (2015). Virtue ethics and nursing: On what grounds? *Nursing Philosophy, 16*(1), 40–50. doi:10.1111/nup.12063

Noddings, N. (1984). *Caring: A feminine approach to ethics and moral education.* Berkeley, CA: University of California Press.

Reasonable Person. (2016). USLegal™ definitions. Retrieved from http://definitions.uslegal.com/r/reasonable-person

Sheets, V. (2005). Licensure discipline: A challenge for boards of nursing—and nurses. *American Journal of Nursing, 105*(7), 83–84.

Tschudin, V. (2010). Nursing ethics: The last decade. *Nursing Ethics, 17*(1), 127–131. doi:10.1177/0969733009352408

Yates, D. (n.d.). *Lystra Eggert Gretter public health advocate and professional reformer 1858–1951.* Retrieved from http://www.truthaboutnursing.org/press/pioneers/lystra_gretter.html#pledge

CHAPTER 14

CARE OF SELF

A Nursing Imperative

The authors acknowledge the vital role of nurses in caring for themselves, their own health and well-being, for the welfare of patients for whom they care, and for a healthy work environment. Nursing is a profession that often involves complex patient care environments, challenging organizational factors, and other high-stress situations that may result in physical and/or psychological impairment if not addressed. In addition to personal consequences, lack of nurses' self-care may contribute to job dissatisfaction and burnout, high rates of nursing turnover, and the predicted ongoing nursing shortage. These factors may ultimately place patient care and safety, as well as the nurse, at risk. That the nurse is to be "engaged in care of self in order to care for others" is one of the assumptions that underlies the essentials of professional nursing (American Association of Critical-Care Nurses [AACN], 2008). In this chapter, nurses' self-care and basic personal self-care strategies are presented to address stress-related issues and problems. Consequences of nurses not caring for self are discussed, including effects on the individual nurse, patients, organizations, and institutions. Organizational strategies are recommended that may contribute to management or avoidance of stress and stress-related problems. Intrapersonal and organizational approaches together may help alleviate some of the identified problems and ultimately help empower nurses individually and as a profession.

This chapter is presented in a somewhat different format from the preceding chapters. Self-reflection questions are integrated throughout to assist in understanding and making decisions about care of self.

OBJECTIVES

After reading this chapter, the learner will be able to:

1. Examine how care of self relates to the concept of nursing agency, presented earlier in this book

2. Discuss basic self-care strategies for nurses as they relate to Orem's (2001) Universal Self-Care Requisites

3. Evaluate the role of intrinsic motivation in self-care

4. Identify strategies recommended to help with compassion fatigue, moral distress, and lateral violence (LV)

5. Recognize the value of the components of emotional intelligence

6. Distinguish between positive and negative effects of stress and provide examples

7. Identify and define various types of occupational stress

8. Analyze various factors that may be related to burnout

9. Differentiate between moral distress and moral dilemma

10. Discuss different ways that individuals can experience and respond to moral distress

11. Discuss theories of causation related to LV

12. Consider the effect of stress on patients and organizations

13. Evaluate organizational strategies designed to reduce stress

14. Become self-aware related to the experience of stress in nursing and develop a personal plan for self-care

KEY CONCEPTS   nursing agency • intrinsic motivation • stress • occupational stress • burnout • compassion fatigue • compassion satisfaction • traumatization • moral distress • lateral violence • emotional intelligence

NURSING AGENCY

A significant recommendation from the Institute of Medicine (IOM; 2010) report on the future of nursing is that nurses should assume leadership roles and be full partners with physicians and other health care professionals in the redesign of health care in the United States. For nurses to authentically participate in this endeavor, they must cultivate their maximum potential, both as individuals and as a group. Nursing is the largest health care profession in both the United States and Canada (AACN, 2011; Laschinger & Fida, 2014). Nurses working at full potential toward a common goal can become a major force for positive change in the design and provision of health care.

How can nurses, individually and collectively, best maximize their potential to become essential participants and leaders in health care redesign? Education is an essential factor. Orem (2001) described educated nurses as essential for nursing, because "the *nurse* is the **agent**" (p. 38) whose actions result in nursing care. Nursing agency comprises the social, interpersonal, and professional–technological capabilities of people educated as nurses to perform professional nursing practice. Nursing agency is "refined and further developed through time with reflective experience and additional education" (Taylor & Renpenning, 2011, p. 21).

Although important, education by itself is not enough. Nurses are well advised to reflect upon their practice, their developed and developing capabilities, and factors that may contribute to or deflect them from their self-empowerment. Nursing is often stressful, but stress does not need to have negative outcomes. When stress is encountered, thoughtful reflection is required to determine what can be changed and what actions are required to bring about the needed change. This often involves taking self-care actions that may ultimately contribute to reduced stress and greater self-empowerment. A nurse interviewed for an article titled "Why America's Nurses Are Burning Out" emphasized that nursing schools should teach that "self-care must come first" (Gupta, n.d.). In the words of the American Nurses Association (ANA, 2015a) Code of Ethics for Nurses, Provision 5, "The nurse owes the same duties to self as to others, including the responsibility to promote health and safety, preserve wholeness of character and integrity, maintain competence, and continue personal and professional growth" (p. 19). At least in this instance, the airlines have it right—put on your own oxygen mask before putting it on others.

NURSES' SELF-CARE

The self-care requisites and capabilities identified in this book apply to the nurse as well as to the identified patient. As in any caregiving relationship, the giver of care must establish some equilibrium between meeting the self-care demands of self and others. Placing more emphasis on one or the other will eventually lead to disequilibrium or distress.

Essentially all authors who addressed the issue of stress in nursing recommended that nurses practice self-care. Nurses may be disinclined to take time out of busy schedules to care for themselves but doing so is essential. Nurses need an opportunity to "rest, recover, and restore balance" (Leiter & Maslach, 2003, p. 95). Basic self-care strategies for nurses are presented in Table 14.1, based on stress-related problems identified in the literature. These strategies are organized by using Orem's (2001) Universal Self-Care Requisites as a framework.

Some additional details may be helpful when trying to implement the suggestions identified in Table 14.1. For example, what does it mean to practice good nutrition? A variety of resources can be accessed online. The U.S. Dietary Guidelines (2010), released in 2011, were designed to help people choose a healthy diet. These guidelines emphasize three major goals for Americans:

- Balance calories with physical activity to manage weight.
- Consume more of certain foods and nutrients such as fruits, vegetables, whole grains, fat-free and low-fat dairy products, and seafood.
- Consume fewer foods with sodium (salt), saturated fats, trans fats, cholesterol, added sugars, refined grains, and processed foods.

Another online dietary resource is provided by the United States Department of Agriculture (USDA) Center for Nutrition Policy and Promotion (CCNP;

TABLE 14.1 Orem's (2001) Universal Self-Care Requisites as Framework for Nurses' Self-Care

Requisite	Related Problems Identified in Nursing	Actions Required to Meet the Requisite
1. Maintenance of sufficient intake of air, water, and food	• Altered eating patterns associated with shift work (Doyle, 2014; Lehman, 2014)	• Practice good nutrition (see guidelines provided). • Avoid excessive caffeine and alcohol; stay hydrated (Krischke, 2011; Lombardo & Eyre, 2011; Responding to Stressful Events, 2005). • Practice deep breathing (Kravitz, McAllister-Black, Grant, & Kirk, 2010).
2. Provision of care associated with elimination	• Gastrointestinal (GI) disturbance • Irritable bowel syndrome	• Exercise • Nutrition • Hydration • Take bathroom breaks when needed.
3. Maintenance of balance between activity and rest	• Shift work contributes to altered sleep patterns. • Less than 11 hours between shifts may contribute to sleep problems and severe fatigue (Doyle, 2014).	• Get enough rest; optimal sleep is 7 to 9 hours (Healthy Sleep, 2015; Kift, 2012; Lombardo & Eyre, 2011). • Take frequent uninterrupted breaks during work shifts (American Nurses Association [ANA] Position Statement, 2014; Kift, 2012). • Take opportunities for physical activity and exercise, e.g., yoga, tai chi, biking, massage (Kravitz et al, 2010; Lombardo & Eyre, 2011; Public Health Agency of Canada, 2016.
4. Maintenance of balance between solitude and social interaction	• Long hours • Fatigue • Conflicting demands between home and work	• Learn relaxation techniques (Kravitz et al, 2010). • Be involved in personally meaningful spiritual practices (prayer, church, meditation, reading, reflection) (Kravitz et al, 2010; Krischke, 2011; Lombardo & Eyre, 2011). • Develop social support; spend time with supportive family and friends (Kravitz et al., 2010; Responding to Stressful Events, 2005). • Be self-nurturing; do something for yourself every day (Mathieu, 2007; Public Health Agency of Canada, 2016).

(continued)

TABLE 14.1   Orem's (2001) Universal Self-Care Requisites as Framework for Nurses' Self-Care *(continued)*

Requisite	Related Problems Identified in Nursing	Actions Required to Meet the Requisite
5. Prevention of hazards to life functioning and well-being	• Shift work and long work hours associated with increased risk for accidents (Sleep Deprivation, 2011) • Lifting heavy patients may lead to injury. • Lack of assistance in doing work	• Acknowledge stressors (Kift, 2012). • Ask for help in performing work activities when needed. • Be aware of changes in habits, attitude, and moods (Public Health Agency of Canada, 2016). • Know when to seek professional help: (a) cannot return to a normal routine; (b) feeling extremely helpless; (c) having thoughts of harming self or others; (d) using alcohol and/or other substances excessively (Public Health Agency of Canada, 2016). • Utilize counseling and employee assistance programs (EAP) (Hendren, 2010; Henry, 2014).
6. Promotion of normalcy	• Shift work and working long hours may interfere with normal socialization.	• As much as possible, continue to participate in usual social and recreational activities (Public Health Agency of Canada, 2016).

USDA, n.d.). Called *Choose My Plate*, this website describes how to arrange food on your plate, usually a small dinner plate, to ensure that you are getting enough of the right foods. Half of the plate should be filled with fruits and vegetables, and the other half should be filled with whole grains and lean protein such as chicken, fish, or vegetable protein. A serving of low- or no-fat dairy should also be included.

How much water should you drink? Recommendations vary, but usually specify at least eight 8-ounce glasses per day, with adjustments made for level of exercise, illness, and outdoor temperature and humidity.

The optimal amount of sleep as identified in Table 14.1 is 7 to 9 hours. But what if you have a problem getting enough sleep or not feeling rested after you sleep? Approximately 18 million adults in the United States have sleep apnea, which has been associated with serious health concerns (Sleep Apnea, n.d.). Symptoms of sleep apnea are headache when awakening and not feeling rested even if you have got an adequate amount of sleep. Snoring is also associated with sleep apnea. Not all people who snore have sleep apnea, but people who have sleep apnea do snore. It is important to be evaluated if you think you might have this problem. In addition, some self-care strategies have been identified to help: (a) lose weight if you need to,

(b) limit alcohol and stop smoking, (c) eat healthy, (d) tend to allergies, and (e) develop a good sleep routine (Sleep Apnea, n.d.).

In regard to sleep in general, having a small (emphasis on small) snack before bed can be helpful. Foods that help sleep are those that contain tryptophan (milk, nuts and seeds, bananas, honey, and eggs) and carbohydrates (cereal with milk, yogurt and crackers, cheese and bread or crackers). Deterrents to sleep include large meals and foods containing caffeine (including chocolate, cola, tea, caffeinated or decaffeinated coffee). It is also important to be aware of medications that might contain caffeine (e.g., pain relievers and cold medication). Although it is tempting to have a nightcap, it is recommended to avoid alcohol 4 to 6 hours before bedtime. Heavy, spicy meals should be finished 4 to 6 hours before bedtime, and protein should be kept to a minimum. Drinking fluids, even water, should be stopped at least a couple of hours before bed, to minimize having to get up during the night. It is important to avoid smoking altogether, but especially before bedtime or during the night, because nicotine is a stimulant. Some general strategies to help with sleep include taking a brief power nap during the day. This has been associated with more alertness, stress reduction, better cognitive function, more patience, and better health. Light exercise, such as going for a walk or doing gentle yoga stretches, is also recommended as is listening to music that you find relaxing.

Another self-care strategy identified in Table 14.1 is to do something daily that is self-nurturing. See Box 14.1 for questions to help you determine what this might mean for you.

Finding a spiritual practice that is meaningful to you is another important way to take care of yourself. Spirituality is a deeply personal experience. Whatever practice or practices you choose should be nurturing and enriching for you. Meditation is one practice that has found its way into modern society and has been found meaningful by many. Some people may be put off by the idea of meditation, thinking that is religious, or too hard, or needs to be done in a certain way. None of these things is true. *Meditation* can be defined as "a practice of concentrated focus upon a sound, object, visualization, the breath, movement, or attention itself in order to increase awareness of the present moment, reduce stress, promote relaxation, and enhance personal and spiritual growth" (Meditation, n.d.). A basic recommendation for those who might want to try meditation but are intimidated by the idea is to start small, 3 to 5 minutes at a time. Find a comfortable way of sitting and close your eyes. Take a couple of deep, cleansing breaths. Then begin to focus on your breath. Take a long, deep breath, slowly count to 7 on the in breath, pause at the top of the breath, and then slowly count to 7 on the out breath. Pause at the bottom of the out breath and then repeat. Simply focus on the breath. If your mind begins to wander, return your attention to the breath. When you are finished, take one final

---

BOX 14.1 Self-Reflection Questions: Self-Nurturing Activities

Think back to when you were a child. What activities did you find especially comforting?

If time was not an obstacle, what activities would you choose to do today that you would find to be self-nurturing? How would you pamper yourself?

deep, cleansing breath and open your eyes. This is the simplest form of meditation, and it can be performed anytime and anywhere. Even just taking two or three deep breaths while standing, with your eyes closed, can be a form of meditation, and is most certainly a way to reduce stress. There are many types of meditation that come from a variety of different traditions and are used for a variety of purposes, but five major classifications have been identified: (a) concentration meditation, (b) mindfulness meditation, (c) reflective meditation, (d) creative meditation, and (e) heart-centered meditation (Self-Guided.com, 2016). Other classifications may be found, and literally thousands of sources are available to explore this topic.

A couple of other strategies not addressed in Table 14.1 on self-care include cultivating the "right" attitude; that is, finding the positive in situations, if at all possible. Are you an optimist or a pessimist? Is the glass half empty or half full? When we find ourselves harboring negative thoughts, that can be an opportunity for cognitive reframing. If we change the way we look at something, we can change the way we experience it. It is important to acknowledge the thoughts and feelings we are having; if we change the thoughts, the feelings will also change, and so will our behaviors (Positive Attitude, n. d.). For example, you pass a colleague in the hall at work, and she looks at you in a way that you interpret as angry. You think, "She must be angry at me for some reason, but I don't know why . . . maybe it's something I did, or maybe I forgot to do something?" You then begin to feel anxious and worried, and become distracted in performing your work. What if instead you noticed yourself feeling anxious because of your thoughts about the experience with your colleague? What if you were to challenge your thinking, and reframed it as, "Wait, maybe she isn't angry with me at all. Maybe she was thinking about something that she felt angry and concerned about, and it had nothing at all to do with me." You notice the feelings of anxiety and worry begin to dissipate, and you are able to return your focus to your work. This is a very simplified presentation of cognitive reframing. Additional resources related to cognitive restructuring and reframing are available online. Another way to deal with negative thoughts and emotions is to process them with a trusted friend or to keep a gratitude journal where you can keep track of things you are grateful for.

And finally, do not forget to laugh! Laughter helps to reduce stress hormones, trigger the release of endorphins, and improve the function of the blood vessels, which may help to decrease pain and prevent heart disease; laughter also adds joy and enthusiasm to life, reduces anxiety and stress, improves mood, strengthens relationships, helps diffuse conflict, and enhances teamwork and group bonding (HelpGuide.org, n.d.). As Orem and Vardiman (1995) suggested, using humor and laughter can help provide insights into both self and others.

Some suggestions to get more humor in your life are identified in Box 14.2.

Those of you reading this book may look at the suggested self-care strategies and think, "I already know that I need to eat well, get enough sleep, and exercise. This is all of the same old advice. But I just don't have time." Or, "After a hard day at work the last thing I want to do is exercise," or, "Exercise and taking time to cook healthy meals feels more like punishment than reward."

Motivational interviewing was suggested earlier in this book as a way to help patients become engaged in self-care. A comparable approach to help engage in one's own self-care is described in the book by Michelle Segar (2015), *No Sweat: How the Simple Science of Motivation Can Bring You to a Lifetime of Fitness*. In essence,

> ## BOX 14.2 Ways to Get More Humor in Your Life, or How to Tickle Your Funny Bone
>
> - Watch a movie or television show that makes you laugh.
> - Go to a comedy club.
> - Read the comics in the newspaper.
> - Hang out with people who make you laugh.
> - Share a good joke or a funny story.
> - Have a game night with friends.
> - Play with your children (roll around with them, finger paint, play with clay).
> - Make time for fun activities (bowling, karaoke).
> - Take a 15-minute recess every day.
> - Do not take yourself too seriously.
>
> Adapted from Laughter (n.d.).

Segar describes how to develop intrinsic motivation for health-oriented behavior change that helps to prioritize one's own self-care in ways that can be successfully and readily sustained. For example, individuals decide to exercise because they "should," or because they need to lose weight to become healthier. To accomplish this, they decide to go to the gym several times a week to use weight machines and the treadmill. This exercise program does not last long, because, in truth, for most people this is not much fun and soon becomes just another task or chore. Using Segar's approach, these same individuals are encouraged to find something that they love to do, and that provides energy for what has meaning in their lives. If going to the gym is still something they choose to do, instead of working out alone on weight machines, if they value social connection, they might choose to join a yoga, aerobics, or strength-training class where they can connect and have fun with others. If as children these people loved to swim, perhaps that is something they can do now after a long day's work, as it provides both relaxation and refreshment, as well as exercise. Or, if spending more time with their children is important, maybe they can reclaim a childhood passion and play touch football, or take the family roller-skating or bicycle riding. The point is to find something you love to do and make time to do it, in addition to taking any and every opportunity to move, because in Segar's words "everything counts." This includes housecleaning (assuming that you are listening to music and dancing or singing loudly as you do it), gardening, or Zumba classes at the YMCA. Segar advocates using the "MAPS" approach, that is, finding the "right" meaning (M) or reasons for doing something; developing awareness (A) of what you enjoy and what gets in the way; giving yourself permission (P) to prioritize your own self-care activities, and forgiving yourself when you do not do it perfectly; and finally, creating a strategy (S) to make it all happen. Also in Segar's words, "What sustains us, we sustain."

Something that may help with all of these issues is a consideration of time management strategies. There are many tips to be found on the Internet and in popular self-help books. One strategy that was originally used by Dwight Eisenhower and popularized by Covey, Merrill, and Merrill (1994) is the Time Management Matrix. See Figure 14.1 for an adaptation of the Time Management Matrix by Covey et al.

In addition to basic self-care strategies identified earlier, more specific approaches have been suggested to address certain stress-related problems that pose potentially serious consequences for nurses, patients, and organizations (e.g., compassion fatigue, moral distress, and LV). Although these and other problems related to lack of nurses' self-care are discussed later in this chapter, specific individual self-care strategies are presented here in an effort to provide an integrated overview of ways in which nurses are encouraged to care for themselves.

It should come as no surprise that the main solution suggested for compassion fatigue is basic self-care (Krischke, 2011). This could involve simple things like eating well, staying hydrated, and taking time for meditation/reflection. See Box 14.3 for additional self-care strategies recommended to help with compassion fatigue.

Since nearly every nursing action reflects the nurse's beliefs and values (Storch, 2004), nurses may experience moral and ethical conflict more often than is readily apparent. Box 14.4 summarizes individual strategies to help deal with ethical issues and moral distress.

Nurses who use positive strategies such as self-care, assertiveness, or collective action to alleviate the effects of moral distress and to proactively address these issues may become more self-aware, and make different choices and decisions in the future (McCarthy & Deady, 2008).

Lateral violence, defined as "nurse-to-nurse" aggression (Embree & White, 2010, p. 167), has received much attention in the literature, and is discussed in some detail later in the chapter. Box 14.5 provides suggestions for strategies to address LV.

FIGURE 14.1   Time Management Matrix

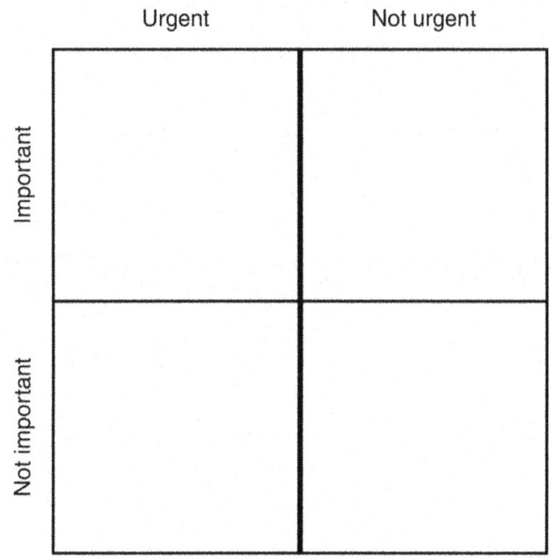

Adapted from Covey et al. (1994).

BOX 14.3 Self-Care Strategies to Address Compassion Fatigue

- Take inventory of work, family, and other commitments.
- Make a list of self-care ideas that would work for you.
- Do something nurturing for yourself every day.
- Delegate (ask for help) both at home and work.
- Have a transition from work to home such as meeting with a friend or taking a walk.
- Learn to say "no" (or "yes") more often.
- Identify what you really want and prioritize these activities.

Adapted from Mathieu (2007).

BOX 14.4 Individual Strategies for Moral Distress

- Take care of your own basic health and social needs (Wallis, 2015).
- Cultivate mindfulness to regulate emotional responses (McCarthy & Deady, 2008).
- Promote "compassionate intention" by engaging in practices that encourage kindness, gratefulness, and generosity among other "prosocial emotions" (Wallis, 2015).
- Refine moral-reasoning skills (Wallis, 2015).
- Engage in honest self-reflection and genuine discourse with others (Burston & Tuckett, 2012; Vogel, 2007).
- Trust your own sense of values and be willing to state them.
- Be assertive when confronting situations that cause distress.
- Participate in institutional ethics committees.

BOX 14.5 General Strategies to Address Lateral Violence

- Develop conflict resolution, assertiveness, and negotiation skills (Blair, 2013; Lachman, 2015).
- Access and utilize institutional information, opportunities, resources, and support (Lachman, 2015; Laschinger, 2011; Roberts, 2015).
- Cultivate emotional intelligence (See Goleman, 2006; Littlejohn, 2012; Salovey & Mayer, 1990).

One of the identified strategies to address LV, emotional intelligence is a set of skills theorized to help people solve problems in constructive or adaptive ways. *Emotional intelligence* has been defined as "the subset of social intelligence that involves the ability to monitor one's own and others' feelings and emotions, to discriminate among them and to use this information to guide one's thinking and actions" (Salovey & Mayer, 1990, p. 189). Five components of emotional intelligence are identified: (a) self-awareness regarding one's own emotions and their effect on others; (b) self-regulation, that is, the ability to suspend judgment and think before speaking or acting; (c) internal motivation, or passion to work for one's own vision of what is important in life as opposed to external rewards such as money or status; (d) empathy, the ability to "put oneself in another person's shoes" and to understand the emotional reactions of others; and (e) social skills, including the ability to find a common ground and establish rapport with others (Goleman's Emotional Intelligence, n.d.).

Finally, obtaining professional counseling, accessing employee assistance programs (EAP), or joining peer support groups may be helpful in addressing stress-related problems. These options have especially been recommended for someone experiencing either direct or indirect traumatization.

STRESS IN NURSING

What, then, are the consequences of nurses not taking adequate care of self? In this section, positive and negative effects of stress are examined. Effects of stress in individual nurses, patients, and organizations are considered.

Although the first known use of the term *stress* (short for *distress*) was in the 14th century, stress itself has existed for millennia. *Stress* can be defined as "a state of mental tension and worry," "a constraining force or influence," or "a state resulting from a stress; especially: one of bodily or mental tension resulting from factors that tend to alter an existent equilibrium" (Stress, n.d.). Stress can be conceptualized as a "relationship between the person and the environment that is appraised by the person as taxing or exceeding his or her resources and as endangering well-being" (Folkman, Lazarus, Gruen, & DeLongis, 1986, p. 572). Stress, a factor long associated with both physical and psychological impairment, is considered an occupational hazard and has been a source of concern in nursing for several decades (Jennings, 2008).

Findings from more than 43,000 nurses from more than 700 hospitals in the United States, Canada, England, Scotland, and Germany from 1998 to 1999 indicated job dissatisfaction, burnout, and intent of nurses to leave the profession (Aiken et al., 2001). Authors of this study suggested major workforce management reforms to ensure satisfactory patient care and an adequate force of nurses for the future. In spite of this and related recommendations by others, recent literature indicates that these problems persist. A "workforce crisis" especially in hospitals was identified, and this crisis is manifested in nursing turnover rates and an ongoing nursing shortage (Jennings, 2008).

Positive and Negative Effects of Stress

Many authors provide physiological evidence to support positive effects of stress (for example, see McEwen, 2008). Some commonly accepted benefits of stress are that it can increase motivation, provide cognitive or mental improvement, and enhance physical performance. Mild or moderate amounts of stress may also contribute to feelings of excitement and creative energy. Excessive amounts of stress, and/or stress that is experienced over long periods, usually has negative consequences. Table 14.2 summarizes commonly recognized signs and symptoms of stress.

After reviewing the content in Table 14.2, see Box 14.6 for critical thinking/self-reflection questions.

Prolonged exposure to stressful situations has potentially serious consequences. Some studies have shown, for example, that "shift work" may contribute to risk for diabetes mellitus (DM) through altered sleeping and eating patterns, associated weight gain, increase in appetite and body fat, and insulin resistance (Doyle, 2014; Shift Work and Diabetes Risk, 2014). Nurses who experience disrupted sleep or sleep deprivation may be at increased risk for development of sleep disorders (Doyle, 2014); accidents and other injuries (Doyle, 2014; Sleep Deprivation, 2011); and impaired cognition and poor clinical decision making (Shift Work and Cognition, 2014; Sleep-Deprived Nurses, 2013). *Shift work disorder* was defined as a combination of difficulty sleeping and excessive sleepiness while awake, which especially affects people who work at night (Doyle, 2014). Other consequences of chronic exposure to stress may be heart disease (Doyle, 2014; Hendren, 2010); alcohol and/or other substance abuse and dependence (Maslach, Schaufeli, & Leiter, 2001; Vahey, Aiken, Sloane, Clarke, & Vargas, 2004); and mental health problems such as anxiety, depression, and low self-esteem.

Types of Occupational Stress

Substantial effort has been made to capture and categorize the experience of occupational stress. Four major types of occupational stress for nurses, and other helping professionals, are extensively reviewed in the literature: burnout, compassion fatigue, traumatization, and moral distress. Multiple authors have described lack of conceptual clarity among these concepts. Violence in the workplace is without question another source of stress for nurses and other health care professionals, and is addressed later in this section.

BURNOUT

Burnout is a phenomenon that occurs in response to chronic job stressors, and it has negative effects on both employee health and workplace well-being. A common understanding of the three components of burnout includes emotional exhaustion, depersonalization or cynicism, and loss of sense of personal accomplishment (Jennings, 2008; Leiter & Maslach, 2003; Maslach et al., 2001). Causes of burnout are primarily associated with work-related environmental factors, such as heavy

---

BOX 14.6　Self-Reflection Questions: Stress

What physical, emotional, cognitive, and/or behavioral symptoms of stress have you experienced? How did you address these symptoms, and were your efforts successful?

TABLE 14.2 Signs and Symptoms of Stress

Physical	Emotional	Cognitive	Behavioral
• Fatigue/low energy	• Anxiety	• Constant worrying	• Overeating or undereating
• Headaches	• Restlessness	• Ruminating	• Procrastination or avoidance of
• Upset stomach	• Feeling overwhelmed	• Racing thoughts	responsibilities
• Aches, pains, tense muscles	• Irritability or anger; easily	• Forgetfulness and disorganization	• Angry outbursts
• Chest pain/rapid heart beat	frustrated	• Lack of focus or motivation	• Nail biting, fidgeting, pacing
• Sleep problems	• Difficulty relaxing	• Difficulty making decisions	• Drug or alcohol abuse
• Change in sex drive/ability	• Low self-esteem	• Poor judgment	• Tobacco use
• Nervousness and shaking	• Sadness or depression	• Pessimism or seeing only the negative	• Social withdrawal
• Dry mouth/difficulty swallowing			
• Clenched jaw and grinding teeth			

Adapted from Mayo Clinic (n.d.); Stress (n.d.); WebMD (n.d.).

workloads, inadequate staffing levels, lack of administrative support, limited resources, and job dissatisfaction (Laschinger & Fida, 2014; Sabo, 2011). Burnout also has been associated with work–family conflict; that is, work can interfere with family responsibilities, or family obligations can interfere with work, especially for those in the "sandwich generation," caring for both children and parents (Jennings, 2008).

Maslach's (1982, 1998) initial theoretical understanding of burnout was expanded through consideration of the person in the context of the work environment. The comprehensive model that was developed explored the amount of "match or mismatch" between the individual and six aspects of the person's work environment: workload, control, reward, community, fairness, and values (Maslach et al., 2001). The model predicts that greater disparity or mismatch between the person and his or her work environment will more likely lead to burnout. A better fit is predicted to result in the individual's engagement with his or her job, and less burnout. This model hypothesizes burnout as a mediator variable, that is, "the mismatches lead to burnout, which in turn leads to various outcomes" (p. 414), such as job dissatisfaction, intent to leave, and actual turnover. The six aspects of work environment included in the model are derived from research related to burnout, and they comprise the "major organizational antecedents of burnout" (p. 414). These factors do not exist in isolation, but they are interactive with each other and with the three dimensions of burnout (exhaustion, depersonalization, and reduced self-efficacy). See Table 14.3 for a summary of these environmental factors, and their hypothesized relationship to burnout.

Individual nurses' choices also contribute to burnout, such as decisions to work overtime, or to work three 12-hour shifts at their primary place of employment and then to work additional hours in other places. These individual decisions are usually not made with a priority of balance and personal self-care in mind, but rather to maximize financial resources. Although this is important, it is essential to consider the overall cost to personal well-being.

Finally, Maslach et al. proposed a change in focus from the negative outcome, burnout, to a more positive aspect of a person's work life, that of engagement (Maslach et al., 2001). A focus on job engagement is more consistent with the strengths-based approach that is gaining influence in current psychology, as opposed to the more traditional primary focus on problems. One way of understanding job engagement is that it is the opposite of burnout, represented by "a sustainable workload, feelings of choice and control, appropriate recognition and reward, a supportive work community, fairness and justice, and meaningful and valued work" (p. 417). Another way to understand job engagement is to consider it a concept to be defined and measured separately from burnout. Using a framework described by Watson and Tellegen (as cited in Maslach et al., 2001), burnout could be classified as having low levels of activation and pleasure, compared with engagement, which would have high levels of activation and pleasure. From this perspective, *job engagement* could be defined as "a persistent, positive affective-motivational state of fulfillment in employees that is characterized by vigor, dedication, and absorption" (p. 417).

COMPASSION FATIGUE

Concepts related to compassion fatigue and vicarious traumatization began emerging in the 1990s (Sabo, 2011). *Compassion fatigue* has been defined as exhaustion

TABLE 14.3 Organizational Strategies to Reduce Stress (Addressing Areas of Work Environmental Factors Related to Burnout)

Workload	• Adequate staffing (Vahey et al., 2004) • Avoid "quick return" scheduling (Doyle, 2014; Fewer Quick-Return Shifts, 2015); limit "extended hour" shifts (ANA Position Statement, 2014).
Control	• Nurse input when designing work schedules (ANA recommendations reported in ANA Position Statement [2014]), work environments, and work processes • Training and education; feeling competent at a job can help reduce stress. • Unit staff meetings for problem solving (Leiter & Maslach, 2003) • Structural empowerment, i.e., provision of "information, opportunities, resources, and support" (Lachman, 2015; Laschinger, 2011; Roberts, 2015) • Positive/authentic leadership (Bamford, Wong, & Laschinger, 2013; Laschinger & Fida, 2014) to support employees' ability to do their work
Reward	• Recognition and reward (Leiter & Maslach, 2003)
Fairness	• Skill development to create a "just culture" (Blair, 2013)
Community	• Nurse leadership committed to stopping lateral violence (Blair, 2013; Roberts, 2015) • Employer encouragement of nurses to be proactive about managing their health, including getting 7 to 9 hours of sleep per 24 hours, managing stress effectively, and developing healthy exercise and nutrition habits (ANA Position Statement, 2014) • Mentorship and buddy programs (Henry, 2014; Leiter & Maslach, 2003) • Retreats, writing workshops, and stress-reduction programs (Hendren, 2010; Henry, 2014) • Creation of space for relaxation (comfortable chairs, music, Reiki, light massage; Hendren, 2010; Lombardo & Eyre, 2011)
Values	• Organization systems developed to assist with ethical dilemmas (Wallis, 2015) • Interprofessional models to address ethical issues (e.g., discuss ethical issues on rounds, weekly unit meetings in which all team members have the opportunity to voice concerns; McCarthy & Deady, 2008; Wallis, 2015); addressing ethical issues as a group "derails any antagonism that might otherwise result from ethics discussion" (Wallis, 2015, p. 20). • Education to improve ethical understanding, ethical skills, and communication (Burston & Tuckett, 2012)

Adapted from Leiter and Maslach (2003).

resulting from a combination of various types of physical, emotional, and spiritual stressors that are associated with caring for patients in significant emotional and/or physical distress (Lombardo & Eyre, 2011). Although empathic caring is essential to the nursing role, it may result in feeling overwhelmed and helpless, especially when the patient does not change or does not get better. The caregiver may engage in self-sacrificing behaviors, that is, caring more for others than for self. Compassion fatigue and also direct or indirect trauma may be associated with demands of working with certain populations, such as pediatric oncology, critical care, mental health, or those experiencing extreme suffering or trauma such as in the emergency department (Sabo, 2011).

Since empathic caring is considered an integral part of the nurse–patient relationship, some authors have taken issue with the implication that empathy can have a negative outcome, instead of resulting in a fulfilling working relationship with patients (e.g., Sabo, 2011). Stamm (2010) developed a model of "Professional Quality of Life" that comprised compassion satisfaction and compassion fatigue. Compassion satisfaction is the pleasure that helpers derive from their work. Compassion fatigue is the negative aspects that result from helping others. Stamm described burnout and secondary traumatic stress as elements of compassion fatigue.

Why some health care workers experience satisfaction and reward in the same work that results in compassion fatigue for others is a question that has not been sufficiently addressed, although at least part of the answer may be found in how nurses do or do not care for themselves. Differences in perception may also be related to personality factors. Nurses exposed to the very same stressors may perceive them very differently, that is, cognitive appraisal of the experience will be different (Jennings, 2008; Lazarus & Folkman, 1984). It seems reasonable to presume that all or most caregivers experience some elements of both compassion satisfaction and compassion fatigue.

TRAUMATIZATION

Vicarious traumatization has been described as an occupational stressor in nursing. This experience varies significantly between and among individuals, due in part to different life experiences, such as personal history of abuse, extreme stressors, or trauma; exposure to use of extremely invasive technology to keep patients alive; and ongoing experience with human trauma and suffering (Sabo, 2011).

Several authors distinguished between direct or primary and indirect or secondary traumatization. Direct or primary traumatic stress may be experienced by people who work with horrific war injuries, those who work in trauma centers, those who are directly in the path of danger (such as firefighters or soldiers), and those who witness violence. Indirect or secondary stress can result from exposure to the trauma of others, such as listening to someone else describe the horror he or she experienced (Kift, 2012; Responding to Stressful Events, 2005; Sabo, 2011; Stamm, 2010). Symptoms/signs of traumatic stress include inability to concentrate, repeated thoughts about a traumatic situation, feeling numb or withdrawn, irritability, keeping busy to avoid thoughts of the traumatic situation, and using alcohol or drugs to relax (Kift, 2012). A person experiencing traumatic stress may or may not meet specific criteria for post-traumatic stress disorder.

MORAL DISTRESS

Moral distress in nursing has been called a "rising concern" (Wallis, 2015, p. 19). Although ideas related to moral distress date back at least as far as Aristotle, the works of Jameton (1984) and Wilkinson (1987/1988) brought the concept to the forefront of nursing. Jameton's original definition of *moral distress* is when a person knows "the right" thing to do, but is not able to act due to administrative or institutional constraints. Jameton distinguished between moral distress and moral dilemma, which is concerned with conflicting ethical principles. There is lack of conceptual clarity about moral distress, which may contribute to the propensity to confound moral distress with psychological and emotional distress (Johnstone & Hutchinson, 2015; McCarthy & Deady, 2008).

In addition to the external factors that may contribute to moral distress, internal or intrapersonal aspects may be involved. In fact, moral distress is often associated with conflict between internal and external values (Vogel, 2007). Someone may disagree with a value imposed by the institution, or expressed by another health care colleague, but choose not to express or act on his or her own values because of fear of recrimination or lack of self-confidence. Furthermore, it may be nurses' perceptions of situations rather than external factors that form the experience of moral distress (Burston & Tuckett, 2012).

It is the internal or intrapersonal aspect of moral distress that led Johnstone and Huthinson (2015) to challenge the underlying assumption that nurses know the right thing to do but are unable to carry it out. There is lack of evidence to support that nurses' moral judgments are always correct. Instead, these authors asserted that judgments are often made on the basis of personal opinion, subjective values, religious beliefs, education, upbringing, and feelings rather than on principles of ethical decision making. These authors acknowledged that there are external constraints but contended that nurses are not powerless to address ethical conflicts. It is true that nurses may not always be right in their moral judgments. However, nurses do have their own identity and experience, choices, and insights. When values based on these factors are voiced, consciously taken into account, and become part of the discourse along with patient preferences and thoughtful consideration of ethical principles, decision-making balance is achieved. Efforts to enact personal and professional values, even if not successful in bringing about change, should not be viewed as failure, but rather as action taken toward individual and professional responsibility and empowerment. See Box 14.4 for ways to increase empowerment in the area of moral distress.

Burston and Tuckett (2012) concluded that three factors are involved in nurses' experience of moral distress: first, the individual traits, experiences, and worldview of the nurse; second, characteristics of the work environment; and third, broad external influences such as economic factors, legal and professional standards, and "third-party expectations" (p. 318). Additional external factors contributing to moral distress, among others, include end-of-life issues and changing technology, resulting in potentially more aggressive treatment of patients with terminal illness (McCarthy & Deady, 2008; Wallis, 2015); lack of resources and inadequate staffing (Burston & Tuckett, 2012; Wallis, 2015); inconsistent or lack of communication among various health care providers, patients, and their families (Wallis, 2015); power differential among health providers (McCarthy & Deady, 2008); and finally, organizational structure and lack of institutional support (Burston & Tuckett, 2012; McCarthy & Deady, 2008). Interaction between individual and structural factors has been proposed as a major force in the development of moral distress (Varcoe, Pauly, Webster, & Storch, 2012).

The experience of moral distress can affect individuals in very different ways. In one study reviewed by McCarthy and Deady (2008), new nurses described the experience of moral distress as disappointment in themselves, uncertainty, and self-blame. Compromising one's own values can lead a person to minimize or deny any wrongdoing, and to ultimately abandon his or her own principles in order to protect his or her sense of self (McCarthy & Deady, 2008). On the other hand, moral distress can make nurses more aware of and reflective on their beliefs and strengthen their resolve to do things differently or better next time.

Moral distress, dilemmas, ambiguity, and uncertainty are also experienced by other health care professionals. Nurses may be predisposed to moral distress because of their proximity or closeness to patients. "When the health care system or health professionals (including nurses) treat patients shabbily, it is a nurse who is at the bedside witnessing the results of that ethical failure and who experience moral distress" (McCarthy & Deady, 2008, p. 261). Jameton (2013) stated that, although all members of health care teams have ethical positions and dilemmas, it is nurses who are much more involved in the emotional aspects of care. The Canadian nurse ethicist Storch wrote (as cited in McCarthy & Deady, 2008), "nurses who are morally engaged are concerned about values, including respect, dignity and quality of care.... Nursing ethics is about being in relationship to persons in care. The enactment of nursing ethics is a constant readiness to engage one's moral agency. Almost every nursing action and situation involves ethics" (p. 255). See Box 14.7 for critical thinking/self-reflection questions related to this topic.

VIOLENCE IN THE WORKPLACE

Multiple sources of stress within nursing have been addressed throughout this chapter. One issue that deserves further attention is violence in the workplace. This can be in the form of violence directed to health care staff from patients, families, visitors, or other health care staff. It is important to recognize that workplace violence can also occur in the form of LV, which is addressed here.

LV is an issue that has received significant attention in recent years. Many related and overlapping terms such as *lateral or horizontal violence, bullying,* and *incivility* are used to describe this concept (Embree & White, 2010; Roberts, 2015). Efforts have been made to distinguish among incivility, bullying, and horizontal/lateral violence, but these differences remain unclear (Lachman, 2015). Within nursing, *LV* has been defined as "nurse-nurse aggression" (Embree & White, 2010, p. 167).

It is estimated that 39% of new nurses in their first year of practice observed bullying in the workplace, and 31% actually experienced it (Lachman, 2015; Laschinger, 2011). Numbers ranging from 46% to 100% of practicing nurses have been reported to experience some form of LV (Lachman, 2015; Roberts, 2015).

The first three provisions of the ANA Code of Ethics for Nursing (ANA, 2015a) define essential values of the nurse, with four interpretive statements relevant to disruptive behaviors in the workplace. (Lachman, 2015). "The Joint

---

BOX 14.7   Self-Reflection Questions: Moral Distress

Have you experienced ethical dilemma(s) or moral distress? How did you resolve it? If still unresolved, how has this affected you and your nursing practice?

Commission (2008) Sentinel Event Alert 'Behaviors That Undermine a Culture of Safety'" (2008) addressed an organization's responsibility to develop standards, a code of conduct, and suggestions to eliminate behaviors that destabilize a culture of patient and staff safety. Finally, standards to make a zero-tolerance policy regarding LV were developed by the AACN (2004, 2005). The six standards are skilled communication, true collaboration, effective decision making, appropriate staffing that matches patient needs and nurse competencies, meaningful recognition, and authentic leadership (AACN, 2005, p. 13). It is important to acknowledge that merely having a policy in place does not change the underlying issues that lead to LV, and does not prevent individual nurses from behaving in ways that perpetuate the problem. Policies are, in some ways, efforts to mandate behavior. They must be supported by genuine efforts to understand the root causes of LV in order to provide effective solutions.

Disagreement exists about what causes LV. Some authors maintained that nurses are an "oppressed group," primarily because of a hierarchical work arrangement with physicians (Blair, 2013; Roberts, 2015). Historically, nursing has essentially been governed by the medical paradigm with its focus on control and cure. A shift to the business model values of efficiency, productivity, and cost control has occurred within recent years. Nurses have often passively adopted values conveyed by the dominant paradigms. As nurses become more aware of how these values affect their own belief systems, health, and well-being, they experience more dissension and conflict within themselves and within the work environment. This disconnect may result in blaming each other, or LV, and/or dissatisfaction with being a nurse (Vogel, 2007). Nurses are not, however, powerless to address these issues. Opportunities for choice and change occur when nurses and other health care providers are willing to engage in thoughtful reflection and genuine dialogue that reveals differences among value systems. Having the willingness to take these actions requires courage and commitment, but it also results in taking responsibility for our own discomfort and taking the first steps into our own place of power (Vogel, 2007).

LV is a multifaceted phenomenon that most likely has multiple causative factors. The importance of understanding root causes cannot be underestimated, but it is beyond the scope of this work. Regardless of causation, serious results of LV, incivility, and bullying have been documented: risk to patient safety, reduced patient satisfaction, decreased nurse job satisfaction, absenteeism, and decreased retention of nurses (Blair, 2013; Roberts, 2015; Roberts, Demarco, & Griffin, 2009). Refer to Box 14.5 for a review of strategies to address LV. See Box 14.8 for critical thinking/self-reflection questions related to LV.

BOX 14.8   Self-Reflection Questions: Lateral Violence (LV)

Have you experienced LV in the workplace? What do you think was the underlying cause? How did you respond? Have you ever initiated LV? If so, what do you think was the underlying cause?

Does your institution have a policy regarding LV? If so, how effective is it? What do you think would make it more effective?

EFFECTS OF NURSES' STRESS ON PATIENTS

Less research has been reported on how nurses' stress affects patient outcomes. Jennings (2008) reported results of studies of the relationship between burnout and increased patient mortality, failure to rescue (Aiken, Clarke, Sloane, Sochalski, & Silber, 2002; Halm et al., 2005), and patient dissatisfaction (Leiter, Harvie, & Frizzell, 1998; Vahey et al., 2004). In the field of mental health services, burnout may interrupt the continuity of patient care and negatively influence the quality of care and patient satisfaction. In addition, burnout and especially emotional exhaustion may result in negative feelings about mental health patients, ultimately resulting in poorer outcomes for people with serious mental illness (Morse et al., 2012). Research reported by Spence Laschinger and Leiter (2006) supported the mediating role that burnout/lack of job engagement plays in patient safety outcomes.

EFFECTS OF NURSES' STRESS ON ORGANIZATIONS

Chronic stress experienced by nurses can also have negative effects on institutions. These can be poor job performance, absenteeism, intention to leave, and turnover; those who do stay in their work situation may have lower productivity and effectiveness, as well as decreased job satisfaction (Maslach et al., 2001).

Nursing Turnover

Nursing turnover is defined and measured in many different ways (Hayes et al, 2006; Kovner, Brewer, Fatehi, & Jun, 2014). Regardless of measures used, high rates of turnover are consistently reported across studies (Kovner et al, 2014; Laschinger & Fida, 2014; Nursing Solutions, Inc. [NSI], 2015). Reasons for voluntary turnover included relocation, personal reasons, career advancement, retirement, education, salary, commute/location, scheduling, and workload/staffing ratios (NSI, 2015). Other reasons for turnover included job dissatisfaction, workload, poor management style, lack of empowerment and autonomy, lack of opportunities for promotion, and work schedules (Hayes et al., 2006). Medical–surgical nursing (20.7%), emergency (21.7%), and behavioral health (30.7%) are the specialty areas with the highest rates of turnover (NSI, 2015). Although more nurses than ever are graduating from nursing programs, the turnover rate for new nurses also is reported as being high. Data from the Robert Wood Johnson RN Work Project indicated that about 17.5% of new nurses leave their first job within a year of starting (Kovner et al., 2014). The meaning of this statistic is not altogether clear, because no distinctions are made between changing positions within the organization, leaving the organization, leaving professional nursing, and working in non-nursing jobs.

It is generally accepted that turnover of registered nurses results in increased cost to the health care system. Approximately 83% of hospitals do not track the cost of turnover, but the estimated cost of turnover for each bedside RN ranges from $36,900 to $57,300, with the average hospital losing approximately $6.2 million (NSI, 2015). Each percentage change in hospital turnover rate would potentially

---

BOX 14.9   Self-Reflection Questions: Turnover

From your experience, what factors do you think are the most associated with nursing turnover? When you have left or changed jobs, what has been your reason or reasons? Are there differences between the "stated" and "real" reasons for leaving a position?

---

either cost or save the average hospital an additional $379,500 (NSI). The cost estimate of nursing turnover varies, depending on geographic area and nursing specialty (Embree & White, 2010). However, it is clear that the cost is substantial. If hospitals are concerned about profit margins, attention needs to be given to nurse retention. See Box 14.9 for critical thinking/self-reflection questions about nursing turnover.

Nursing Shortage

Some disagreement exists about whether or not there is, or is projected to be, a nursing shortage. Vacancies of 10% or more were reported by 24.2% of hospitals, with an overall RN vacancy rate of 7.2% (NSI, 2015). The overall national RN vacancy rate is estimated to be 8.1% (AACN, 2014). Nursing shortages are projected in the coming years due to the numbers of aging baby boomers who will need health care, expanded access to health care secondary to the Affordable Care Act (ACA), aging of the workforce, and nursing programs struggling to produce enough graduates (AACN, 2014; ANA, 2015b). To the contrary, the Healthcare Staffing Report (January, 2015) cited the U.S. Health Resources and Services Administration (HRSA) in predicting an excess supply of nurses in the United States by 2025. This report cited a "muted" effect of the ACA on demand for nurses. Regional shortages are still projected, especially in the South and West. This predicted nursing surplus is based on the "skyrocketing" number of new graduates, and assumes that the number will remain constant and that these new nurses will stay in the profession. The authors of the Healthcare Staffing Report acknowledged the possible growth in demand for nurses that may come from new health care delivery models, with focus on managing effects of chronic illness and prevention of acute health issues.

The nursing shortage may not have fully manifested as of yet, due primarily to impending retirement of a large cohort of nurses who are themselves baby boomers (AACN, 2014; Nurse Residency Programs, 2015). Newer nurses will need to fill the void, and this reinforces the need for hospital retention strategies. Although the overwhelming majority of hospitals (89.1%) view retention as a "key strategic imperative," just more than one third (36.4%) report having a formal retention strategy (NSI, 2015).

Negative effects of the nursing shortage include nurses working long hours under often stressful conditions that can result in fatigue, injuries, and job dissatisfaction/burnout. In these conditions, nurses are more inclined to make medical errors and other mistakes (ANA, 2015b). Some studies have shown that increased workloads are associated with higher hospital readmission rates and higher rates of infection. Inadequate nurse staffing has been associated with higher mortality rates; also, inadequate staffing has been reported by nurses to reduce quality of care (AACN, 2014).

ORGANIZATIONAL STRATEGIES TO REDUCE STRESS/BURNOUT

Although various types of occupational stress have been identified in this chapter, some stress-reduction strategies may be applicable across different types of stress. The majority of authors recommended a combination of intrapersonal and organizational approaches to stress reduction (Awa, Plaumann, & Walter, 2010; Laschinger & Fida, 2014). In Table 14.3, organizational strategies are suggested to help reduce stress in nursing. Advocating for these approaches is something that should be of concern not just to nurse managers but also to all nurses.

As mentioned earlier in this chapter, formal retention strategies need to be developed by organizations (NSI, 2015). New graduate residency programs may also be important. These programs are on the rise, with 36.9% reported in 2011 and 45% reported in 2013 (Future of Nursing Campaign for Action, 2015). NSI (2015) reported that 76% of hospitals in their study reported using new nurse residency programs with 80% perceived effectiveness.

Authentic leadership is a relatively new concept in nursing literature. It is defined as "a positive relationship-focused leadership style that emphasizes self-awareness, honesty and transparency, behavioral integrity, and consistency" (Laschinger & Fida, 2014, p. 20). Authentic leadership has been associated with work engagement as described by Maslach et al. (2001). Nurses who work for managers who demonstrate authentic leadership characteristics report a better fit with their work environment and greater work engagement (Bamford, Wong, & Laschinger, 2013; Laschinger & Fida, 2014). Authentic leadership qualities need to be encouraged and developed within organizations. Nurse leaders need to advocate for resources to help them develop authentic leadership practice.

When organizations implement strategies to address burnout and other occupational stress, positive outcomes may be realized: increased retention, decreased turnover rates, increased performance, and increased patient satisfaction and quality of care (Henry, 2014).

SUMMARY

The intent of this chapter is to emphasize the importance of nurses caring for themselves. This is critical for the health and well-being of the individual nurse, for optimal patient care, and for a healthy and productive work environment. Nursing can be a highly stressful profession. How individual nurses perceive stressful situations, and how they choose to implement self-care activities, is paramount in determining positive versus negative effects of stress.

In this chapter, basic self-care strategies are presented, using Orem's (2001) universal self-care requisites as an organizing framework. Consequences of not caring for self are discussed. In addition to individual self-care strategies, organizational approaches were discussed to help prevent and alleviate stress. Both of these approaches are essential in addressing stress-related problems in nursing and other helping professions.

Those of you reading this book are or will become nurse leaders of the future. What commitments are you willing to make in regard to your own self-care? How will you endeavor to change the work environment for yourselves and others? The future of nursing depends on your individual and our collective answers to these questions.

LEARNING ACTIVITIES

Use the MAPS approach identified by Segar (2015) to help you on your own personal journey to self-care, health, and well-being. Reading Segar's entire book is strongly recommended.

MEANING: FIND A REASON THAT MOTIVATES YOU

1. **Understand that the wrong "why" for doing something is because you *should*.**
2. **Make a list of "personal projects"**—five most important things that you are currently engaged in or thinking about doing. These will most likely reflect who you are and what you care about the most.
3. **Focus on something that really gets you excited!** Brainstorm before narrowing it down to one. Do you want to swim the English Channel or walk across England? Do you want to hike the Grand Canyon or run a marathon? Have you always wanted to learn horseback riding? Think of things that would be fun for you. And then choose one to focus on for now.
4. **Build some freedom into your goals.** For example, if you decide that running is what you want to do, allow yourself to "dance, skip, stop to look at a bird or a flower" (Ferguson, n.d.), or do anything else you feel like doing along the way.

AWARENESS

1. **Spend some time noticing what it is that you enjoy.**
2. **Pay attention to what you are doing now.** If your goal is to start walking more, buy a pedometer or another kind of activity monitor and chart the total number of steps/miles that you walk each day.
3. **Notice how you feel when you do some activity you enjoy.** When you go running, bike riding, skating, swimming, walking, or whatever activity you choose, how do you feel afterward? Do you feel more or less stressed than you did earlier?
4. **What might get in the way of moving toward your chosen activity or goal?** Lack of awareness about this often results in sabotaging success. For example, if you know that you tend to eat "comfort food" when feeling stressed, it is good to be aware of what causes you to feel stressed and what symptoms you experience. You can then choose to do something else to

(continued)

LEARNING ACTIVITIES (*continued*)

relieve stress. Or, you can choose to eat comfort food. At least you will be making a conscious choice and will have the opportunity to own your decision!

5. **Do you really have "no time"?** Complete the Time Management Matrix (Figure 14.1) and think about this again. In regard to physical activity, remember that everything counts. Make it a "treasure hunt" to find hidden opportunities to move: taking the stairs at work, marching in place as you watch television, and even going shopping.

PERMISSION

1. **Give yourself permission to prioritize your own self-care activities.**
2. **Give yourself permission to celebrate your victories, both short term and long term.** Recognize how good you feel after taking a yoga class. Take a hot bath or sit in the Jacuzzi after a long run. Get a massage. Identify some small rewards that you can enjoy along the way, and plan a big reward for achieving a major milestone.
3. **Ask for support.** Pick your support person/people carefully. Choose those who accept you as who you are right now, those who help you feel good when you are with them. Tell them what you are trying to accomplish and ask whether they would be willing to support you in your goal. Tell them specific things that they can do to help you (Ferguson, n.d).
4. **Forgive yourself when you do not do it perfectly.** It is okay to just take a break sometimes. And it is okay to negotiate your plans with life circumstances as they arise. And, if what you are trying to accomplish is just not working, take time to reevaluate. Remember that no matter what happens, you have not failed, and you have gained some important information along the way. And, it is okay to change your mind about the activity that you want to pursue.

STRATEGY: HOW TO DEVELOP SUSTAINABLE CHANGE

1. **Act based on internal rather than external reasons—shift from "performance" goals to "learning" goals.** Rather than trying to exercise for 50 minutes 6 days a week, or lowering your cholesterol numbers (performance goals), aim for mastering new tasks such as learning how to be more active on any given day and under various circumstances (learning goals). This helps us "integrate and sustain" new behaviors in our busy lives (Segar, 2015).
2. **Take the lifelong view.** Work toward developing habits that result in a healthier lifestyle over the long haul rather than achieving quick results.
3. **Use sustainable self-care strategies as a way to achieve overall well-being.** Taking good care of one's self provides fuel for what has meaning in our lives.

(*continued*)

LEARNING ACTIVITIES (*continued*)

4. **Focus on integrating one new behavior change or activity at a time.** Doing this will help prevent you from becoming overwhelmed and giving up altogether. Once you have mastered one thing, for example, taking the dog for a walk each day, then aim for another.

5. **Develop consistency rather than focusing on quantity.** Start with small, weekly behavioral goals.

6. **Move from theory (what you have learned) to practice.** Learn through doing by integrating new behavior into many different aspects and circumstances of life.

References

Aiken, L. H., Clarke, S. P., Sloane, D. M., Sochalski, J. A., Busse, R., Clarke, H., … Shamian, J. (2001). Nurses' reports on hospital care in five countries. *Health Affairs, 20*(3), 43–53.

Aiken, L. H., Clarke, S. P., Sloane, D. M., Sochalski, J., & Silber, J. H. (2002). Hospital nurse staffing and patient mortality, nurse burnout, and job dissatisfaction. *Journal of American Medical Association, 288*(16), 1987–1993. doi:10.1001/jama.288.16.1987

American Association of Critical-Care Nurses. (2004). *Zero tolerance for abuse position statement.* Retrieved from www.aacn.org/wd/practice/docs/zero_tolerance_for_abuse .pdf

American Association of Critical-Care Nurses. (2005). Standards for establishing and sustaining healthy work environments: A journey to excellence. *American Journal of Critical Care, 14*(3), 187–197. Retrieved from www.aacn.org/healthywork

American Association of Critical-Care Nurses. (2008). The essentials of baccalaureate education for professional nursing practice. Retrieved from www.aacn.nche.edu/ education

American Association of Critical-Care Nurses. (2011). *Nursing fact sheet.* Retrieved from http://www.aacn.nche.edu/media-relations/fact-sheets/nursing-fact-sheet

American Association of Critical-Care Nurses. (2014). *Nursing shortage.* Retrieved from http://www.aacn.nche.edu/media-relations/fact-sheets/nursing-shortage

American Nurses Association. (2015a). *Code of ethics for nurses with interpretive statements.* Silver Springs, MD: Author.

American Nurses Association. (2015b). *Nursing shortage.* Retrieved from www.nursing world.org/nursingshortage

American Nurses Association Position Statement. (2014). ANA releases new position statement on nurse fatigue. *Medscape.* Retrieved from www.medscape.com

Awa, W. L., Plaumann, M., & Walter, U. (2010). Burnout prevention: A review of intervention programs. *Patient Education and Counseling, 78*(2), 184–190. doi:10.1016/j.pec .2009.04.008

Bamford, M., Wong, C. A., & Laschinger, H. (2013). The influence of authentic leadership and areas of worklife on work engagement of registered nurses. *Journal of Nursing Management, 21,* 529–540. doi:10.1111/j.1365-2834.2012.01399.x

Blair, P. L. (2013). Lateral violence in nursing. *Journal of Emergency Nursing, 39*, e75–e78. http://dx.doi.org 10.1016/j.jen.2011.12.006

Burston, A. S., & Tuckett, A. G. (2012). Moral distress in nursing: Contributing factors, outcomes and interventions. *Nursing Ethics, 20*(3), 312–324.

Covey, S. R., Merrill, R., & Merrill, R. R. (1994). *First things first: To live, to learn, to leave a legacy.* New York, NY: Simon & Schuster.

Dietary Guidelines. (2010). Retrieved from www.health.gov/DietaryGuidelines

Doyle, K. (2014). Short rest periods between shifts linked to shift work disorder. *Reuters*, July 3, 2014. Retrieved from www.reuters.com/article/2014/07/03/us-shift-workers-nurses-health-idUSKBN0F81V920140703#WfVoxvj4PzuRXz7v.97

Embree, J. L., & White, A. H. (2010). Concept analysis: Nurse-to-nurse lateral violence. *Nursing Forum, 45*(3), 166–173.

Ferguson, T. (n.d). Self-care: Ten guidelines for developing a personal self-care plan. Retrieved from www.healthy.net/Health/Article/Ten_Guidelines_for_Developing_a_Personal_Self_Care_Plan/992/4

Fewer Quick-Return Shifts. (2015). Fewer quick-return shifts improve nurses' recovery. *Medscape*. Retrieved from www.medscape.com/viewarticle/846799

Folkman, S., Lazarus, R. S., Gruen, R. J., & DeLongis, A. (1986). Appraisal, coping, health status, and psychological symptom. *Journal of Personality and Social Psychology, 50*(3), 571–579.

Future of Nursing Campaign for Action. (2015). Campaign progress: Dashboard indicators. Retrieved from http://campaignforaction.org/dashboard

Goleman, D. (2006). *Emotional intelligence: Why it can matter more than IQ* (10th ed.). New York, NY: Random House.

Goleman's Emotional Intelligence. (n.d.). Daniel Goleman's five components of emotional intelligence. Retrieved from www.sonoma.edu/users/s/swijtink/teaching/philosophy_101/paper1/goleman.htm

Gupta, S. (n.d.). Why America's nurses are burning out. Retrieved from http://www.everydayhealth.com/info/v1ss/nurse-burnout

Halm, M., Peterson, M., Kandels, M., Sabjo, J., Blalock, M., Braden, R., … Topham, D. (2005). Hospital nurse staffing and patient mortality, emotional exhaustion, and job dissatisfaction. *Clinical Nurse Specialist, 19*(5), 241–251. doi:10.1097/00002800-200509000-00007

Hayes, L. J., O'Brien-Pallas, L., Duffield, C., Shamian, J., Buchan, J., Hughes, F., … Stone, P. W. (2006). Nurse turnover: A literature review. *International Journal of Nursing Studies, 43*(2), 237–263.

Healthcare Staffing Report. (January, 2015). *No more nurse shortage? Surplus projected for 2025.* Retrieved from www.staffingindustry.com/Research-Publications/Publications/Healthcare-Staffing-Report

Healthy Sleep. (2015). New recommendations to achieve healthy sleep. *Medscape*. Retrieved from http://www.medscape.com/viewarticle/847220

HelpGuide.org. (n.d.). Laughter is the best medicine. Retrieved from www.helpguide.org/articles/emotional-health/laughter-is-the-best-medicine.htm

Hendren, R. (2010). Seven strategies to reduce nurse burnout. Retrieved from www.healthleadersmedia.com/content/NRS-252471/Seven-Strategies-to-Reduce-Nurse-Burnout

Henry, B. J. (2014). Nursing burnout interventions: What is being done? *Clinical Journal of Oncology Nursing, 18*(2), 211–214.

Institute of Medicine. (2010). *The future of nursing: Leading change, advancing health.* Retrieved from http://books.nap.edu/openbook.php?record_id=12956&page=R1

Jameton, A. (1984). *Nursing practice: The ethical issues.* Englewood Cliffs, NJ: Prentice-Hall.

Jameton, A. (2013). A reflection on moral distress in nursing together with a current application of the concept. *Bioethical Inquiry, 10*, 207–308. doi:10.1007/s11673-013-9466-3

Jennings, B. M. (2008). Work stress and burnout among nurses: Role of the work environment and working conditions. In R. G. Hughes (Ed.), *Patient safety and quality: An evidence-based handbook for nurses.* Rockville, MD: Agency for Healthcare Research and Quality. Retrieved from www.ncbi.nlm.nih.gov/books/NBK2668/

Johnstone, M., & Hutchinson, A. (2015). "Moral distress"—time to abandon a flawed nursing construct? *Nursing Ethics, 22*(1), 5–14. doi:10.1177/0969733013505312

Kift, L. B. (2012). Nurses on the front line: Warning signs and tips to manage your stress. Retrieved from www.nursetogether.com/nurses-on-the-front-line-warning-signs-and-tips-to-manage-your-stress

Kovner, C. T., Brewer, C. S., Fatehi, F., & Jun, J. (2014). What does nurse turnover rate mean and what is the rate? *Policy, Politics, & Nursing Practice, 15*(3–4), 64–71.

Kravitz, K., McAllister-Black, R., Grant, M., & Kirk, C. (2010). A psycho-educational intervention for stress reduction and the prevention of burnout. *Applied Nursing Research, 23*, 130–138.

Krischke, M. M. (2011). Expert tips to fight compassion fatigue. Retrieved from http://www.compassionfatigue.org/pages/nurseconnect.pdf

Lachman, V. D. (2015). Ethical issues in the disruptive behaviors of incivility, bullying, and horizontal/lateral violence. *Urologic Nursing, 35*(1), 39–42.

Laschinger, H. K. S. (2011). Job and career satisfaction and turnover intentions in newly graduated nurses. *Journal of Nursing Management, 20*(4), 472–484.

Laschinger, H. K. S., & Fida, R. (2014). New nurses burnout and workplace wellbeing: The influence of authentic leadership and psychological capital. *Burnout Research, 14*, 19–28. http://dx.doi.org 10.1016/j.burn.2014.03.002

Lazarus, R. S., & Folkman, S. (1984). *Stress, appraisal, and coping.* New York, NY: Springer.

Lehman, S. (2014). *Shift work linked to greater diabetes risk.* Retrieved from http://www.medscape.com/viewarticle/830564

Leiter, M., Harvie, P., & Frizzell, C. (1998). The correspondence of patient satisfaction and nurse burnout. *Social Science & Medicine, 47*, 1611–1617.

Leiter, M. P., & Maslach, C. (2003). Areas of worklife: A structured approach to organizational predictors of job burnout. *Emotional and Physiological Processes and Positive Intervention Strategies Research in Occupational Stress and Well Being, 3*, 91–134. doi: 10.1016/SI479-3555(03)0300-8

Littlejohn, P. (2012). The missing link: Using emotional intelligence to reduce workplace stress and workplace violence in our nursing and other health care professions. *Journal of Professional Nursing, 28*(6), 360–368.

Lombardo, B., & Eyre, C. (2011). Compassion fatigue: A nurse's primer. *The Online Journal of Issues in Nursing, 16*(1), 3. doi:10.3912/OJIN.Vol16No01Man03

Maslach, C. (1982) *Burnout: The cost of caring.* Englewood Cliffs, NJ: Prentice-Hall.

Maslach, C. (1998). A multidimensional theory of burnout. In C. L. Cooper (Ed.), *Theories of organizational stress* (pp. 68–85). Oxford, UK: Oxford University Press.

Maslach, C., Schaufeli, W., & Leiter, M. (2001). Job burnout. *Annual Review in Psychology, 52*, 397–422.

Mathieu, F. M. (2007). Transforming compassion fatigue into compassion satisfaction: Top 12 self-care tips for helpers. Retrieved from www.compassionfatigue.ca

Mayo Clinic. (n.d.). Stress symptoms: Effects on your body and behavior. Retrieved from http://www.mayoclinic.org/healthy-lifestyle/stress-management/in-depth/stress-symptoms/art-20050987

McCarthy, J., & Deady, R. (2008). Moral distress reconsidered. *Nursing Ethics, 15*(2), 254–262.

McEwen, B. S. (2008). Central effects of stress hormones in health and disease: Understanding the protective and damaging effects of stress and stress mediators. *European Journal of Pharmacology, 583*(2–3), 174–185. doi:10.1016/ejphar.2007.11.071

Meditation. (n.d.). *The free dictionary.* Retrieved from http://medical-dictionary.thefree dictionary.com/Meditation

Morse, G., Salyers, M. P., Rollins, A. L., Monroe-DeVita, M., & Pfahler, C. (2012). Burnout in mental health services: A review of the problem and its remediation. *Administration in Policy and Mental Health, 39*(5), 341–352. doi:10.1007/s10488-011-0352-1

Nurse Residency Programs. (2015). Nurse residency programs: Rolling out the welcome mat. *Medscape.* Retrieved from www.medscape.com.

Nursing Solutions, Inc. (NSI). (2015). 2015 National healthcare retention & RN staffing report. Retrieved from www.nsinursingsolutions.com

Orem, D. E. (2001). *Nursing: Concepts of practice* (6th ed.). St. Louis, MO: Mosby.

Orem, D. E., & Vardiman, E. M. (1995). Orem's nursing theory and positive mental health: Practical considerations. *Nursing Science Quarterly, 8,* 165–173.

Positive Attitude. (n.d.). Develop a positive attitude for stress relief. Retrieved from http://stress.about.com/od/positiveattitude/a/reframing.htm

Public Health Agency of Canada. (2016). *Responding to stressful events: Self-care for caregivers.* Retrieved from http://www.phac-aspc.gc.ca/publicat/oes-bsu-02/caregvr-eng .php

Roberts, S. J. (2015). Lateral violence in nursing: A review of the past three decades. *Nursing Science Quarterly, 28*(1), 36–41.

Roberts, S., Demarco, R., & Griffin, M. (2009). The effects of oppressed group behaviors on the culture of the nursing workplace: A review of the evidence and interventions for change. *Journal of Nursing Management, 17,* 288–293.

Sabo, B. (2011). Reflecting on the concept of compassion fatigue. *Online Journal of Issues in Nursing, 16*(1), 1.

Salovey, P., & Mayer, J. D. (1990). Emotional intelligence. *Imagination, Cognition and Personality, 9*(3), 185–211.

Segar, M. (2015). *No sweat: How the simple science of motivation can bring you to a lifetime of fitness.* New York, NY: AMACOM Books.

Self-Guided.com. (2016). The five types of meditation techniques. Retrieved from http://www.self-guided.com/types of meditation.html

Shift Work and Cognition. (2014). Shift work impairs cognitive function. *Medscape.* Retrieved from www.medscape.com/viewarticle/834583

Sleep Apnea. (n.d.). Obstructive sleep apnea: 5 self-care strategies. Retrieved from www.webmd.com/sleep-disorders/sleep-apnea/sleep-apnea-self-care

Sleep Deprivation. (2011). Sleep deprivation in medical caregivers has deadly results. *Medscape.* Retrieved from www.medscape.com

Sleep-Deprived Nurses. (2013). Tired, sleep-deprived nurses may regret clinical decisions. *Medscape.* Retrieved from www.medscape.com/viewarticle/818499

Spence Laschinger, H. K., & Leiter, M. P. (2006). The impact of nursing work environments on patient safety outcomes: The mediating role of burnout engagement. *The Journal of Nursing Administration, 36*(5), 259–267. doi:10.1097/00005110-20060 5000-00019

Stamm, B. H. (2010). *The concise ProQOL manual* (2nd ed.). Pocatello, ID: ProQOL.org.

Storch, J. L. (2004). Nursing ethics: A developing moral terrain. In J. L. Storch, P. Rodney, & R. Starzomski (Eds.), *Toward a moral horizon* (pp. 1–16). Toronto, ON, Canada: Pearson.

Stress. (n.d.). *Merriam-Webster dictionary online.* Retrieved from www.merriam-webster .com/dictionary/stress

Taylor, S. G., & Renpenning, K. (2011). *Self-care science, nursing theory, and evidence-based practice.* New York, NY: Springer.

The Joint Commission. (2008). Sentinel event alert "behaviors that undermine a culture of safety". Retrieved from http://www.jointcommission.org/sentinel_event_alert_ issue_40_behaviors_that_undermine_a_culture_of_safety

USDA Center for Nutrition Policy & Promotion. (n.d). Choose my plate. Retrieved from www.choosemyplate.gov/

Vahey, D. C., Aiken, L. H., Sloane, D. M., Clarke, S. P., & Vargas, D. (2004). Nurse burnout and patient satisfaction. *Medical Care, 42*(2 Suppl), 1157–1166. doi:10.1097/01 .mir.0000109126.50398.5a

Varcoe, C., Pauly, B., Webster, G., & Storch, J. (2012). Moral distress: Tensions as springboards for action. *HEC Forum, 24,* 51–62.

Vogel, L. (2007). Willingness and its relevance to nursing. *Advances in Nursing Science, 30*(3), E73–E83.

Wallis, L. (2015). Moral distress in nursing. *American Journal of Nursing, 115*(3), 19–20.

WebMD. (n.d.). Stress symptoms: Effects of stress on your body. Retrieved from http:// www.webmd.com/balance/stress-management/effects-of-stress-on-your-body

Wilkinson, J. M. (1987/88). Moral distress in nursing practice: Experience and effect. *Nursing Forum, 23*(1), 16–29.

APPENDICES
NURSING SITUATIONS AND CASE STUDIES

Mrs. Smith appears throughout the text as a paradigm case to illustrate many of the concepts presented. Part IV includes a summary of comments about Mrs. Smith and her health and self-care concerns. Additional scenarios are presented to illustrate other concepts. Some have a more detailed analysis, whereas others serve as data for you to consider in clarifying or developing your understanding.

There is no specific format for developing and analyzing nursing situations, or for writing case studies beyond using the elements presented in the book. In some instances, one might want to begin with a systems analysis, clarifying the roles and relationships of those involved in the particular situation of concern. From a nursing perspective, these will be described in terms of health and self-care, looking for the health outcomes sought and self-care requirements or limitations. When there is an identified patient, you might begin by examining the basic conditioning factors (BCF).

In many of these narratives, as you read them you will begin to see connections, familiar patterns, and come-to-ready conclusions. Start with that and then move on to a deliberate analysis. How do you know this? What is it about this situation that resonates with you? Remember the discussion on tacit knowing, tacit maps from Chapter 3? Through your prior experiences and reflections, you can move ahead. As this is a learning experience, take time to reflect on this. Think about the concepts that are presented in the text. What can you learn about this situation?

How might it give clarity to your practice? What kind of questions, theoretical and practical, does it raise for you? Share your reflections with your colleagues; their different background may bring to light ideas about your practice.

APPENDIX A: PRIMARY HEALTH CARE CLINICAL SITUATION

The focus of this clinical situation is on assisting the patient with self-management of her chronic disease. This includes development of self-care agency and helping the patient monitor her own progress. There are also considerations of identifying and negotiating self-care demands and patient participation.

MS. GREENE

Ms. Greene is a 55-year-old Caucasian who came to the clinic 8 months ago. She had been seeing a local MD for management of her health care since her diagnosis of type 2 diabetes 15 years ago. She was put on metformin and Levemir. Comorbidities include hypothyroidism, restless leg syndrome, hyperlipidemia, depression, dyspnea, and obesity.

Ms. Greene lives alone, was formerly married, and has no children. Her sister, who lives nearby, is her primary support system. She is currently unemployed and receives health care assistance through Medicaid. Whatever financial support she receives, if any, is minimal. She has in the past and this previous month not taken medication because of lack of money.

When first seen by the nurse practitioner (NP), Ms. Greene had been out of her metformin for at least one month. She still had a supply of synthroid and diazepam as well as a supply of insulin that she had accumulated.

The NP sees her responsibility as melding the allopathic medicine responsibilities with a nursing perspective. The NP agreed to work as long as Ms. Greene was willing to do the necessary work to regain control of her diabetes. Ms. Greene agreed, and the nurse–patient relationship was established. On the first visit, her Hg A1C was 13.8. She worked and was able to get her A1C down to a level of 10, showing good progress. The goal is an A1C of 7 or lower. At that time, she left the United States and traveled to Italy for 3 months, where she continued to do well, getting lots of exercise from walking. On her return, she was faced with some family stress and began eating "everything." Her A1C was 13.5, and her blood sugar averaged 349.

The NP started her on Levemir 40 units/day. She was to check her blood sugar in the morning. If it was above 140, she was to add 1 unit each night. The NP said "morning tells you what to do at night." She would also take Humulin 3 units before each meal. The NP scheduled her for a return visit in 1 week. She did that to emphasize the importance of testing and increasing the insulin dose. The program established with the NP made sense to Ms. Greene. On the return visit, the NP noted that she was following the prescribed routine and scheduled the next visit in 2 weeks.

Other comments that the NP noted were that Ms. Greene had the capabilities, information, and skills to manage her diabetes but did not have the skills to manage the changes in the home situation. She also lacked resources to buy medication. The NP was able to set her up with a drug plan that would provide her with medications at a reduced price. There is also the issue of diet; lacking finances usually leads the person to eat high-carbohydrate and high-fat foods. Fresh vegetables and lean proteins are out of her price range. One of the issues that the NP dealt with was that Ms. Greene was unaccustomed to the use of assistive services. Many people react negatively to needing help; concomitantly, they seem to tumble into a lack of willingness to do the work of self-care. Managing this requires vigilance and work on the part of the NP. The local food bank was able to help satisfy the hunger, but the foods available were not the best for controlling blood sugar. There were few low-glycemic index foods available.

The NP saw her role as helping the patient to take actions to regain glycemic control and avoid negative effects. The patient's perspective was the avoidance of symptoms of hypoglycemia and eating at a low cost. Together, they designed a plan that would fit with her abilities and limitations. The NP focused on developing a treatment plan that would get the A1C down to an acceptable level. It would require frequent visits to the clinic for the patient to check blood sugar levels, and to encourage, guide, and redirect her. For meaningful results, A1C is measured every 2 to 3 months to gauge progress to meeting the goal of A1C of 7 or lower. In addition, the NP would work to help her accept that the management of diabetes could function as a means to a healthy, productive life.

The NP noted the self-care deficit as the "inability to sustain over time the level of self-care management needed to achieve positive outcomes."

The major theories supporting the practice of this NP include:

- Self-care deficit nursing theory

- Harm reduction model

- Cognitive learning theory

- Theories about the effect of poverty and social conditions of living on people

- Human growth and development theories

- Medical and pharmacological theories

She identifies the tenets underlying her practice as:

- Respect for dignity and autonomy of people

- Acknowledgment that patients are the agents of care

- Goal to establish a partnership with the patient
- To be a positive helping agent

Of importance to this NP is negotiation of the therapeutic self-care demand with the patient. Using the process described in this book to identify the demands, the optimal set of behaviors to achieve optimal health outcomes, the NP establishes an ideal therapeutic self-care demand (TSCD). The problem is that the patient might have a different view. The nurse must identify what the patient is willing and able to do. Nursing in primary care is coaching. The goal, to meet the ideal TSCD, is a process that occurs over time and is accomplished through renegotiation and expansion on initial negotiated TSCD.

The NP referred Ms. Greene to the diabetes clinical nurse specialist for more in-depth assessment of capabilities, dispositions, and knowledge of her diseases. She began by conducting a detailed history with a focus on the eating habits, current self-care system, social history, and knowledge of the disease and its management. The patient plan includes the following:

- Ms. Greene will test glucose at least once a day
- She will try to prepare at least one meal a day, limiting eating out
- Seek counseling at the clinic to assist with managing family stress, appointment to be set up; she will keep the appointment
- Apply for assistance with paying for medication and supplies with help from clinic staff
- Return to clinic in one month

(Personal communication from E. Geden, RN, BC-FNP, PhD, Family Nurse Practitioner, November 2015.)

APPENDIX B: CHILD HEALTH SITUATION

Developmental requisites are of obvious importance when working with children. Issues of meeting universal and health care requisites are significant, especially when a child is in ill health. The dependent-care system and family system are important in the detection of illness and in establishing the appropriate care system for the child.

BETTY

Betty H is a 7½-year-old Caucasian girl who was recently hospitalized with a brain tumor (suprasellar germinoma). She had a 4-month history of symptoms. Conservative medical treatment is planned with radiation therapy.

Betty lives with her mother, father, and two sisters, ages 5 and 10, on a 170-acre farm near a small Midwestern town. She talks about her farm animals quite a bit and wants to get home to play with them and see whether they remember her.

She likes school and has several friends who live nearby.

Mrs. H stays with Betty nearly all the time. She is a college student but has dropped her class load until Betty is better. Her husband is a construction supervisor. He is very supportive and is able to be at the hospital frequently. He along with family members and friends are caring for the two sisters at home. They have a good health plan and with Mr. H's good job they have no financial concerns.

Four and a half months ago, Betty developed headaches and intermittent vomiting, occurring usually after breakfast. Her parents saw no particular pattern and were not concerned. When the vomiting became more frequent, Betty was checked by her local doctor and treated for recurrent otitis media. The vomiting stopped, as it was suspected to be of viral origin. When the vomiting recurred, she was assessed for gastrointestinal pathology and a cranial CT scan was carried out. The cause of her symptoms was not determined. The headaches became a daily concern, and the vomiting progressed to many times throughout the day. Betty also developed ataxia, photophobia, sluggish left pupil, polyuria, polyphagia, and polydipsia. She lost 12 pounds during this time.

She was again hospitalized and had a repeat CT scan. A tumor of the third ventricle was discovered. Betty's condition continued to deteriorate with the onset of confusion 1 week after hospitalization. A peritoneal craniotomy was performed, a biopsy was taken, a ventricle-peritoneal shunt was placed, and a central line was inserted for medications and TPN. The diagnosis of germinoma was made from the biopsy sample.

This particular brain tumor is situated beneath and behind the optic chiasma. It usually displaces, infiltrates, and spreads along the optic nerves into the hypothalamus, hence the presenting symptomatology. Since surgery and placement of the shunt, Betty has become more alert, is able to participate in her own hygiene, is mobile, and has an increasing appetite. Radiation therapy was planned for the near future but because Betty again became confused after surgery, it was started earlier.

Mrs. H notes that Betty has been very self-sufficient and participated in most of her own care except when she has periods of confusion. After surgery, Betty began letting others do things that she was capable of doing.

At present, Betty has become very "tired" from lack of sleep, the disease process, or her treatments. She is awakened several times during the night when the nurses come to check on her. Mrs. H is particularly concerned about Betty's lack of sleep, her eating, and the side effects of her medications.

The doctor says she could go home and return to the hospital for daily radiation therapy.

Discharge planning should include attention to the following:

- Requisites of concern on discharge include:
- Managing medications
- Managing side effects of treatment
  - Balancing rest and activity
  - Balancing solitude and social interaction
  - Promotion of normalcy
  - Promotion of age-appropriate developmental activity
  - Overcoming effect of illness and treatments on development
  - Reestablishing normal sibling relationships and normalizing Betty's place in the family—resuming educational programs/activities
- Assessment of self-care agency of Betty
- Assessment of person making up the dependent-care system (in particular Mrs. and Mr. H)
- Assessment of potential for normal family functioning while integrating Betty's care into family system
- Plans for follow-up regarding earlier assessment and planning information

APPENDIX C: MENTAL HEALTH

Mental health and illness issues lead us to questions about the self-care agency of the individual. It is necessary to carefully assess the foundational capabilities and dispositions to determine the ways in which the patient is able to participate in self-care activities. Assessment will also look at the existent self-care system and its effectiveness. Community variables and social determinants of health are frequently of concern in relation to the individual managing self-care in the presence of mental health issues. Identification of community systems in operation that facilitate or limit self-care is an important component of the assessment process. Action may be required at various levels within the community, and thinking about these should be part of the consideration of possible courses of action. In the following situation, the need to promote safety is paramount for the patient and to the community. There are cultural concerns and biases that affect the development of the interdisciplinary care system.

MR. G

Mr. G is a 56-year-old African American man who was brought into the psychiatric emergency department (ED) by the police, who had found him running in the street trying to stop traffic. When asked why he was doing this, Mr. G spoke very rapidly, saying he had heard the voice of God telling him that a major disaster was coming and that he needed to warn people to take shelter. Mr. G said he also thought he could prevent the disaster by climbing to the top of the highest building he could find and by offering himself as a sacrifice. He was planning to do this after he warned as many people in the street as he could. Mr. G had not slept for several days and had not eaten, because he "didn't have time" and had "more important things to do." He was pacing rapidly in the confined area of the ED and said he would have to leave soon, because lots of people were going to die. When asked whether he had been drinking fluids, he said he drank lots and lots of Coca-Cola, because it helped him stay sharp and focused on his mission since he could no longer afford the "other stuff." He said he had used "another kind of coke a few times, not the kind you drink but the kind you smoke, you know the smokin' coke but it was a joke because they took all my cash money, and I didn't have none and I was broke, you know, smoke broke and hoke joke." When asked whether there was someone they could call to be with him, Mr. G continued to pace, saying his wife had kicked him out of their home 6 months ago, because he was "going through a rough patch" and stayed in bed for days at a time. He lost his job at the Auto Parts store where he had worked for 3 years. His wife was an elementary school teacher, who was helping to raise two grandchildren since their grown daughter who was divorced was going back to school and needed help. "She told me if I was just going to be a lazy bum and not help out I could just leave. So I went to stay with my mother but you can't call her because she is old and sick." His father had died from a stroke approximately 10 years ago. Mr. G said that his daughter did not want much to do with him, but his adult son and his wife sometimes helped him out with money, transportation, and other needs. When asked about medications used in the past, Mr. G said, "I was on something for a long time, it started with an L or maybe it was an L M N O P...." When asked whether it might have been Lithium, Mr. G said, "That was it, but I stopped taking it because I started feeling good and didn't think I needed it any more. And it slowed me down too much and I couldn't keep up with all my projects." When asked to sit down for a brief physical exam and to have his blood drawn, Mr. G became agitated, stating, "I don't think you know how important my mission is. I should have gone a long time ago, I need to go now." He calmed a bit with reassurance from the nursing staff. He would not allow his blood to be drawn, stating, "I think you are part of the conspiracy that's going to bring about the disaster, you might be wanting to poison me." He did, however, allow his blood pressure to be taken, and the reading was 162/96. Other than being somewhat thin and dehydrated, Mr. G's physical health seemed relatively stable at this time.

It was decided by the treatment team that Mr. G. should be placed on 72-hour emergency hold because of his risk for harm to self, that is, running in traffic and planning to jump off a high building. When informed of this, Mr. G became anxious and agitated, stating repeatedly that he had important work to do. One of the nurses walked with Mr. G as he paced, saying she understood that he had work to do, but they just wanted to help him eat and get some rest because they were concerned for his well-being. Mr. G finally said he supposed he could stay for a little while but that he would have to leave soon.

Mr. G was given a medical diagnosis of bipolar I disorder, manic episode, and was started on lithium carbonate 600 mg three times a day. Mr. G agreed to this, only because it had "helped him some in the past" and he did not want to fight with anyone anymore. He was also started on Olanzapine 20 mg one time daily. It was decided that Mr. G's blood pressure would be monitored three times a day while he was hospitalized to determine the need for blood pressure medication.

APPENDIX D: MRS. SMITH

All aspects of the self-care theory are presented within the text. The focus is on her changing self-care system and factors that condition it. What are the community's responsibilities, if any, to assist impaired elderly? The health deviation and universal self-care requisites take precedence in cases of emergency care. As the patient is recuperating, attention will be paid to the developmental requisites. In many cases where the patient is elderly, the self-care agency, though once adequate and developed, may be declining.

BASIC CONDITIONING FACTORS

Mrs. Smith is a 65-year-old divorced woman with one son, John. He is 30 years old and unmarried, lives in the same city, and has a supportive relationship with his mother. There is no other information available regarding the extended family. Her physical appearance is described as being tall and lean, possessing sallow skin tone and dark hair. She recently retired from working as an administrative assistant in a small company. While working there, she became computer proficient. She has her own computer and Wi-Fi at her home. She lives and functions independently in the family home where she has lived for 35 years. Her home is in an urban area, with bedrooms on the second floor. The entry has three steps and no handrail.

She makes her own decisions about finances and other personal matters and has done so since her divorce 20 years ago. She participates in several group activities such as playing bridge with friends. She describes herself as spiritual but not religious. She speaks English, and can read and write though an idiopathic tremor makes writing difficult for her. She is confident that she will be able to manage any changes in her system of living as she ages. She has not had regular checkups by a practitioner, as she was uninsured through her employer. She is a U.S. citizen and on her 65th birthday registered for Medicare. She has a supplemental insurance plan with the American Association of Retired Persons (AARP). Mrs. Smith is a high school graduate. She learned her skills on the job. She is an avid reader.

While working in her house one day, she fell and fractured the head of the right femur. She was able to call first responders and was transported to the hospital where surgery would be performed. X-rays revealed that in addition to a hip fracture, Mrs. Smith had osteoporosis. This probably was a problem in her current health situation.

Environmental factors conditioning Mrs. Smith's demand now are a function of being in the hospital and her health state. She is neither able nor allowed to manipulate her environment.

At this time, her health state is that of a person with a fractured hip and with osteoporosis. She is in the hospital awaiting surgery. She received analgesia and is on bedrest until the surgery can be performed. Her son is with her, and both understand her need for nursing to meet her self-care. She is beginning to understand that she will need assistance not just during the hospitalization but also in the rehabilitation phase of recovery. A significant percentage of individuals who sustain a hip fracture have increased mortality for up to one year. Often, the individuals who survive hip fracture do not return to their pre-fracture functional status or living arrangements.

Mrs. Smith's prior experiences within the health care system are limited. She was hospitalized for the birth of her child but has had no other acute illness. She has experienced the usual seasonal illnesses. How the health care system will condition Mrs. Smith's demands and access to services to help her meet those demands varies greatly by the political/social/cultural system within which she resides. If she lives in the United States, she would be eligible for Medicare and with a supplemental insurance policy, most, if not all, of her hospital costs could be met. The benefits available to her are dependent on the specific insurance program in which she is enrolled. Within the Canadian system, Mrs. Smith would have fewer concerns as to follow-up care and payment. In both systems, a social service person would most likely be the one to make the arrangements for follow-up care. The nurse would want to be involved, as some of the decisions as to type of care or specifics of care relate to the nursing care needed.

Mrs. Smith lives a comfortable life. She has a modest pension, social security, and some investments that are for her retirement. Her monthly resources are adequate to meet her needs with some left to add to savings. She is trying to establish good health practices, though her usual pattern had her eating fast food meals or frozen-prepared meals. She does not drink alcohol or smoke. Her home is in an urban area, with bedrooms on the second floor. The entry has three steps and no handrail. Since she retired, time is not an issue. Mrs. Smith was considering finding part-time or seasonal work to supplement her retirement funds. This plan will likely be altered due to her current health condition.

Mrs. Smith views herself and her son as her family. She has no other close relatives. Her father and mother both died of heart disease at the ages of 70 and 75, respectively. Mrs. Smith's son, John, who will be helping her at home, has had little personal experience with illness or injury. He works as an information system technician and has good problem-solving ability related to his work.

She was admitted to the emergency room where her care was transferred to the orthopedic surgeon. Pressure gradient stockings were applied immediately after admission. After surgery, she will spend probably 3 days in the acute-care setting, after which she will be discharged to either home or a rehabilitative facility. Patients with pre-existing joint disease, medium/high activity levels, and a reasonable life expectancy should have total hip replacement as the primary treatment.

Mrs. Smith's self-care demands and capabilities are conditioned first and foremost by her health state and health system factors. Her mobility and comfort are conditioned by her injury and medication received to relieve her pain. Her son's presence is having a negative effect on her as he is having difficulty in controlling his responses to her injury. If he is not able to control his response to her injury and impending surgery, Mrs. Smith may be directing her energy and attention to solacing him rather than working on understanding and accepting her own health situation. As the nurse–patient relationship develops, more information about many of the BCF can be acquired through interaction with her or perhaps with her son.

Mrs. Smith's requisite for maintaining an adequate intake of air is conditioned by the fact that she is on bedrest and has received medications that may depress respiration. When monitored, her respirations are normal and it is determined that the demand is being met.

Up until her injury, Mrs. Smith's requirements for intake of food were adequate to meet her basic energy needs. Her diet was insufficient in factors affecting calcium intake and utilization as manifest by the osteoporosis. Her diet will now be supplemented with high-energy protein preparations containing minerals and vitamins. (Vitamin D supplementation, injected or given orally, suppresses parathyroid hormone, increases bone mineral density, and reduces falls after hip fracture in previously independent elderly women.)

Perioperative complications include acute confusional state (delirium), narcotic sedation, and hemodynamic fluctuations. There are comorbidities associated with immobilization, such as urinary tract infection (UTI), atelectasis, pneumonia, and thromboembolic events. All patients undergoing hip fracture surgery should receive antibiotic prophylaxis. Mrs. Smith received thromboprophylaxis using fondaparinux for 28 days starting 6 hours after surgery. (Fondaparinux injection comes as a solution [liquid] to be injected subcutaneously [just under the skin] in the lower stomach area. It is usually given one time a day for 5 to 9 days or sometimes for up to about 1 month.) It should be given at around the same time every day. An annual infusion of zoledronic acid is associated with a reduction in the rate of new clinical vertebral and non-vertebral fractures and may improve survival after a low-trauma hip fracture. Current guidelines for management of hip fractures may be found at www.mja.com.au/journal/2010/192/1/evidence-based-guidelines-management -hip-fractures-older-persons-update

The diet of hip fracture patients in rehabilitation should include high-energy protein preparations containing minerals and vitamins. Mrs. Smith needs to improve/maintain circulation while on bedrest. Compression device therapy was begun on her admission to prevent thromboembolitic problems. Immobilization or limited mobility presents other hazards.

Mrs. Smith's fluid requirements are increased after the surgery. She was NPO before the surgery. Until she was able to retain fluids postsurgery, intravenous (IV) fluids were used to maintain her intake and output. As soon as she was able to tolerate oral liquids, her intake was switched to oral.

Until Mrs. Smith is mobile, her elimination is problematic. She should have an output of urine that is compatible with her intake. Her bladder needs to be emptied regularly to prevent retention or incontinence, both of which are hazardous. Once she starts receiving solid food, she should have a bowel movement within 2 days.

In the immediate postoperative period, Mrs. Smith required an increase in rest. As she moves to the rehabilitation phase of her recovery, she will continue to have needs for recuperative rest and also an increase in the amount of activity.

As Mrs. Smith processes the meaning of her injury and future recovery, the nature of her social interactions will change. She will have needs for more purposive social interactions—people to help her with her mobility, support as she works through the rehabilitation process, and attempts to reestablish her independent living. These requisites require Mrs. Smith to contemplate her current situation and draw some conclusions as to what kind of changes she might need or want to make. Mrs. Smith successfully transitioned through adult developmental stages. As she returns home, she probably will need to engage in some other activities that help her move forward, given her recent retirement and injury. As Mrs. Smith works to regain her independence, she also needs to recognize her developmental and safety needs. Are there hazards, such as throw rugs, in the house? Is she realistic in accepting her limitations and the need to work for recovery?

Mrs. Smith recognized her need for assistance after her fall. By calling 911, she sought appropriate assistance. She might have called her son to help but he would neither be able to transport her nor be able to provide pain relief.

Mrs. Smith attended to her condition by agreeing to have hip surgery. After surgery and postoperative recovery, she will have to attend to rehabilitation. Depending on how that progresses, she will have to make adjustments to her diet and need to modify her activity and rest.

In designing the discharge plan for Mrs. Smith, the nurse will list the things that need to be done, such as therapeutic exercise of her hip, eating three meals with high protein and calcium, taking pain medication before therapy and before bed, resting in the afternoon for at least 1 hour, and drinking water at meals and at least one glass in between each. Other guidelines include not drinking water after the dinner meal except as needed for taking medications, keeping the incision clean and dry using warm water, cleansing at the sink until the wound heals, and showering when approved by the MD. Observe for signs of infection, such as redness around the incision, or other unusual signs. Return at appointment times, and maintain contact information for the care coordinator, nurse practitioner, or physician.

Mrs. Smith will need to make adjustments in many aspects of her daily life, at least until her rehabilitation is completed. One of these will be to manage the osteoporosis medication and monitor its effects. For a time, Mrs. Smith will need assistive devices such as a walker or a cane. Time will tell whether she has other mobility issues. These requisites require Mrs. Smith to contemplate her current situation and draw some conclusions as to what kind of changes she might need or want to make. Mrs. Smith has a requisite to maintain an adequate intake of food. What does that mean to an elderly woman recovering from surgery after a fall? What should be the distribution of nutritional elements, such as protein, calcium, vitamins, fiber, and the like?

Postoperatively, Mrs. Smith is not to strain the hip joint with heavy lifting or other unusual activities. Specific techniques of body posturing, sitting, and using an elevated toilet seat can be extremely helpful. She is not to cross the operated lower extremity across the midline of the body (not crossing the leg over the other leg) because of the risk of dislocating the replaced joint. Nor should she bend at the waist. When lying on the nonoperated side, she should use a pillow between the legs in order to prevent the operated lower extremity from crossing over the midline. She will attend outpatient physical therapy for a period while incorporating home exercises regularly into her daily living.

The nurse will help Mrs. Smith decide how she will accomplish these tasks, what other concerns she might have now and in the near future, and ways to adjust her environment to protect her, such as removing scatter rugs, installing handholds for the toilet, and adjusting the height of chairs and the bed for ease of sitting and rising.

Mrs. Smith was instructed to look for signs of infection, including swelling, warmth, redness, or increased pain in or around the surgical site, and to notify the doctor's office immediately if these changes were noted or if there was injury to the hip. If Mrs. Smith develops an infection that is amenable to antibiotics, the action required is to take the antibiotic. The action system to accomplish this includes that a person has the knowledge and understanding of the symptoms of an infection, recognizes these symptoms, knows he or she must visit a health care provider to get a prescription, visits a health care provider and gets a prescription, goes to a pharmacy to get the prescription filled, reads and understands the instructions for taking the medication, understands signs and symptoms of undesirable side effects, integrates/plans for taking the medication as directed, takes the medication, assesses the results of taking the medication, and reports to the health care provider if the antibiotic is not effective or there are undesirable side effects.

Mrs. Smith was told to notify any caregivers that she has an artificial joint. Antibiotics are recommended during any invasive procedures, whether surgical, urological, gastroenterological, or dental. Infections elsewhere in the body should also be treated to prevent seeding of infection into the joint. This is important, because bacteria can pass through the bloodstream from these sites and cause infection of the hip prosthesis.

The first few weeks were difficult because of exhaustion, limits to mobility, little help at home, poor appetite, and so forth. The exhaustion led to difficulty in concentrating, difficulty in sleeping, and generally struggling with not being as strong and active as earlier (www.medicinenet.com/total_hip_replacement/article.htm).

Initially, Mrs. Smith and her son were a nuclear family. However, given that both are adults and do not live in the same residence, the nature of the family has changed. They are a relational dyadic family. There is no other information regarding extended family or close friends in supportive roles. There appears to be a close relationship between Mrs. Smith and John. It would help to know whether John was assisting his mother out of a sense of duty or of affection, as this will condition his participation in her care, both now and in the future.

Mrs. Smith and her son do not constitute a community. They do, however, exist as subsystems of a number of communities. Each one has the local community within which they live and work. Mrs. Smith's community includes the small groups to which she belongs, her neighborhood, and the area she uses to access services such as banking, health care, and so forth. It is the community that provided the first responders for her injury. Her community values the health and safety of its members. Were those services not available, her story might be quite different.

Mrs. Smith is likely to require or benefit from home nursing. Which services are available to her depends on the community where she resides. The availability of home care services might be limited by the insurance or funding sources that she can access. She has Medicare and a Medicare supplement policy that will provide some financial assistance, though these plans have limits imposed on things such as length of stay or which providers she might be able to use.

Mrs. Smith is a member of a definable population: women older than 65, elderly, living alone, and with limited discretionary income for health care. After her injury, the population can be further denoted as elderly women with mobility limitations after hip replacement.

APPENDIX E: DESCRIPTION OF A POPULATION FROM A NURSING PERSPECTIVE

The use of a description of a population, as discussed in Chapters 9 and 12, facilitates the production and control operations. When wanting to design nursing or health care programs for specific groups or cohorts of patients, making the characteristics of the group explicit facilitates the program planning. A detailed description, validated by members of the targeted group, is the first step.

IDENTIFIED POPULATION

The geriatric clinical specialist has as one of her focuses the populations whose inpatients are 75 years of age and older who are at high risk for complications that are associated with their treatment regimen. This population can be divided into several subpopulations, one of which will be defined.

Primary Organizer

The main concern about this population are persons being discharged on a complex medication regimen who do not have a dependent-care agent in the home to assist them.

Although the aged benefit when medications are used judiciously, they may also demonstrate altered or unexpected responses to medication. This incidence of drug-induced side effect and adverse interactions rises steadily with age and complexity of drugs prescribed.

Factors that contribute to the complexity of a medication regimen include:

- The number of medications in the regimen
- The availability of the medications
- The decision-making processes that are necessary to carry out the regimen
- Ability and willingness to follow additional directions as prescribed

- The mechanical actions to be performed in taking the medications
- Understanding the expected outcomes and possible side effects and interactions of medications and other substances

Basic Conditioning Factors

Age/gender. All of the clients in this population are 75 years of age or older. Roughly 97% of them are male.

Developmental state. Clients are adjusting to decreasing physical strength and health as well as to retirement and reduced income. Furthermore, most of them are adjusting to illness or death of a spouse or significant other.

Conditions of living. Poor nutritional status is a common occurrence in the population due to immobility, apathy, reduced income, lack of knowledge, lack of oral health, and decreased taste discrimination.

Family system factors. Due to illness/death of spouses and mobility of offspring, most of the clients in this population do not have a strong immediate family support system. If dependent care is needed, family members are often either unavailable or unwilling to assume dependent-care agent responsibilities. Thus, when those clients need help with their medications, the help may not be available. This leaves them at risk for medication-related problems.

Health state. The incidence of multiple acute and chronic diseases for which medications are prescribed is quite high for this population. Some of these illnesses alter the clients' mobility, sensory ability, comfort status, and orientation status, thus affecting self-care ability.

A significant factor is that all of the clients in this population are dealing with their own illnesses along with the illness or death of a spouse or significant other that is likely to induce bouts of depression. People experiencing depression are less likely to follow prescribed medication regimens.

Health care systems factors. All of these clients are admitted to the hospital for their health care needs. On discharge, they will be followed by a community health nurse.

Relevant life experience. Most of the clients were prescribed medication before admission to the hospital. For these people, there is a potential that they will continue to take their old medications along with the newly prescribed ones, which increases the chance of drug interactions, side effects, and overdoses.

The clients who were not prescribed medications before admission are not accustomed to taking routine medications.

Foundational Capabilities and Dispositions

Sensory and learning capabilities. Sensory losses with aging affect all sensory organs. Due to loss of sight and hearing, many of the clients have difficulty understanding written and verbal instructions. An altered sense of touch along with decreased fine motor capabilities in this population makes opening medication containers difficult.

Attention and memory. Most of the clients in this population will forget at one time or another to take their medications as prescribed. As long as symptoms are present, they attend to the need to take the medication. However, when symptoms are no longer noticeable, they may not attend as fully and forget whether the medication was taken. Thus, they omit either a dose or an extra one.

Those clients who do remember to take their medications consistently admit to using a documentation system that serves as a reminder.

Ability to manage self. Frequently, a spouse is responsible for overseeing many of the patient's physiological needs. Taking on the aspect of self-care is a major adjustment. The patient needs to be able to manipulate the medications and packaging.

Universal Self-Care Requisites

Prevention of hazards. Complex drug regimens have a high potential for errors in administrations that are associated with adverse drug reactions. Elderly patients have a decreased tolerance to medications that are associated with slow metabolism of drugs.

Promotion of normalcy. Dependency interferes with promotion of normalcy.

Health Deviation Self-Care Requisites

These patients need to be able to carry out prescribed measures and need to understand how and when to take medications.

Awareness of side effects. There is a need to know side effects of medications and actions to take to avoid side effects. Be aware that over-the-counter drugs may react adversely with prescribed medications.

Living with effects of pathological condition. Deal effectively with chronic illness; follow prescribed medication regimen.

Self-care limitations: In general, people in this class exhibit:

- Limited ability to maintain attention and vigilance regarding medication regime
- Limited, controlled use of physical energy
- Knowledge about medication regime
- Limitations in sensory functions
- Limited support system

Self-Care Deficit

A *self-care deficit* in this population is defined as "insufficient knowledge and limited ability to operationalize self-care with respect to taking prescribed medications on discharge."

Method of helping: Teaching, guiding, supporting

As the nurse considers how to design a program for this population, what kinds of antecedent knowledge are necessary? There would be detailed knowledge of the pharmacodynamics of the major categories or drugs in use with this population, which drugs are used, and the frequency of combinations of drugs. This could be determined by a retrospective chart review. There would have to be knowledge of teaching/learning theory, especially as it relates to adult learners. Adult development theory would be useful. Remembering that we want to take a holistic view of the situation, data on socioeconomic status, mental status, and comorbidities are also needed.

What kind of programs might be designed from this information? One aspect might be that of monitoring or surveillance of medication-taking behaviors, providing means that aid the patient: provide alarms to remind patient to take medication; have pharmacist prepackage medications by day/time; locate medications conveniently (e.g., a.m. meds in bathroom, noon meds in kitchen); schedule time to record effects of medication. Perhaps phone calls by nurses, or computer-based technologies for reporting and surveillance, could be developed. Are there different living arrangements possible? Are there resources in the community that could be mobilized?

As the nurse begins to gather such data, using principles of complexity and systems, patterns begin to emerge. From these patterns, solutions or design aspects begin to form.

INDEX

Lightning Source UK Ltd.
Milton Keynes UK
UKOW04f1437181016

285580UK00002B/42/P